Maria Mesner/Gudrun Wolfgruber (Eds.)

The Policies of Reproduction at the Turn of the 21st Century

Bruno-Kreisky International Studies, vol. 6

Maria Mesner/Gudrun Wolfgruber (Eds.)

The Policies of Reproduction at the Turn of the 21st Century

The Cases of Finland, Portugal, Romania, Russia, Austria, and the US

StudienVerlag

Innsbruck
Wien
Bozen

© 2006 by Studienverlag Ges.m.b.H., Erlerstraße 10, A-6020 Innsbruck
e-mail: order@studienverlag.at
Internet: www.studienverlag.at

Corporate design by Kurt Höretzeder
Layout and Cover: Studienverlag/Christine Petschauer

Distributed in North America and South America and the rest of the world excluding Austria, Germany, and Switzerland by: Transaction Publishers, Rutgers – The State University,
35 Berrue Circle, Piscataway New Jersey, 08854-8042, USA, www.transactionpub.com

This book is printed on acid-free paper.

Bibliographic information published by Die Deutsche Bibliothek
Die Deutsche Bibliothek lists this publication in the Deutsche Nationalbibliographie;
detailed bibliographic data is available in the Internet at http://dnb.ddb.de

ISBN-10: 3-7065-4088-6
ISBN-13: 978-3-7065-4088-9

The German version of this book has also been published by Studienverlag:
"Kinder kriegen – Kinder haben. Analysen im Spannungsfeld zwischen staatlichen Poli-
tiken und privaten Lebensentwürfen". ISBN 3-7065-4073-8

Contents

Russia

Austria

Editors' Preface

Starting from the political field of reproduction, the processes accompanying child-bearing and child-rearing, the authors of this publication explore the significance that "gender" – as both a social attribute and as a category of discrimination – has had in different societies since the 1960s and still has today. We have asked the scholars assembled here to write about countries that appear suitable to us, due to different social, economic and political developments, for representing a very broad spectrum of reproduction policies: Finland as a North European welfare state; Portugal as a former military dictatorship with a comparatively late democratisation and opening up to the outside; selected exemplary countries on the other side of the former "Iron Curtain", such as Romania and Russia; and the USA as an example from outside Europe. In keeping with an emancipatory aim linked with a criticism of essentialist conceptions of gender and with "the refusal [...] to serve the status quo" (Scott 2001), the authors address issues of reproduction and generativity in relationship to and overlapping with categories of discrimination such as gender, "ethnic affiliation" / "race" and social affiliation (Gehmacher and Mesner 2003). At the same time, the articles demonstrate the very different approaches and diversity of methods in gender studies (see Gehmacher and Mesner 2003; Bauer and Neissl 2002a). This publication assembles sociological, historical, political science and anthropological approaches and combines them, we think, in a meaningful way.

This publication is based on a comprehensive concept of reproduction: in German, this concept refers to the tasks and processes that serve the "private" mental and physical regeneration of human beings, which are frequently posited as a complementary opposite to public gainful employment. The English word reproduction, on the other hand, refers more to the process of human procreation. This collection of articles is intended to enable a consideration of both aspects together, that of procreation and that of reproduction, with a focus on childcare. The themes of the articles are the meanings, power relations and structural and social framework conditions both of child-bearing and child-rearing. In this way, we hope to unsettle the frequently asserted dichotomy between "natural" procreation and the "social sphere of reproduction". The "biological" side of reproduction – childbearing, which is often presumed to be "natural" – and child-raising, i.e. care-giving tasks, are presented as two sides of one and the same coin, as two aspects that can ultimately not be separated from policies. The articles in this publication address both the question of who is entitled to decide which groups of persons should have children in which circumstances and under which conditions, and the question of resources that are made available to different groups of persons for care-giving work. This includes issues of the gender-specific effect of policies that aim to regulate human generativity: access to and practices of contraception and abortion, and the discussion of the legal regulation of modern reproduction technologies. What is evident here is how different welfare state policies that regulate the meanings and consequences of childcare construct and reproduce assumptions about and consequences of gender attribution.[1]

Though they focus on reproduction, the individual articles also illustrate that the relevant norms and practices in the respective specific national contexts cannot be separated from norms and practices in the realm of gainful employment. In addition, they also prove to be closely linked in many ways with issues of political representation.

Most of the articles deal with a period of time beginning in the 1960s. This reflects the idea that the formation of a second women's movement in the late 1960s in Central Europe and the USA had a central altered impact in terms of the significance of gender, and represented a caesura in the public discussion of gender roles. This assumption is simultaneously affirmed and relativised by the articles collected here. It is once again evident that it is difficult to make generalisations and that comparative perspectives can have a relativising effect. In many Western European and North American countries, the legal prohibition against abortion was the pivotal point of debates, as for instance in the USA and Austria. In other countries, though, such as Portugal, which underwent a late and rapid political party development following the end of the military dictatorship in 1974, or former state socialist regimes such as Russia and Romania, or Finland, which had a relatively early democratic constitution and a largely egalitarian gender contract, the discussions followed a different course, and not only due to women's different opportunities for articulation and participation.

The confrontation with the respective reproduction and gender policies in other/ "foreign" countries always poses a challenge, provokes thinking about how to deal with what is one's "own" and what is "foreign", as well as questions about and arising from difference. Sometimes there is no lowest common denominator that can be distinguished as a result, patricularly if one wants to avoid the danger of blurring the specific effects of reproduction policies in their respective national context on single individuals. Our intention with this publication is therefore also to suggest a change of perspective, to enable a new view of what is "one's own", of the familiar and the unfamiliar, of what is "foreign". Lastly, we also hope to contribute in this way to "relativising and dynamising what is taken for granted in the present" (Bauer and Neissl 2003b, 9).

The individual articles show that socially and politically defined criteria of belonging and exclusion and unequally distributed opportunities for access determine how individuals regulate procreation and (have to) take responsibility for care work. This applies to belonging to the "nation", to the state and welfare state, to possibilities of access to social benefits that are provided (care facilities and financial benefits) and to the employment market. Though it manifests itself in different ways, a set of problems arises here, again and again: the effects of the reduction of social welfare state offers, a stronger tie between social rights and belonging to the employment market, and the impacts of economic globalisation and neo-liberalism on the relation between gender and reproduction.

Ritva Nätkin shows how it became possible, in the process of seeking Finland's independence from Russia, for women to become participants in the nation through the concept of social maternalism and to demand initial welfare state regulations within the framework of a pro-natalist qualitative population policy as well as on the basis of a welfare feminism (see Banks 1981). Nätkin addresses the results of intensive welfare state policies, in which responsibility is given to the state; one effect was that the delegation of equality issues to the state merely resulted in a swing from a maternalist to a family discourse. In keeping with this, *Teija Hautanen* finds that reproductive tasks and child care continue to be a central component in the current Finnish gender agreement. Her article investigates why in Finland, unlike many Western European countries, it was not the legalisation of abortion that was most controversially and vehemently discussed, but rather the question of child care and child care facilities. On the basis of these debates, which appeared to be gender-neutral in the way they were conducted, Hautanen demonstrates how welfare state policies with the goal of equality are not sufficiently effective and continue to regard women as being primarily responsible for reproduction.

Virgínia Ferreira shows that it is most of all a "diffuse feminism" that is to be held responsible for the fact that in the newly formed political parties in Portugal in the mid-seventies, (almost) anything could be discussed except abortion. Due to the strong role of the Catholic church, in the constellation of family policies, social policies and women's issues, the family continues to remain at the centre of social-political measures and debates. The decision to have children thus falls into a field marked by substantial gender-specific and social inequality, a largely segregated labour market and an inadequate infrastructure of public child care facilities. *Sílvia Portugal's* article examines the question of how those affected deal with these burdens and how the lack of sufficient state child care facilities is compensated in a semi-welfare state. Traditionally, it is family networks that ensure "compatibility", i. e. care work and primarily female, mostly unpaid reproduction work. In other words, the costs of the welfare state society are still borne by women.

Whereas the clerical-dictatorial regime in Portugal impeded a public feminist debate on reproductive rights for a long period of time, in state socialist regimes questions of reproduction, abortion and birth control were situated primarily in the context of the interests of nationalist population policies. Currently, feminist concerns are being formulated cautiously, but they are being answered again with an emphasis on national interests. In Romania and Russia, current debates over abortion are closely linked with health policy initiatives due to the economically precarious situation. Issues related to reproduction are discussed more in terms of "public health" rather than of individual or feminist concerns. *Adriana Baban's* article examines how the right to health becomes a precondition for the participation of women in all social, political, economic and family contexts within the framework of current debates on human rights. At the same time, health policy measures specific to women are closely tied to women's reproductive rights. Baban illustrates how current social policy measures centre around state and national self-representation rather than a woman's right to her body. *Livia Popescu's* article also examines women's health costs as negative effects of a maternalist social policy legacy from the socialist era. The author blames the lack of criticism of gender roles in the private sphere for the continued definition of women as being responsible for child care and household work, which additionally has a negative impact on the health of women and children.

Michele Rivkin-Fish addresses how the public debate on reproduction after the end of the Soviet era focused on two interrelated arguments: the problem of low birth rates and the resultant danger of a "demographic crisis," and complaints about progressive moral decay in the family and sexual life (especially of women). Here the author identifies surprising continuities beyond the regime change. *Yelena Kulagina's* article outlines the socio-economic problems that families are currently confronting in the course of overall social transformation processes. She identifies the persistence of traditional gender images and gender roles in conjunction with a general economic crisis and insufficient social security as the cause of an increasing gender asymmetry; here, the sphere of reproduction is therefore dependent on a woman's own resources.

The question of why and how the US American debates on reproduction rights, which first attained greater significance after the legalisation of abortion, have formed the arena for conflicts between liberal and conservative ideas about family, personal freedom, state intervention, the relationship of religion versus politics, sexual morality and social welfare, is the topic of the article by *Linda Gordon*. She sketches out a long line of development from the liberalisation of abortion laws, through the evolution of the pro-life movement, to debates on teenage pregnancy as a new theme of the 1980s, and the events of the present day. *Ann Orloff* examines the implications of the US American policy of regulating access to service offers in the sphere of care facilities exclusively through participation in the labour market. Her article analyses the current social aid reform as a model of social welfare that is based on the goal of full employment.

The controversial "family policy" measure of the "child care allowance," introduced in Austria in 2002, was the subject of vehement political debates; the question of whether and to what extent this measure actually represents a new crossroad in Austrian reproductive policies in a historical perspective is the subject of the article by *Maria Mesner*. This article focuses on the ideological orientations and objectives of the political actors and on the gender models that are given preference through these political proposals. The Austrian debate on new reproduction technologies is also marked by an interest in supporting traditional family structures. *Aurelia Weikert's* article examines the development of political and public discourses on new reproduction technologies since the 1970s and asks which groups of actors have had a crucial impact on determining the legal developments. She focuses on how originally feminist demands for self-determination over one's own body in analogy to debates on the legalisation of abortion have been inverted into their opposite in conjunction with specific political interests who attempt to make use of female generative potentials.

The articles by *Maria Wolf* and *Johanna Gehmacher* are to be regarded as concluding commentaries on the theme of this publication. They address issues that link the individual articles on specific countries and identify research gaps and perspectives: Gehmacher emphasizes the conjunction of gender and nationalism, and Wolf does the same from a technology-critical feminist perspective.

On the one hand, the conclusion of a publication such as this one always answers questions. At the same time, however, it also opens up perspectives on other questions and approaches that have hardly been raised yet, much less discussed, and which are beginning to emerge on the horizon. In this sense, it was striking that the mere endeavour of making contact with international experts on reproduction issues suggested a speculation that became increasingly concrete in reading the articles. It appears that in scholarly discourse as well, the field of reproduction is a typically female one. There were hardly any male scholars who have focused on reproduction policies to be found. Parallel to this, in the texts included here, it is almost exclusively women who appear as (potential) care-givers, whereas men are rarely named as being responsible for children, represented at best as "absent" or as agents of state policies or a state symbolised as male. This leads to the question whether the absence of male actors is to be seen as the singular result of the specific topic of research or also as an expression of traditional gender role attributions within scholarly discourse, that repeat gender-specific attributions in the assignment to fields of research. An assignment of this kind naturally has consequences for the research perspective and the research results, including gaps in research and blind spots that could be starting points for further analyses and interpretations: for example, "family" frequently becomes the unquestioned site of reproduction. Future analyses and research projects must reserve the right to question the specific constitution of the group so designated and thus to take alternative forms of living and sexual orientations into consideration.

Another important field of research is that of ethnic differences. Due to increasingly growing trans-national movements of voluntary or involuntary migration, issues linked to migration and integration policies and categories of ethnic and cultural affiliation take on even greater significance. These issues are in conflict with rhetorics of national homogeneity that is not called into question.

The comparative perspective suggested by the individual articles particularly raises questions of divergent processes over the course of time, very different caesurae that explain continuities and discontinuities. It would be worth analysing the different meanings and consequences that caesurae can assume, such as the symbolic years of 1968, 1989, 1945, etc. More numerous and more detailed analyses of (dis)continuities in terms of elite groups and hegemonic attitudes and interpretations of society would also be interesting.

In order to enable the analytical comparison and thus the theoretical and empirical discussion without leaving the particular perspectives of the nation-state unquestioned and hence posited as absolutes, it would be desirable to form research teams with representatives from different national contexts. However, this step must be left up to other activities and projects. We hope that the present publication can serve as a basis for future analyses and the impulse to motivate endeavours of this kind.

The present publication assembles revised papers from the conference "The Gender of Politics: The Example of Reproduction Policies in Austria, Finland, Portugal, Romania, Russia and the US", which took place from 13–15 March 2003 in Vienna, organized by the *Bruno Kreisky Archive Foundation* together with the editors.

We are grateful to the National Bank for the crucial financial support that made both the conference and the subsequent publication of this book in both English and German possible. We would also like to thank the *Bruno Kreisky Archive Foundation* for providing the needed infrastructure and the *Kreisky Forum* for providing the venue for the conference. For the work involved in the delicate translations, the careful editing and the editorial supervision of the articles, thanks are due especially to Aileen Derieg and Pat Blashill. We are also grateful to Elisabeth Brandl for organisational and administrative support.

Naturally, our very special thanks go to the authors for their willingness to engage in discussion and the often elaborate revisions of their articles.

In conclusion, we would like to thank all the people not mentioned here by name, the friends, family and colleagues, who helped and supported us throughout the preparation and publication of this book.

Maria Mesner, Gudrun Wolfgruber
Vienna, May 2006

Note

1 The applicability of Gøsta Esping-Andersen's welfare state theory model proves problematic, however, as the category of gender, regional conditions and the significance of religious movements are not taken into consideration. Cf. Mesner 2002, 6ff.; Esping-Andersen 1990; more recent comparative studies on the social and welfare state also lack a view of the category of gender; cf. Kaufmann 2003.

References

Banks, Olive. 1981. *Faces of Feminism. A study of Feminism as a Social Movement.* Oxford: M. Robertson.

Bauer, Ingrid and Julia Neissl (eds.). 2002a. *Gender Studies, Denkachsen und Perspektiven der Geschlechterforschung.* Innsbruck: Studienverlag.

Bauer, Ingrid, and Julia Neissl. 2002b. Weigerung den Status quo zu bedienen. Das kritische Potential der Gender Studies. In Ingrid Bauer and Julia Neissl (eds.) *Gender Studies. Denkachsen und Perspektiven der Geschlechterforschung*: 7–15. Innsbruck: Studienverlag.

Esping-Andersen, Gøsta. 1990. *The Three Worlds of Welfare Capitalism.* Princeton, N.J.: Princeton University Press.

Gehmacher, Johanna, and Maria Mesner. 2003. *Frauen- und Geschlechtergeschichte. Positionen/Perspektiven.* Innsbruck: Studienverlag.

Kaufmann, Franz-Xaver. 2003. *Varianten des Wohlfahrtsstaats. Der deutsche Sozialstaat im internationalen Vergleich.* Frankfurt/Main: Suhrkamp.

Mesner, Maria. 2002. Überlegungen zu Geschlecht und Reproduktion in der zweiten Hälfte des 20. Jahrhunderts: Finnland, Österreich, Portugal, USA. In Andrea Griesebner and Christina Lutter (eds.) *Die Macht der Kategorien (=Wiener Zeitschrift zur Geschichte der Neuzeit 2/2)*: 6ff. Vienna/Innsbruck.

Scott, Joan W. 2001. Die Zukunft von gender. Fantasien zur Jahrausendwende. In Claudia Honegger and Caroline Arni (eds.) *Gender. Die Tücken einer Kategorie*: 39–63. Zurich: Chronos.

Teija Hautanen

Every Child's Right to Public Day Care in Finland

Introduction

Public provision of day care has been taken for granted in Finland for over thirty years now, and the first "day care generations" have already become mothers and fathers. A great deal of debate has been carried out about day care all through its history, and we can hence conclude that the Finnish day care system was built through many battles.

This presentation will deal with the history and present situation of Finnish day care. At the moment, all Finnish children under school age have the right to day care, irrespective of whether their parents work or not. I will now explain how we have come to this situation, what "battles" have been fought and what the consequences of these battles have been.

Childcare arrangements are always related to gender policy. The conditions of childcare are set according to what is considered appropriate from a gender political point of view. On the other hand, care arrangements per se construct gender. I will approach the theme from this particular point of view and, when doing so, I will consider children's day care services as a significant part of the Finnish gender contract, as do many other researchers within women's studies.

"Gender contract" is a concept that Rantalaiho (1994, 10–15), among others, has suggested should be used when the welfare state and gender are being analysed simultaneously. Nordic researchers within women's studies have used it to describe the unspoken rules, reciprocal responsibilities and rights that define the relations between men and women. Gender contract is by no means a static state of affairs, but is constantly being negotiated. These negotiations have most often been specifically about women's position. Rantalaiho emphasizes that it is the redefinition of women's citizenship that characterises the changes in the gender contract.

Women's Gainful Employment and Day Care Services before the 1960s

For a long period, i.e. until the 1960s, Finland was a relatively poor and agrarian country full of small farms. Women's labour contribution was needed at home farms, and it was also valued by various NGOs as well as the state. Farm wives were considered to have an important role in securing the livelihood of family households and in promoting well-being. This is why Rissanen (2000, 26–27), for example, notes that the farm wives on Finnish farms cannot be regarded as housewives. According to him, the "farm wife policy" can be seen as the first Finnish contract on the division of labour between the genders. The day care issue, however, was not part of farm wife policy".

Yet many women were gainfully employed at that time. They worked as servants or hired hands in the country, and in industry or various services in cities and towns. Jallinoja (1980, 225–230) concedes that, generally speaking, Finnish women started to work outside the home quite early on, but adds that it was nonetheless relatively uncommon for married women to work outside the home before the Second World War. It is noteworthy, though, that not all the working women who had children were married; some had had children out of wedlock, some had been widowed or become single parents for other reasons, and this had made them look for employment. According to labour statistics, only about ten percent of the female labour force of industry and some other fields were married in the first decade of the 20th century. Until 1950, as many as 34 percent of the gainfully employed women in cities and towns were married. Jallinoja assumes that it was during the war that wage work of women with families became more common. It is after all a common phenomenon that increasing numbers of women go to work during war years.

After the war, in the 1950s, as many as 45 percent of the gainfully employed women were married. This figure was the highest in the Nordic countries (Anttalainen 1986, 34). In many other Western countries, women opted to stay at home again after the war, but in Finland the change was permanent.

Day care services developed slowly in Finland before the 1970s, in spite of the fact that the first kindergartens were founded as early as the 1880s. These first kindergartens were funded by private interests, such as charitable and religious organisations, workers' associations and factories. In 1927, Parliament passed a decree about state subsidies to kindergartens. The most essential justification in the government's proposal was its concern for children. This new decree was the beginning of state funding and supervision, even if it was not yet the beginning of general municipal day care. The parliamentary proceedings reveal that even then, in the 1920s, the same conflicts that are still topical today flared up when child day care was being discussed: the child's place and the woman's duty as children's caregiver became a political issue. The next time that Parliament legislated about child day care was in 1936 as part of the new Child Welfare Act. With this act, municipalities were obligated for the very first time to found and maintain institutions that would support children's upbringing in homes, or else create such circumstances that would enable various organisations to found day care institutions. However, municipalities were not allocated separate funding for these activities, nor did the act include any sanctions, so it did not cause very much development in practice (Rauhala 1996, 105–109).

Kurikka (1993) has studied Finnish day care policies from their beginnings to the 1980s. She says that if we look at the early development of child day care, we cannot find an interest of women that would have been the one and only issue. It is true that women of that time had in common a wish to influence reproduction policies, but the emphasis and demands varied from one group of women to another. For working women, employment was an economic necessity, and they wanted more time together with their families, whereas the middle and upper class women fought for their right to education and good jobs. However, in the early 1920s, social democratic women made the societal provision of day care their central goal. One of the reasons behind this was a strong wish to detach day care from the idea of bourgeois charity work (Kurikka 1993, 56–65).

The Changes of the 1960s and the Passing of the 1973 Law on Child Day Care

Finland underwent a major structural change in the 1960s and 1970s. In a short period of time, a poor agrarian country developed into a modern industrial and service state. Our economic development was among the fastest in the world. New housing, factories, hospitals, schools etc. were built in great numbers. The Finnish countryside grew more and more quiet, people migrated in huge numbers to cities and towns, and many even emigrated abroad. Besides this structural change, there were many cultural and socio-political changes, as there were elsewhere in the world at that time.

The gender contract changed too. Julkunen (1994, 190–192) calls the new contract a "wage work contract". As the name implies, normalising women's wage work is at the core of this contract. The gainful employment of wives and mothers in particular had often been defined as a social problem before, and now it became women's right, part of emancipation and the foundation of their independence. The new contract underlined the similarity of men and women and extended even to the use of language. Instead of women, people talked about persons, parents, spouses, equality and family. The equality movement maintained a strong confidence in the state, and the new gender contract was cemented by the many societal political reforms of the period.

Arranging child day care was a central goal for the actors of the new gender contract. The number of wives and mothers in working life increased even before there was a proper day care system (Julkunen 1994, 195). In the 1960s and the 1970s, the increased need for a labour force was more often met by employing women rather than by employing men (Jallinoja 1980, 231).

Lack of day care services was catastrophic, and day care thus became a central topic in the socio-political debate of the 1960s. It was then that the emotionally-loaded phrase "latchkey kids" was coined to describe children who were left alone on weekdays. Some of the children were actually left at home alone because it was so difficult to arrange day care. Some were taken care of by domestic workers or close relatives. Care arrangements were often unstable.

Even though it was still common in the 1960s to regard mothers' wage work negatively, the day care issue was seen as an important one by many quarters. The issue motivated different women's associations to join forces, including the women's organisation Association 9 (Yhdistys 9) (part of the radical movement), traditional child welfare organisations, political-party women's associations, and the women of the labour movement. Public discussions as well as governmental planning machinery (in many instances the same individuals were active in both) saw the state as the central solution to the issue: the state had to adjust to women's gainful employment. The role of the state in these discussions was to provide funding and supervision to guarantee a nation-wide congruity of the activities (Rauhala 1996, 164–168).

According to Anttonen (1999, 26) there were many conflicts in the political discussions of that time. While the women activists of the left wing and even some of the right-wing conservative Coalition Party backed the development of day care services, the development of home care was seen as a central goal among agrarian parties, and they got some support for this from the Coalition Party. And employers' organisations, which were close to the political right, supported the development of day care services. There was thus a dividing line between the political actors: some favoured the "farm wife policy," others the "wage work policy".

Child day care became a government issue in 1970, and the draft bill for an act on child day care was brought before Parliament in 1972. The preparation of the act seems to have progressed without many conflicts, while its discussion in Parliament has been described as exceptionally stormy and emotionally charged. The "battle lines" were not between men and women in Parliament; instead, the tension was strongest between the left-wing and the agrarian parties (Rauhala 1996, 172–173).

Kurikka (1993, 92–94) writes that, despite the emotional charge, there was not a single member of Parliament who would have directly opposed the draft bill. It was regarded as a necessary reform, but the representatives of the centre and the right-wing in particular took the floor to speak in favour of home care – besides supporting day care services. They gave much attention to the proposed "mother's wage", which would have enabled mothers to stay at home to care for their children. There was also a great deal of discussion about whether day care outside the home would be harmful for a child's development or not.

The proponents of day care won and the Child Daycare Act was passed in 1973. The act displays a confidence in governmental planning and supervision, which was thought to promote regional equality in particular. The goal of the act was to provide day care to everyone who desired it. In this way, day care was defined as a universal social service, for which parents paid a fee that was adjusted according to their earnings. The goal at that point was that the state and the municipalities would be responsible for 80 percent of the operating costs and the families for 20 percent (Kurikka 1993, 174).

After the act took effect, the number of day care services rapidly increased. During the first decade after the law was enacted, an increase in the number of day care opportunities was made possible chiefly by an increase in family day care. Välimäki and Rauhala (2000, 397) describe municipal family day care as a special, Nordic form of day care, in which the local authority places the provider of a social service, the childminder, in her or his own home. These childminders were able to take care of their own children and their household in their own homes, which, according to Välimäki and Rauhala, was one of the central motivations for individuals seeking to become municipal family day care providers.

However, there were not enough opportunities for day care, and children were assigned to municipal day care according to their parents' income. This meant that there was no room for children of the well-to-do families in municipal day care establishments. For this reason, Anttonen (1999, 27) remarks that, in practice, day care did not become a universal service targeted to all families at this point, as was the intention of the act.

Day Care Became the Subjective Right of Children under School Age in 1996

The period of time from the 1960s to the end of the 1980s is often described as the construction period of the Finnish welfare state. Finland was doing fine economically, and there was a political consensus about carrying out socio-political reforms. In the 1980s, no one disputed the values of justice and equality yet, and the welfare state enjoyed wide support (e.g. Anttonen and Sipilä 2000, 43).

Parliament continued to talk about support for home care (more on this in the next section) even after the Child Daycare Act had been passed. Another matter that aroused discussion was that, due to the limited capacity of the day care system every child was not guaranteed an opportunity, even though the parents needed it. The law package that came into effect in 1985 after Parliament's passage has been called a historical compromise. It reconciled the views of different interest groups. Those in need of day care services were guaranteed it for children under three years of age, and those who took care of children under three at home were granted a right to monetary compensation (Anttonen 1999, 43).

The beginning of the next decade brought a severe economic recession with mass unemployment to Finland. Although it did not last many years, one result was that our state economy still emphasizes thrift and an endless need for saving today. While people in the 1980s joined forces to develop social policy together, the 1990s brought a new discourse: the public sector was now a greedy monster that had become much too large and devoured too much money. Even though Finland is doing extremely well today economically, it seems that we have irretrievably lost our previous eagerness to develop the welfare state, as there seems to be little interest in the matter, even within the left-wing.

However, in spite of the recession and its consequences, the discussion on the development of child day care continued in the 1990s. Some of the themes were the size of the fees, and pre-school education for six-year-olds. Left-wing parties strongly suggested that the right to day care should be extended to all children under school age, i.e. under the age of seven. As early as 1990, the government submitted a draft bill suggesting the extension of the right to day care to all children under school age, but its passage was postponed because of the recession. However, the women's network (founded in 1991), which operates within Parliament and which transcends party boundaries, worked actively in favour of the extension of the right to day care, and the amendment finally took effect at the beginning of 1996. It has been said that this amendment is the result of long battles – "the fight" lasted for many years between the left and the right wing.

Children under three thus attained a "subjective right" to day care first, and this right was then extended in 1996 to cover all children under the age of seven. The phrase "subjective right" means that municipalities do not have any discretionary power regarding the provision of day care. The spirit of the law is that it is the parents who define the need for care. A municipality cannot deny them day care service because of inadequate funding, but instead has to see to it that families have access to municipal day care, which is either provided or monitored by the local authority. If either one of the parents cannot go to work because day care service is not available for the child, the parents have the right to seek indemnification for their economic loss (Heikkinen 1998, 24; Suoninen 1996; Tuori 2000, 261–262).

Finnish nationality is not a prerequisite for a child or parents to have the right to municipal day care. Instead, one needs to have an official Finnish home municipality. When a person has a home municipality, he or she is entitled to municipal health care and social services. The fact that one is currently living in Finland does not necessarily mean that she or he has a home municipality, because local authorities need to be convinced that the residence in Finland is permanent in nature.

Because parents now have the right to define their need for childcare services, the fact that they are not able to care for a child themselves (because of work or studies for example) is no longer the only reason for enrolling a child in day care. This has caused a great deal of discussion. The right of an unemployed person to use public day care services has been considered dubious, and similar accusations have been targeted at mothers who bring an older child to day care while staying at home with a baby (Lehto 1998, 419).

Vainio (2004) has studied letters to the editor dealing with the right to day care in Finnish newspapers. On the basis of her study, we can conclude that the arguments of those who oppose the wide coverage of day care are, to a large extent, familiar with the history of day care. They claim, for example, that a home is always a better care place for a child than a care institution that just makes the children go with the crowd. Some of the writers accuse the parents who use day care of being selfish. The fact that unemployed persons take their children to day care causes a torrent of criticism about the wasting of taxpayers' money, about insensitivity toward children, and about the parents' wish to have an easy life. However, there are also some among the writers who find this possibility justified. Unemployment is often seen as a burden to family life, and a going to day care is thought to bring stimulation and regularity to a child's life.

A great majority of Finnish municipalities have coped well with the requirements of the amendment, but they are nevertheless its most prominent opponents. The increasing share that day care requires from their overall social and health care services budgets constitutes a major problem. For day care services, parents pay a fee which varies depending on their income (18–200 € a month, including meals), but the fees only cover approx. 10–15 percent of the real expenses (Lehto 1998, 420). The high expenses of day care tend to lead to cuts in other areas of social services, such as services for the elderly. The Association of Finnish Local and Regional Authorities has therefore urged that the right to full-day care service should be linked with parents' working or studying or with social and educational justifications (e.g. Komminaho 1997, 3).

In 1997, around the same time that the amendment to the Child Daycare Act took effect, a support system for private care was launched, which meant that an allowance was paid for children under school age, who were taken care of by a private day care provider. This care provider could be a private day care centre, a private childminder or a caregiver employed by the family (Anttonen 1999, 69). As yet, private day care does not compete with municipal day care, but instead chiefly supplements municipal services. An increase in private day care services may nonetheless be one possible development trend in Finland, because today's Finnish society tends to favour solutions that operate according to market mechanisms, so therefore not only big state firms but also social and health care services are being privatised.

The latest day care reform took place in 2001, when the municipalities were obligated- to arrange pre-school education for all six-year-old children. The part-time, pre-school education is voluntary and free of charge. It has been arranged as part of the municipal school system or day care services.

Finnish Paid Family Leave

In the following I will briefly introduce the present family leave in Finland, since this has a significant impact on the age of children that are taken to day care outside of their home. At the moment, a child can be cared for at home by his or her own parents with the support of two systems: the parents can at first take maternity, paternity and parental leave, and then childcare leave.

One of the reforms of the 1960s was the maternity allowance system, which came into effect in 1963. The maternity leave it provided was short: less than two months. Many changes have been made to the system over the years. In 2003 the "leaves" and allowance were as follows: maternity allowance was paid to the mother for 105 workdays, beginning 30 workdays before the due date at the latest; parental allowance was paid for 158 workdays, payable to either the mother or the father; paternity allowance was paid to the father for 18 workdays during the time the mother receives maternity or parental allowance, and for an additional one to twelve workdays, in case it is the father who is on parental leave on the last twelve workdays of the parental leave period. The paid allowance is adjusted according to the recipient's income, and in practice, amounts to approximately 60 percent of her or his earnings. If the person claiming the allowance has not been earning any income, she or he receives the minimum daily allowance of 11,45 € for each workday.

With the help of the daily allowance adjusted for earnings, a parent thus has the opportunity to care for her/his child at home until the child is about ten months old. After that, the parent can take a childcare leave until the child is three years of age. If the parent has had a steady job before taking these leaves, the law requires that she or he may return to the same job after the leave is over.

Anttonen (1999, 42–43) writes that the childcare leave and the child home care allowance that the caring parent is entitled to during the period of childcare leave were both part of the 1980s compromise, which sought to "give a little to everyone." This was the outcome of the debate, begun in the 1960s, about how to take care of young children: support was given to both day care and home care. According to Anttonen, this compromise is related to the 1980s rhetoric promoting the freedom of choice. The idea was that each family should have the right to choose which was the best day care form for them, and society should support this freedom of choice. Not even the political right, says Anttonen, was in favour of the idea that the care of young children should be a private matter. All the parties concurred that public power should help pay for the costs incurred by day care.

The amount of the child home care allowance has varied. At the moment it is 252 € a month for the care of one child under the age of three. The system includes additional benefits which the family is entitled to according to the number of children, and low-income families are entitled to a supplementary benefit as well. In 1998, for example, families received an average of approximately 360 € a month in child home care allowance (Anttonen 1999, 58). Besides this allowance paid by the Social Insurance Institution, some of the larger municipalities pay their own benefits to the parents of children who are cared for in their own homes.

Parents are entitled to claim a continuation of the childcare leave in the form of a partial childcare leave until the end of the year in which the child begins school. This means that they have the opportunity to work less than 30 hours a week and receive a small compensation (approximately 60 € a month) for the reduction in their pay due to shorter working hours. This right to a partial childcare leave will soon be extended to cover the child's first two school years. However, it is uncommon to opt for a partial childcare leave, and people are poorly informed about it. Finnish working life has traditionally been based on full-time employment. The possibility of increasing the number of part-time jobs has arisen quite recently; this would make it easier for parents to combine work with family life. People have been concerned about the lonely afternoons of small school children, and it is hoped that extending the coverage of partial childcare leave would relieve this situation.

Use of Day Care Services and Finnish Stay-at-home Motherhood

When a child is taken care of at home during paid family leaves or after them, the care-giver is nearly always the mother. The proportion of working mothers increases rapidly at the point when the child turns three. It is, however, very rare for the mother of a baby to go out to work, and approximately 70 percent of the one to two-year-old children are still cared for at home. Childcare leave ends when the child turns three, and as many as more than half of all three-year-old children are in day care (Sauli 2000, 133–134).

The fact that some parents take their children to day care even though one or both of the parents is at home has aroused many opinions and arguments. Statistics show, however, that this practice has not become much more common after the 1996 amendment. In 1998, for example, about five percent of all the children in day care came from families in which neither one of the parents worked. The figure was the same even before the amendment (Sauli 2000, 137). Focusing on the mothers' situation, in turn, nearly 84 percent of the children of jobless women were cared for solely at home (Vaajakallio 1999, 40).

If we look at things historically, city and country people have had a different attitude toward day care. This distinction can still be seen in practice. Babies are cared for at home both in cities and in the country, but the older the child gets, the bigger the difference: about 80 percent of six-year-old children are in day care in cities and towns, while the figure in the country is only about 50 percent (Sauli 2000, 135).

Anttonen's (1999, 70–92) interpretation is that, judging from statistics, home care of children is very common in Finland in spite of the right to day care. She maintains that the childcare leave and the child home care allowance are factors that have contributed to a change in the norms of taking care of small children in this country. Society, professionals and the parents themselves have begun to perceive it as the normal state of affairs that a child is cared for at home during his or her first years. Anttonen also compares Finland with the other Nordic countries, and concludes that Finland and Norway are home-care countries to a much higher extent than Sweden and Denmark. However, Finnish mothers do not stay at home for long. Instead, most of them return to working life or studies or register themselves as unemployed after a few years.

If we compare Finland with the other Nordic countries, employment in Finland tends to be full-time employment with weekly working hours of 35 to 40. Even though women go back to work earlier in Sweden and Denmark, they work part-time more often than Finnish women do. In 1991, for example, over half of the gainfully employed Swedish mothers of children under school age held a part-time job, while the corresponding figure in Finland was ten percent (Julkunen 1995, 93).

Discussion

In the above, I have described the development and present situation of the Finnish day care system. If I sum up the political processes, I can say that public day care of good quality and extensive availability has been an important goal to the left-wing parties. The agrarian parties and the right-wing parties have often opposed it. On the other hand, issues concerning public day care have also brought together women from different political positions.

Child day care has become a universal social service targeted at all families who live permanently in Finland, and we no longer dispute its importance. Women's gainful employment is a norm to us these days and, at the same time, an indicator of equality. Stay-at-home motherhood has nevertheless not disappeared, since it is common for mothers to take care of small children at home during their first years. This solution is supported by many professionals in education. We can think that the women's wage work contract and the stay-at-home motherhood contract live side-by-side, or better yet, overlap.

Even though child day care is characteristically a women's issue and an issue that impacts women's lives in particular, this matter has not been specifically emphasized in Finland in the implementation of day care policies. Kurikka (1992, 179) maintains that the demands made with regard to day care in Finland have seldom been raised from a women's rights perspective. The day care issue was first a child discourse issue and, from the 1970s on, a family discourse issue. Typically, the Finnish family discourse has seen families as fixed entities and similar to each other, and it has not been common to look inside the families and see gender or diversity there, such as ethnic differences (e.g. Forsberg 2003, 7–15).

Day care policies are by no means an exception. Since the building of the welfare state started in the 1960s, it has not been common to use expressions which emphasize women's points of view or the benefits that women get from the reforms. The state-led equality policy has ruled the discussions and its façade is gender neutral. Behind this gender neutrality lies the rhetoric of hegemonic normative individualism. It dominates the Finnish welfare state practices as well as the rhetoric of politics, education and media discussions. According to Ronkainen (2002, 96), it consists of a moral code which means that a person should be treated without particularities (without bodies, gender, ethnicity, etc.) Women have of course benefited from this when acting in the public realm, but on the other hand normative individualism easily hides gender-specific problems and consequences.

The discussion on day care has not ended. Some of the themes that often come up are day care groups that are too big and the number and educational qualifications of staff in day care centres. The need for day care as such is hardly questioned, although people may complain about its quality. The proponents of home care do not oppose public day care very loudly either, but stress the possibility for parents to have a real freedom of choice instead. They want to raise the size of child home care allowances and get the pension issue resolved for the parents – in practice, mothers – who take care of their children at home.

References

Anttalainen, Marja-Liisa. 1986. *Sukupuolen mukaan kahtia jakautuneet työmarkkinat Pohjoimaissa*. Helsinki.

Anttonen, Anneli. 1999. *Lasten kotihoidon tuki suomalaisessa perhepolitiikassa. Sosiaali – ja terveysturvan tutkimuksia 52*. Helsinki: Kansaneläkelaitos.

Anttonen, Anneli, and Jorma Sipilä. 2000. *Suomalaista sosiaalipolitiikkaa*. Tampere: Vastapaino .

Forsberg, Hannele. 2003. Kriittistä näkökulmaa jäljittämässä. In Hannele Forsberg and Ritva Nätkin (eds.) *Kriittisen perhetutkimuksen jäljillä*: 7–15. Helsinki: Gaudeamus.

Heikkinen, Erja. 1998. Subjektiivisin oikeus. Päivähoitopalvelut paineiden alla. *KuntaSuomi 2004 – tutkimuksia nro 11*. Helsinki: Suomen kuntaliitto.

Jallinoja, Riitta. 1980. *Suomalaisen naisasialiikkeen taistelukaudet*. WSOY.

Julkunen, Raija. 1994. Suomalainen sukupuolimalli – 1960-luku käänteenä. In Anneli Anttonen, Lea Henriksson, and Ritva Nätkin (eds.) *Naisten hyvinvointivaltio*: 179–201. Tampere: Vastapaino.

Komminaho, Alpo. 1997. Päivähoito-oikeus – sosiaalitoimen käenpoika. *Sosiaaliturva* 21/1997.

Kurikka, Minna. 1993. *Päivähoidon politiikan naispolitiikka. Valtio-opin pro gradu – tutkielma. Politiikan tutkimuksen laitos.* Tampereen yliopisto.

Lehto, Juhani. 1998. Muuttuuko pohjoismainen sosiaali – ja terveyspalvelumalli? *Yhteiskuntapolitiikka* 5–6 (63): 413–424.

Rantalaiho, Liisa. 1994. Sukupuolisopimus ja Suomen malli. In Anneli Anttonen, Lea Henriksson, and Ritva Nätkin (eds.) *Naisten hyvinvointivaltio*: 9–30. Tampere: Vastapaino.

Rauhala, Pirkko-Liisa. 1996. Miten sosiaalipalvelut ovat tulleet osaksi suomalaista sosiaaliturvaa? *Acta Universitatis Tamperensis ser A* vol 477. Tampereen yliopisto.

Rissanen, Tapio. 2000. Naisten ansiotyömallin muotoutuminen. Työnteon, toimeentulon ja lasten hoidon järjestäminen Suomessa 1920–1980-luvuilla. *Sosiaalipolitiikan pro gradu-tutkielma.* Tampereen yliopisto.

Ronkainen, Suvi. 2002. Genderless gender as victimising context: the Finnish case. In Maria Eriksson, Aili Nenola and Marika Muhonen Nilsen (eds.) *Kön och våld I Norden. Report from a conference in Køge, Danmark, 23–24 November 2001. TemaNord 2002*: 545. København: Nordisk Ministerråd: 95–108. http://www.norfa.no/_img/1._Victimisation.pdf.

Sauli, Hannele. 2000. Lasten päivähoito. In Leena Kartovaara and Hannele Sauli (eds.) *Suomalainen lapsi. Väestö 2000/7*: 133–138. Helsinki: Tilastokeskus.

Suoninen, Lea. 1996. Miten päivähoitolaki menikään? *Sosiaaliturva* 4/96.

Tuori, Kaarlo. 2000. *Sosiaalioikeus.* Helsinki: Werner Söderström Lakitieto.

Vaajakallio, Laura. 1999. Päivähoito ja pienten lasten vanhempien työssäkäynti. *Hyvinvointikatsaus. Tilastollinen aikakauslehti* 3/1999: 37–41.

Vainio, Anne. 2004. «Laitos aina lapsille viimeinen vaihtoehto». Subjektiivinen päivähoitooikeus ja vanhemman työttömyys Aamulehden yleisönosastokirjoituksissa 1996–97. *Pro gradu-tutkielma, Sosiaalipolitiikan ja sosiaalityön laitos.* Tampereen yliopisto.

Välimäki, Anna-Leena, and Pirkko-Liisa Rauhala. 2000. Lasten päivähoidon taipuminen yhteiskunnallisiin murroksiin Suomessa. *Yhteiskuntapolitiikka* 5 (65): 387–405.

Ritva Nätkin

Contradiction between Gender Equality and Protection of Motherhood: Reproduction Policy in Finland

Finland is a small, sparsely populated country between the east and the west. In European comparisons, Finland was an agricultural country for a long time, and was urbanised, industrialised and modernised rapidly after the Second World War. After the 1960s, the country also prospered. The population's ethnic background and religious and cultural fabric are relatively homogeneous. At least this is what people wanted to believe during the Finnish project for national independence, which began in the 19th century, and in the non-governmental organisations which began to construct a civil society at that time (see Pulkkinen 1998; Alapuro 1987). Finland gained independence from the Russian Empire in 1917. The influential elite in Finland was small at the time (see Rantalaiho 1994) and the same people, both women and men, were active in NGOs, committees, government, etc. That is why the state is said to be understood as almost the same as (civil) society. According to its positive image, we Finns were proud of our independent survival and prosperity between the superpowers. According to its negative image, we are said to be the backwoods of a uniting Europe, suffering from a national archaism and a lack of proper manners, and from hard drinking and its by-products (for more on stigmatised Finnishness, see Apo 1998). When the upper class is narrow, national unity may manifest itself as a one-level culture where there is no room for difference (Alapuro 1998). On the other hand, Finland was a class society in the 20th century, which could be seen on the political level.

It has been said of Finnish women that they have always worked next to men, either on farms or, increasingly after the Second World War, in paid employment outside the home. Compared with the rest of Europe, the role of housewives and stay-at-home mothers remained rather weak. It was just in the 1930s, 1950s and again in the 1990s that Finnish women cared for their own children at home in greater numbers. At the same time, the male breadwinner role has also been weak; women and often mothers of young children have been in full-time employment and participated in providing for the family. Feminist researchers in Finland (see Gordon, Komulainen, and Lempiäinen 2002) debate whether the Finnish woman is especially "strong"–whether she has, based on her role as a breadwinner, a lot of power, and if so, power to do what. Or is she just the "workhorse" because of her double duty as a worker and a mother, which would be a more realistic interpretation in a poor and sparsely populated country. The interpretation of strength also emphasises women's wide participation in social action. In Finland, women were active participants in the popular movements at the end of the 19th and early 20th centuries which resulted in the birth of the nation state, equal and simultaneous suffrage for women and men and women being elected to the national parliament. It has been said that in an agrarian society, the work of both sexes has been appreciated and that this has also shown in social participation. Women have built the welfare state in their own domain (see Marakowitz 1993; Anttonen, Henriksson, and Nätkin 1994) as both citizens and professionals. The Martha Organization has been a particularly central force since the early 20th century in the construction of social motherhood, i.e. maternalism: it had a large membership, as did temperance societies, working class women's organisations and religious organisations. The maternalist orientation of the women's movement and politics was stronger than the individualistic (i.e. women's rights organisations) until the 1960s. (See Sulkunen 1990, 1987; Jallinoja 1983; for the rest of Europe see Bock and Thane 1991.)

That Finnish women are hard-working and the male breadwinner role is weak can partly be explained by the wars fought on Finnish soil (the Civil War in 1918 and the wars against the Soviet Union in 1939 and 1941–45), the heavy casualties of those wars, and the country's sparse population. According to the wartime and post-war population propaganda, there were "too few of us"; the country had to be both reconstructed and repopulated. Every family was to produce 4–6 children so that the Finnish population would not decrease. The baby boom generations were born at the end of the 1940s. The nationalistic emphasis on the united population who survived was strong at that time, and it can be regarded as the life force of the welfare state which developed later. The Finnish welfare state, which is presently associated with the Nordic model, is a nationalist construct that has been developed along with the building of the nation.

Population politics has been a central nationalist project in Europe in the 20th century (see Hobsbawm 1990). If nationalism is defined as a nation's right to a nation state, the definition also works the other way round: the nation state has to have a sufficient population. In Finland at the time of the Second World War, the population question was regarded as a question of the nation's fate because the size of the population threatened to decrease. The size of the population had already been a cause for concern in the 1920s, and this resulted in professional and political action to remedy the situation. A central actor was the Population and Family Welfare Federation of Finland, which NGOs founded in 1941 to promote population increase and to control 'the quality' of the population. Representatives of the nationalist movement, different political parties and professional organisations took part in the work of the Population and Family Welfare Federation; it joined both women and men. The maternity welfare system, which operates under local or municipal health authorities, was largely developed by this NGO.

The homogeneous Finnish culture is also evident in reproduction policy. There are few countries where basic health care covers expectant mothers as extensively as the Finnish maternity and child health centre in Finland. It could be said that visiting these health centres is a moral, even patriotic, duty for the Finns. Homogenous guidance for the homogenous nation is prevalent in the health centres; at any one time there is just the one truth about how things should be done. After the wars, many such services and benefits which had substantial national significance were instituted. A maternity package containing childcare items was the "state's gift to Finnish mothers" (Nätkin 1997, 78) and maternity and child health centres continue to be a service which almost all expectant mothers use (see Kuronen 1993). Maternity welfare and particularly the centres both still invoke the nationalist and population policy meaning with which they were created.

In this article, I pay special attention to population policy and The Population and Family Welfare Federation of Finland as part of reproduction policy, because this is what I have researched (Nätkin 1997). There are two other large NGOs in Finland that deal with reproduction, family policy and family work. The largest is the (General) Mannerheim League for Child Welfare, established in 1920, whose purpose was to reunite the Finnish population after the Civil War and safeguard all children's well being. Its political colour was – at least at the beginning – white, but it was independent of political parties and was at first associated with the Finnish Red Cross. Another large NGO – which started by focusing on unwed mothers and their children but has later concentrated on violence against women and mothers' substance abuse – is the Federation of Mother and Child Homes and Shelters. It was founded in 1945 and its political colour is red (or pink) because it was founded by the Social Democratic Women's Organisation. Among the different organisations, this one is most clearly a women's organisation (not feminist but maternalist), at the same time as it promotes the position of marginalised groups and families. The Population and Family Welfare Federation of Finland (nowadays The Family Federation of Finland) is a federation representing different NGOs, and it specialises in professional education and research more than in the family work which is characteristic of the two organisations mentioned earlier. Its political colour was green, especially at the time it was founded (its first chairperson belonged to the Agrarian Party, which is politically in the centre, and more conservative than the present-day Green Party). The non-governmental organisations have preceded the welfare state in experimenting with different types of operations in reproduction and family policy. Some of these operations have later become municipal or state institutions and some have remained in the NGO domain. The non-governmental organisations still complement the welfare state (the third sector, funded partly by The Slot Machine Association) though, at the same time, they are rather close to the state and local authorities. Apparently, because of the wars fought in the 20th century, the state and the NGOs close to it took on reproduction and population policies and family work, and there was not as large a role left over for church, communities or charities as there is in many other European countries.

Two Concepts: Protection of Motherhood and Gender Equality

Protection of motherhood is an essential concept in The Population and Family Welfare Federation's texts and other population policy texts as well as in professional (doctors' and midwives') journals that I have researched. What was meant by this concept was to protect mothers from a multitude of threats. At present, the most important threats are disease, poverty, different kinds of "risks" and the marginalising and stressful elements of working life. In the first decades of the 20th century, protection of motherhood included protecting mothers against men's sexuality and double standards, which was emphasised by the women's movement, or protecting mothers against race decay, which was promoted by professionals interested in eugenics or quality of the population. The emphasis on protecting motherhood varied depending on who the author was, his or her ideals, and the nature of the current debate. After the Second World War, protection of motherhood began to be concerned with fighting poverty and disease and confronting the demands of working life. This emphasis reflects the fact that from 1940–1970, mothers also became paid workers.

Two veins of emphasis can be discerned in the protection of motherhood: on the one hand, guarding the relationship between the mother and the child, while, at the same time, taking care of the mother and protecting the child, which necessitates that mothers and children are regarded somewhat separately. The categories of mother and child have increasingly diverged in professional texts as one approaches the present day. Child protection and medicine are both inclined to place the child in the foreground, at least in relation to a poor or unwed mother, or a mother with social problems, whereby the mother just becomes a breeding ground for the child.

In protection of motherhood, the woman and the child are seen as being in the inner chamber of the nation, as the nation's conscience or moral backbone – as some sort of nature. Protection of motherhood includes control, paternalist guardianship and eugenics. Population policy also includes a strong idealisation of motherhood and glorification of motherhood's value. The mother is the crucial person when decisions about population increase are made. Along with population policy, the mothers' welfare and well-being become national property. Nira Yuval-Davis (1997) writes that one of the most essential tasks of women in nationalist projects is to act as biological reproducers and generators of new population. Population policy also concentrates on women as they have the capacity to give birth (see Hatje 1974; Nätkin 1997) to the extent that one may talk about nationalising the female body. The scientific discoveries and procedures that had to do with giving birth and child care, and the propaganda and education that they entailed, were so compelling that it can be said that an ordinary mother was, in the context of population policy, a metaphorical soil for nationalistic aims. I think that in Finland this soil was over-exploited and its nourishment was neglected because the mothers were left on their own to burn out with their large families and the double duty of paid work and child care.

The spirit of protection of motherhood was paternalistic but also maternalistic. Motherhood was glorified, controlled and cultivated by both female and male professionals. The vice-chairperson of the Population and Family Welfare Federation, and the "state midwife," Leena Valvanne wrote about the work of a midwife in a maternity and child health centre where the work focused on expectant mothers: "I was like a sower who was able to sow the seed on cultivated fertile soil" (Valvanne 1986, 160). I regard this male metaphor as illustrative of the fact that female professionals were, like male professionals, militant actors in the pursuit of population policy goals (health care similarly employed a number of military metaphors – see Henriksson 1994).[1] The tone of duty which was used to bind ordinary women becomes apparent, for example, in relation to the rhetoric applied in connection to abortion, where women's "self-sacrificial mother's love" was appealed to as women's "natural" task. The Population and Family Welfare Federation, which in the 1950s and 1960s was granted the right to issue statements on abortion, denied most women's applications to terminate their pregnancies (Nätkin 1997, 29). The relationship between the sexes was very asymmetrical, as fathers were not appealed to in this way.

The concept of equality really only surfaced in the 1960s. However, its roots can be found further back in history. In Finnish society equality can be thought to emerge from the partnership of the sexes in agrarian work and from the trail-blazing partnership that had to do with national survival (see Rantalaiho 1994). In this kind of partnership, the relationships between the sexes are complementary, they supplement each other, and there is a clear division of labour between the sexes. Another source of the equality ideal can be found in socialist fellowship between women and men, where women were to be liberated from both private work and housework – which was regarded as bourgeois – and to participate in social action like men. The primary goal in socialist thinking is not equality between the sexes but equality between social classes and regions. This emphasis can also be seen in the social sciences which arose in the 1970s. The third historical source for gender equality concerns the debates in the women's movement where women were seen as individuals and equal rights with men were required. The demand for equality that surfaced in the 1960s entails two concepts of equality: the ideal of the similarity of the sexes, and the concept of different but equal. In the ideal of similarity, men were seen as the norm that women should strive for. In regard to the ideal of different but equal, feminist researchers debate whether difference means hierarchy, complementary roles or something else between the sexes. Some feminist researchers talk about "respecting gender/sexual difference".

On the basis of the concepts of protection of motherhood and gender equality, two competing, ideal types of family can be constructed: the symmetrical and the asymmetrical. In the asymmetrical ideal type, protection of motherhood, the mother and the child are almost entwined in the core of the family and the nation, and in the private sphere, and they are protected. The mother nurtures and the father protects and puts food on the table. The man moves – as a father, professional or a citizen – more on the outskirts of the family and in the public domain as a citizen in the labour market. Protection of motherhood is a strong concept in both population policy and medical discourse. In the symmetrical gender equality ideal type, the woman and the man are individuals who both have a role in the privacy of the family and in the public domain and labour markets. Parenthood is shared and there are two careers. There is a wish to regard the man and the woman as either completely similar or different but as having equal rights. There is also a tendency to see the child more and more as an individual having citizen's rights, such as the right to day care. These ideal types, which are largely based on heterosexuality, are not only family models, but also reflect women's and men's position in society which has, in the national project, has been regarded as having a family-like constellation.

Protection of motherhood has been stronger and come earlier than equality in reproduction policy. Equality and emphasis on individuality come up in professional texts in the 1950s and in politics in the 1960s. Ilpo Helén (1997) has analysed the changes in Finnish professional texts over time and discovered both an emphasis on individuality and a demand for communality. According to Helén (1997, 343–346) the female gender has three phases, for example in (the Population and Family Welfare Federation's) professional texts on marriage counselling. When, at the end of the 19th century, the basis for married life was sexual virtue (the man's honour and the woman's motherhood), which nationalism demanded, at the turn of the century and between the wars the main emphasis was on "healthy reproduction" i.e. national hygiene instead of moral ideals. It was important for the vitality of the nation that the man or the woman had the qualities and life force to reproduce healthily.[2] Since the late 1950s, marriage counselling has emphasised the individual whose psyche was coached to satisfactory married life and parenthood. The happiness and equilibrium of family members were the basis of the welfare society formed from "home, family and the child/ren". The language used in professional texts is increasingly gender neutral.

Instead, symmetrical family ideals and gender relations, such as shared parenthood, seem to be impossible in professional texts. Jaana Vuori (2001) has researched family guidebooks and other texts on parenting published in Finland in the 1980s and 1990s. In these texts the father is the active agent and the mother a taken-for-granted character in the background who however has the final responsibility for childcare and family life. In the background of focusing on the father is the fact that sex role activists (such as Association 9) and welfare professionals started at the turn of the 1960s and 1970s to draw fathers into the family and fatherhood. They wanted to ease the double duty of mothers consisting of full-time paid work outside the home and family responsibilities. The consequences were twofold. On the one hand, the model of the so-called new, caring and active father was created. On the other, mothers gained an extra task: to include the father in parenting in the name of equality and shared parenting.

Including the father and the father's rights is a strong programmatic goal in the Finnish welfare state: in health, social services and, increasingly, in legal practice. Kirsti Kurki-Suonio (1999) has conducted comparative law research on custody disputes and the child's care after divorce in California, Germany, the UK and Finland. Joint custody is the dominant practice in all researched countries and is justified by the child's welfare and best interests and equality. Feminist scholars are critical of joint custody if it is carried out in a way that is too automatic and clear-cut. The relationship between the sexes is very asymmetrical: the fathers only have rights to their children, but the mothers are left with the responsibility for care. On the basis of Finnish legal cases, the feminist researchers' criticism is also based on the fact that joint custody rulings do not take into sufficient account the fathers' violence, alcoholism and neglect, but highlight their rights. As a programmatic goal, the ideal of equality and gender neutrality can thus also turn against women.

Challenges to Reproduction Policy

At the time of the Second World War there was a general concern for the health and quality of the population in Finland, which caused a number of family laws to be passed. The work that NGOs started resulted in the creation of municipal and national benefit and service systems. The first family policy assistance system was the maternity grant in 1938 followed by municipal maternity health centres and midwives' posts in 1944 and the child benefit in 1948. The maternity welfare system, which this system can be called, includes the maternity grant or package, municipal maternity health centres and midwives and today also maternity hospitals and the maternity clinics that operate in these hospitals created at the end of the 1950s. The maternity welfare system also includes paid maternity leave and a maternity allowance (now called parental leave and parental allowance), which began in 1963 and which is an income transfer system.

According to data from journals in the 1940s, 1950s and 1960s which I have analysed, the debate on maternity welfare dealt with, among other things, syphilis, abortion, contraception, sterilisation, giving birth at hospitals, care for premature babies and increasingly as well as with mothers' labour market participation and the possible mother's wage. In the 1970s additional popular topics were added: parenting, breast-feeding, foetal diagnostics and at-risk pregnancies. Those participating in these debates are usually professionals, but ordinary people and political organisations also take part in some cases.

One of the most dangerous threats to the baby's health was syphilis, which was already discussed by maternity welfare professionals in the 1930s and which became more common in Finland during the war. Paediatricians noticed that the child's congenital syphilis could be prevented if the mother was treated during the first three months of the pregnancy. The municipal maternity health centre network, established in the mid-1940s, began to solve this problem by screening all expectant mothers. The mothers were drawn to maternity centres by the maternity grant that was either paid out in cash or given as a maternity package, and at the same time the mothers were obligated to take a blood test for syphilis. At the time, a midwives' journal characterised the syphilis prevention that was carried out in the maternity health centre network as "a beautiful story" in which medicine, so to speak, saved the baby in the womb of the syphilitic mother and got the disease under control. The creation of the network of maternity health centres was largely based on preventing syphilis. Preventing syphilis was outside a layperson's expertise and a sexual taboo; problems such as syphilis were hardly discussed. Professionals – in this case, doctors and midwives – modernised Finland at the same time as they were promoting the health of mothers and their babies. All attention was paid to the mother, although the contagion mostly came from men.

However, on the basis of my data, by far the most debated and contradictory issue after the war was illegal abortion. The situation among the citizens was explosive. Many more abortions were performed than are today: after the war, the estimate is 30,000 per year, and most of these were illegal. The Population and Welfare Federation delegated by the National Board of Health issued statements on abortion in which it interpreted the first 1950 law on abortion, but usually abortion only on medical grounds, or denied it. In the texts that I have analysed, the Federation's "work against abortion" is very prominent, and abortion was regarded almost as an unpatriotic act. There were huge regional differences inside the country. There were large families (10–15 children per family) in the north and east of Finland, often in religious communities. Smaller families (with two children) and more modern attitudes were found in the southern part of the country, evident for example in attitudes towards abortion, contraception and contraceptives. The Finns were in a very unequal position as regards abortion and availability of contraceptives. The poor families with many children in the countryside were characterised by the word "raggedy".

Abortions were not regarded as a direct threat to the unborn child's health and welfare but more as a threat to population growth. The mothers' health was at stake because the quackery involved in illegal abortions caused "fevered miscarriages" and permanent infertility. In the Population and Welfare Federation's centres (called 'marriage centre' or 'social problems centre') the doctors tried to oblige mothers seeking abortion to carry the pregnancies to term, because the society with its family policy benefits had "done so much". Women were strongly made liable. The doctors persuaded the mothers seeking abortion to give birth to "one more baby" before they were granted permission to contraception or sterilisation. The doctors also medicalised the women's wish to terminate the pregnancy by interpreting it as first trimester depression that could be treated (see Nätkin 1997, 127–133). Many children were born in very risky social conditions and there was a lot of social distress. The problem of abortion and its solutions had a number of competing constructs; it was debated whether medical, eugenic, criminal or social indications were grounds for granting abortion. The equality perspective is crystallised in the social indication.

The question of abortion also pitted ordinary people's expertise – evident in the women's wish to limit the birth rate and number of children in their families – against professional expertise and expectations of population growth each other. In a way, "quack" doctors represented the middle ground between lay and professional expertise. But the question of abortion also divided the doctors' consensus. Doctors in private practice outside maternity welfare services and other doctors familiar with women's everyday realities, such as psychiatrists, granted statements on abortion on social grounds even before the 1971 law, and they interpreted the 1950 law differently than the Population and Family Welfare Federation. Social scientists, psychologists and researchers of law also joined the generally heated abortion debate in the 1960s.

Feminist arguments highlighting women's rights to their own bodies were not used in this debate. To some extent the educated younger generation of women, who were clearly different from the women representing maternalist politics and who were against abortion, talked about equality between the sexes, but mostly they appealed to equality between different regions and social groups. The most active group of women lobbying politicians to accept the social indication were the Communist women (Finnish Women's Democratic League). This group was not active in the large NGOs that dealt with family and reproduction policy, as mentioned earlier, because at the time those groups were founded, this organisation was illegal and underground. However, after the war it had parliamentary influence.

Abortion is the most interesting of the reproductive controversies in that it clearly also reflects world politics. That abortion was regarded as unpatriotic had something to do with the fact that it was seen to refer to socialism and the Soviet Union (the former and present Russia). Finnish reproduction policy was influenced by Germany (emphasis on protection of motherhood) and Sweden (emphasis on equality and modernisation), but people in Finland were nevertheless constantly aware of the (negative) impact of their eastern neighbour.

The abortion controversy was solved by the relatively liberal Abortion Act in 1971. Counselling on contraception began at this time and protection of motherhood was improved and both these were enacted in the Public Health Act in 1972. Legislation enabling forced sterilisation was repealed. The Day Care Act of 1973 also belongs to the cluster of family legislation of the early 1970s. Unlike in other Nordic countries, abortion is granted in Finland only if the doctor agrees but in practice abortion is free. The doctor takes into account social indications. The health service system guarantees social rights (see Shaver 1994) and reproductive choice in this regard. It is characteristic of the Finnish homogeneous culture and consensus that the debate and controversy ended with the compromise made at that time.

Equality was not promoted in the 1960s and 1970s only by those in favour of free abortion, but also, in their own way, by the activists and female professionals in the maternalist women's movement. For example, midwives opposed pervasive medicalisation in which the state, bureaucracy and medicine effectively adopted the newborn baby and separated the mother and the child and all family members. The "state midwife" Leena Valvanne began a "battle for the father in the delivery room" where the father was drawn into the reproductive process in the name of shared parenthood.

Newer themes in the maternity welfare debate after the 1970s have, among other things, foetal screenings, the mother's smoking and health habits, substance abuse and depression. The mothers' substance abuse (alcohol and drugs) surfaced as a theme in the 1980s and 1990s, and professionals in maternity welfare and decision-makers still debate it. It has been discovered that the use of alcohol or drugs exposes the foetus and causes damage or withdrawal symptoms for the newborn baby. By means of foetal diagnostics developed in the 1970s, many of the risks threatening the welfare and health of the foetus can be prevented, but effective preventive measures are still being developed for the increasing problem of substance abuse. It is clear that medicine alone is incapable of solving this problem and the focus should not be, as it is in today's debates, only on the mother and the baby. It is a question of at-risk pregnancies and births that require a lot of intervention, but the risks are caused by social as well as medical factors. In the everyday practice of maternity hospitals, the mother and baby exposed to substance abuse require treatment for heightened risks, because drugs are often connected with HIV or hepatitis infections, premature births or ruptured placenta. Isolated rooms, protective gear and unprejudiced attitudes, free of fear and shame, are needed.

It seems to be very difficult in Finland, unlike in Sweden and Norway for example, to intervene in mothers' substance abuse and offer them specialised services. This may have to do with the ideal of equality and the Finnish woman's independence, but also with the fact that Finnish mothers have been left to manage on their own. There is a debate on the legitimacy of different intervention strategies: is the intervention forced or persuasive, are the mother and the child treated together or are they separated (as a way to save the child from the mother)? (Forced) sterilisation is not discussed these days, but abortion is actually imposed on mothers suffering from substance abuse. The third sector NGOs, such as the Federation of Mother and Child Homes and Shelters, try to treat the mother and child (and sometimes the whole family) together, but the traditional municipal child protection attempts to save the child from the mother's care.

The latest and most controversial reproduction policy in public discussion and parliamentary law preparation processes is the right of single and lesbian women to publically funded fertility treatments. There is no law concerning assisted conception, new reproductive technologies and (in)fertility treatment in Finland. The ethical norms of the medical profession alone are regulating the work of private doctors or professionals of the NGOs. The legislative process regulating the use of gametes and embryos in medical fertility treatment which began in 1987 has not yet come to an end. The status quo allowing all couples and individuals free access to fertility treatment still prevails. The "best interest of the child" is declared to be the primary guiding principle. The Population and Family Welfare Federation has been providing these services to single and lesbian women for quite some time, but now there is a threat that these services may become prohibited or even illegal.

Anu Pylkkänen (2003) has analysed this legislative process and notes that over the years, the tension has revolved around two basic issues: one's eligibility and the donor's anonymity. Opinions have been divided on whether other than established heterosexual couples should have access to the treatment, and on whether the child should have the right to know the identity of the donor. Surrogacy has been condemned quite unanimously, thus barring the possibility for infertile and gay couples to have a child that is partly of their own biological origin. Pylkkänen (2003) defines three different styles of argumentation in these debates. The first is a liberal one aimed at securing the freedom of private and individual rights, restricting them only from the child's perspective, if needed. The second is the "anti-discrimination perspective" looking at the ways in which different groups and individuals are treated by the law in the name of equality. The third is a conservative one wishing to secure traditional family patterns and the position of males in families. A common slogan in the debates and the statements of the majority of the Legal Affairs Committee (which gave its report in February 2003) was "the fact that there are already too many fatherless children in the society".

Change of Eras

Gender equality and protection of motherhood can be regarded as competing discourses or fluctuating political focuses with varying predominance. After the 1970's gender equality emphasis, the women's movement again raised the issue of women's particularity/difference. Even the reproduction policy controversies turned out to be rather complicated with regard to intricate aspects of protection of motherhood and gender equality.

Protection of motherhood and gender equality can also be seen as eras where the early 1970s are a turning point. The era of nationalist population policy when protection of motherhood was a central ideology lasted from the 1920s to the 1970s. In the 1970s, this changed to an era of family policy in welfare which does not include as many pro-natalist elements promoting increased birth rates and the ensuing obligations. Having children is now the person's own (and the spouse's) choice within the matrix of heterosexual marriage. The essentiality of protection of motherhood and the mother's care were questioned and replaced by gender-neutral shared parenthood and labour market motherhood. Although the hegemonic discourse on parenthood and family is gender neutral, it is the subject of a lot of feminist critique, women's and critical men's studies, and politics.

Anu Pylkkänen (2003) claims that since the abortion reform in the 1970s, there has been neither reproductive responsibility nor restrictions on who is entitled to procreate, and there has been a tendency to emphasise reproductive freedom and even reproductive rights, even if the discussion seldom uses these conceptions. The responsibility is needed especially in the case of assisted conception and new reproductive technologies. I believe responsibility is also required of both parents in the case of substance-addicted mothers, as a way of securing the welfare or best interest of the child. Pylkkänen claims that there is not enough discussion in Finland concerning fatherhood in practice and the real welfare of children. It is perhaps belated modernisation, the short history of the bourgeois family, and the rapid move from agrarian circumstances to an egalitarian, dual-breadwinner society which makes it difficult to analyse the changes in family and privacy when discussing legislative reforms.

The Norwegian researcher Merete Lie (2002) analyses how the new reproductive technologies change the relationship between nature and culture, women and men. When medical reproductive technologies are illustrated in newspapers and magazines, in the forefront there is a doctor holding a baby. The mother is placed behind him, more distant and unclear. The father is rarely present. Lie asks if science is the metaphorical father of the child? The foetus has, to an increasing extent, come to be understood as a separate being partly because of technological developments, such as ultrasonic scans, in-vitro fertilisation and other new reproductive technologies. There is a growing tendency to regard the foetus as an independent patient or (male) individual who has an existence apart from the mother and has citizen's rights. Riitta Burrell (2003) says that this pro-life inspired tendency is, however, alien to the Finnish culture and legal tradition.

At the turn of the 1970s, Finland also encountered other changes besides tendencies to reproductive freedom. It opened up culturally to international influence and immigration. The tone of the debate emphasising national survival changed and it began to include more global perspectives. People became aware of the imminent population explosion. Whereas population policy at first aimed to increase the number of original and genuine Finns, immigrants became admissible later on. Voices began to be heard saying that Finland should not be populated only by those born in Finland, by people who look and act like us. In the name of solidarity, our borders should be open to people who already exist in the world. Finland continues to apply rather strict policies concerning the residence of foreign nationals in the country. The number of immigrants is considerably smaller than in Sweden, for example.

Welfare state thinking emphasises universality and equality and Finland became, in the 1980s, a part of the Nordic welfare state model that is partly constructed upon these principles. The idea of universality is not totally new, however; it has its roots further back in the history of Finnish social policy. Population policy had created the basis for universal social policy by taking the whole nation as its target instead of just the relief of the poor. Universality has to do with social citizenship and social rights whereby nationality gives rights to income support and basic services. Universality is said to be possible only if there are relatively consistent value systems, if service needs are uniformly defined, if there is a trust in experts, and if individuals are regarded as belonging to the community (Anttonen and Sipilä 2000, 185).

There were elements of a backlash in the 1990s. Finns were faced with new challenges to survival after the economic recession in the early 1990s at the same time as Europe was integrating. Anneli Anttonen and Jorma Sipilä (2000, 46–49) claim that the ethos of lonely survival is an agrarian leftover in Finnish society from subsistence economy. This has been mixed up in the 1990s, however, with both neo-liberalism and European family ideals and (post)modern individualism demanded by the markets. A backlash is also evident in conservative reactions to the discussions concerning (in)fertility treatment. There is also a struggle over the role of the welfare state in integrating Europe, especially where feminist researchers and women's movement activists have taken a stand to defend it.

As Europe integrates, feminist researchers and many other Finnish women are worried about the fate of Finnish welfare, especially as regards health and social services, and women's rights. Integration is shadowed by fears that Finnish women will be removed from working life into traditional tasks in the home at the same time as social security and services are cut back to the level they are in Central and Southern Europe due to liberal economic thinking and Catholic family orientation. It is thought that the system of male breadwinners and housewives prevalent in Europe is also gaining ground in Finland. The fear is that even if there is no conscious choice about this in Finland, market forces and their emphasis on "national competitiveness" will inevitably result in this. On the other hand, no European Union regulations can bind the member states to change their social security and family policies, which are quite different in each European country. The social dimension of the European Union only aims at securing the minimum level of social rights (see Hantrais 1995). Chiara Bertone's (1998) research on the Danish women's movement at the time of the decision to join the European Union shows a similar situation: the European Union is regarded as a threat to Nordic equality and women's positions.

Feminist researchers refer to a "women's welfare state" or the Nordic "women-friendly welfare state" (Anttonen, Henriksson, and Nätkin 1994) when they discuss that system of services and income transfers which, as a part of the national (heterogeneous) welfare state construction, supports women's efforts to combine family and working life, and which shares women's responsibility for caring for children and for care in general. This is partly regarded as a women's achievement and therefore defendable. The utopian idea is that because of this, women will not end up in a worse position than men on the labour market due to motherhood and caring. Women are accustomed to relying on the state and municipalities – for example, in arranging day care for children – to the extent that researchers regard the state as women's "ally" (Anttonen, Henriksson, and Nätkin 1994). According to the criticism this has provoked, the utopia of alliance comes from the Finnish "state feminism" and illusion of equality. As a strategy for emancipation it is said to concentrate too much on motherhood and not to allow enough room for, or even see, difference. It is also said to be nationalistic and groundlessly superior in its relation to others. However, it is a good goal for reproduction policy.

Notes

1   In my dissertation (Nätkin 1997) I analysed the politics of four influential women of The Population and Family Welfare Federation: Rakel Jalas, Elsa Enäjärvi-Haavio, Martta Salmela-Järvinen and Leena Valvanne, and found a maternalist discourse which was common to them despite the fact that they had many class and generational differences. I define maternalism as a political movement and a way of thinking which binds together women and children and their interests in (welfare)politics. Gisela Bock and Pat Thane (1991) see maternalism as one of the trends of feminism in the European women's movements and they also connect maternalism with the birth of the welfare states. Maternalism had influence in the early decades and middle of the 20th century in Europe (and in the USA, see Koven & Michel 1993). According to Bock and Thane, it lost its significance in the 1960s. According to Bock and Thane, maternalism appeared in the parliamentary activity of women in most European countries. It also appeared as an active counter-force in totalitarian states (Hitler's Germany, Franco's Spain and Mussolini's Italy) and their anti-natalism during the Second World War. It was often connected to population or pro-natalist policies which aimed to increase the birth rate, but it cannot be identified with them.

2   Healthy reproduction often meant race hygiene and the segregation and classification of populations. Anti-natalist tendencies were not, however, very strong in Finnish population policy and welfare systems, perhaps because of the sparse population and the unity of the surviving nation. Compulsory sterilisation was possible according to the Sterilisation Law of 1935, but in my data doctors complained that the sterilisations were not carried out. In Rakel Jalas's (a doctor and one of the influental women of the Federation) theory, individual hygiene corresponded with mental and social hygiene in the society and a healthy individual corresponded with a healthy society. She talked about weak and strong individuals, and even about 'the dregs of society' who share an uncontrollable sexual instinct. She promoted, for example, the sterilisation of weak individuals. The effect of the race improvement theory (eugenics) of the 1930s and the survival challenges caused for the Finnish people by the Winter War can be seen in her writings. Also maternity welfare clearly seems to have had a race hygienic root, and maternalist arguments were from time to time merged with race hygienic arguments in the speeches of some women pioneers of maternity welfare. If the women's action, such as the protection of motherhood, were not taken into account, active women (like Rakel Jalas) would later be seen in an unfavourable light. The health services undertaken by child and maternity welfare centres were defined by the contemporaries'positive race hygiene'.

References

Alapuro, Risto. 1998. Sivistyneistön ambivalentti suomalaisuus (The ambivalent Finnishness of intelligentsia). In Pertti Alasuutari and Petri Ruuska (eds.) *Elävänä Euroopassa. Muuttuva suomalainen identiteetti* (Alive in Europe. Changing Finnish identity). Tampere: Vastapaino.

Anttonen, Anneli, and Jorma Sipilä. 2000. *Suomalaista sosiaalipolitiikkaa* (Finnish social policy). Tampere: Vastapaino.

Anttonen, Anneli, Lea Henriksson, and Ritva Nätkin (eds.). 1994. *Naisten hyvinvointivaltio* (Women's welfare state). Tampere: Vastapaino.

Anttonen, Anneli. 1994. Hyvinvointivaltion naisystävälliset kasvot (The women friendly face of welfare state). In Anneli Anttonen, Lea Henriksson, and Ritva Nätkin (eds.) *Naisten hyvinvointivaltio* (Women's welfare state). Tampere: Vastapaino.

Apo, Satu. 1998. Suomalaisuuden stigmatisoinnin traditio (The tradition of stigmatising Finnishness). In Pertti Alasuutari and Petri Ruuska (eds.) *Elävänä Euroopassa. Muuttuva suomalainen identiteetti* (Alive in Europe. Changing Finnish identity). Tampere: Vastapaino.

Bertone, Chiara. 1998. Contructing a women's perspective on the European Union: the Danish Debate. *NORA, Nordic Journal of Women's Studies*, Vol. 6, Number 2: 108–121.

Bock, Gisela, and Pat Thane (eds.). 1991. *Maternity and Gender Policies: Women and the Rise of European Welfare States 1880s–1950s*. London and New York: Routledge.

Burrell, Riitta. 2003. *Äitejä ja sikiöitä* (Mothers and foetuses). Väitöskirja.

Gordon, Tuula, Katri Komulainen, and Kirsti Lempiäinen (eds.). 2002. *Suomineitonen, hei. Kansallisuuden sukupuoli* (Hello Suomi-girl. The gender of nationality). Tampere: Vastapaino.

Hantrais, Linda. 1995. *Social Policy in the European Union*. London: McMillan Press Ltd.

Hatje, Ann-Katrin. 1974. *Befolkningfrågan och välfärden. Debatten om familjepolitik och nativitetsökning under 1930- och 1940-talen* (Population policy and welfare. Discussion about family policy and population increase in 1930s and 1940s). Stockholm: Almänna Förlaget.

Helén, Ilpo. 1997. *Äidin elämän politiikka. Naissukupuolisuus, valta ja itsesuhde Suomessa 1880-luvulta 1960-luvulle* (The politics of mother's life. Female gender, power and self-relationship). Helsinki: Gaudeamus.

Henriksson, Lea. 1994. Ammatillisen sisaruuden uudet jaot – sota terveystyön taitekohtana (The new divisions of occupational sisterhood – the war as a turning point of health work). In Anneli Anttonen, Lea Henriksson, and Ritva Nätkin (eds.) *Naisten hyvinvointivaltio* (Women's welfare state). Tampere: Vastapaino.

Hobsbawm, Eric. 1990. *Nations and Nationalisms since 1780. Programme, Myths, Reality*. Melksham: Cambridge University Press.

Jallinoja, Riitta. 1983. *Suomalaisen naisliikkeen taistelukaudet. Naisasialiike naisten elämäntilanteen muutoksen ja yhteiskunnallis-aatteellisen murroksen heijastajana*. Helsinki: WSOY.

Koven, Seth, and Sonya Michel (eds.). 1993. *Mothers of a New World: Maternalist Politics and the Origin of the Welfare States.* New York and London: Routledge.

Kurki-Suonio, Kirsti. 1999. *Äidin hoivasta yhteishuoltoon – lapsen edun muuttuvat oikeudelliset tulkinnat* (From maternal care to joint custody – the changing legal interpretations of the best interest of the child). *Suomalaisen lakimiesyhdistyksen julkaisuja A-sarja* No. 222. Helsinki.

Kuronen, Marjo. 1993. *Lapsen hyväksi naisten kesken. Tutkimus äitiys – ja lasten-neuvolan toimintakäytännöistä* (For the child's good together with women. A research concerning the practices of maternity and child health centre). Stakes, Tutkimuksia 35. Helsinki.

Lie, Merete. 2002. Science as Father? Sex and Gender in the Age of Reproductive Technologies. *The European Journal of Women's Studies,* vol. 9 (4): 381–399.

Marakowitz, Ellen Louise. 1993. *Gender and nationalism in Finland: the domestica-tion of the national narrative.* New York: Columbia University.

Nätkin, Ritva. 1997. *Kamppailu suomalaisesta äitiydestä. Maternalismi, väestö-politiikka ja naisten kertomukset* (Struggle for Finnish motherhood. Maternal-ism, population policy and women's narratives). Helsinki: Gaudeamus.

Pulkkinen, Tuija. 1998. *Postmoderni politiikan filosofia* (The post-modern philoso-phy of politics). Helsinki: Gaudeamus.

Pylkkänen, Anu. 2003. *Law proposal on fertility treatment in Finland: contested meanings of family, gender and relationships.* A paper presented in a Seminar "Family relationships and intimacy in a globalizing world", in Rauma, Finland 4th–6th September 2003.

Rantalaiho, Liisa. 1994. Sukupuolisopimus ja Suomen malli (The gender contract and Finnish model). In Anneli Anttonen, Lea Henriksson, and Ritva Nätkin (eds.) *Naisten hyvinvointivaltio* (Women's welfare state). Tampere: Vastapaino.

Shaver, Sheila. 1994. Body rights, social rights and the liberal welfare state. *Critical Social Policy,* Issue 39: 66–93.

Sulkunen, Irma. 1987. Naisten järjestäytyminen ja kaksijakoinen kansalaisuus. In Risto Alapuro et al. (eds.). *Kansa liikkeessä*: 157–172. Helsinki: Kirjayhtymä.

Sulkunen, Irma. 1991. *Retki naishistoriaan.* Helsinki: Hanki ja Jää.

Valvanne, Leena. 1986. *Rakkautta pyytämättä. Valtakunnankätilö muistelee* (Love without asking. Statemidwife is looking back). Helsinki: Tammi.

Vuori, Jaana. 2001. *Äidit, isät ja ammattilaiset. Sukupuoli, toisto ja muunnelmat asiantuntijoiden kirjoituksissa* (Mothers, fathers and professionals. Gender, rep-etitions and variations in the experttexts). Tampere: Tampere University Press.

Yuval-Davis, Nira. 1997. *Gender & Nation.* London: Sage Publications.

Sílvia Portugal

Women, Welfare State, and Welfare Society in Portugal

Welfare State and Welfare Society

In the European context, Portugal seems to be one of the countries in which both the institutionalisation of social rights and the equipping of the state with the necessary instruments for the exercise of a coherent social policy occurred later and were more problematic. This fact is related to historical circumstances that influenced the evolution of Portuguese society throughout the 20th century, and especially in its second half: first, the persistence of a dictatorial regime until the beginning of the 1970s, which delayed the modernization of the administrative apparatus and the establishment of citizenship rights; and second, the lateness of the de-ruralization of Portuguese society, that is to say, its industrialization, its urbanization, and the expansion of the service sector (Hespanha, Ferreira, and Portugal 1997).

The so-called "Estado Novo", ruled for nearly half a century by Salazar, adopted a model of social regulation adverse to the development of consistent social policies. It staked itself to what we can call "familism", a conservative ideology supported by the rural condition of a large part of the population, which permitted the maintenance of social support based on family and community solidarity and on weak expectations in relation to consumption and quality of life (Hespanha, Ferreira, and Portugal 1997).

It was only after the establishment of the democratic regime in 1974 that the first systematic programs directed toward constructing a welfare state were developed. This was reflected in the growth of the public expense of welfare, which has continued to increase until now. However, this increase occurred during an international economic crisis, exactly when more developed welfare states had begun to confront the need to adopt more restrictive measures.

As a consequence, the expansionism felt after the change of regimes was followed by a phase of budget restraint after 1982 which prevented Portugal from approaching the model of state-produced welfare that characterized many European countries (Mozzicafreddo 1992). Besides the low level of state expenses in the social domain, the measures adopted had a weak reach and were relatively inefficient. In 1960, only 36 percent of the population potentially within the then-existent social welfare system benefited from it. This rate increased to 76 percent in 1980, and 87 percent in 1990 (Carreira 1996). Nevertheless, this evolution did not prevent a large portion of the population, particularly those who were placed in the margins of the formal labour market, from being relatively excluded from state welfare. As Andreotti et al. show, even though the levels of social expenditure have been increasing during the last two decades, the pattern of its internal distribution remains uneven and completely unbalanced in favour of pensions, giving few resources to active labour policies, housing or social exclusion. A comparative perspective between the North and the South of Europe shows very clearly the allocation of expenditure and the overwhelming weight of insurance and contribution-based welfare provisions in South European countries (Andreotti et al. 2001, 46).

The differences between the Portuguese reality and the model of advanced capitalist societies have led Boaventura de Sousa Santos to characterise the Portuguese state as a semi-welfare state (Santos 1993, 46) whose insufficiencies are partly balanced by strong community ties. The author states that "in Portugal a weak welfare state coexists with a strong welfare society" (Santos 1993). The welfare society can be defined as a configuration of "networks of relationships of inter-knowledge, mutual recognition, and mutual help, based on kinship and community ties, through which small social groups exchange goods and services on a non-market basis, and with a logic of reciprocity" (Santos 1993, 46). The debate raised by the welfare state crisis in developed countries led to the (re)discovery of this welfare society – that is, to the idea that the informal welfare networks and, above all, the family, are an important element in social support, and therefore need to be taken into account when discussing the total production of social welfare.

The attribution of responsibilities and sharing of welfare between the public and the private sectors have become key issues. This became problematic precisely when, under the pressure of the welfare state crisis, the possibility of transferring certain services and duties which had been covered by public policies to the sphere of the family had to be faced.

In view of current social and demographic changes, the constraints on the action of family social networks are increasing. In southern European countries, and specifically in Portugal, the increasing entry of women into the labour market, the decrease in fertility and the consequent reduction in the size of the family, the increase in life expectancy, and demographic ageing are some of the factors which make it imperative to (re)think the family's role in welfare provision. As we can see in Table 1, the social and demographic changes of the last three decades in Portugal are extremely significant, not only because of their impact on the lives of families, but also because of the rapid pace at which they have occurred.

Table 1: Social indicators, 1960–2001

	1960	1970	1981	1991	1997	2001
Women's activity rate (%)	13.0	19.0	29.0	35.9	43.0	44.9
Fertility rate (‰)	24.1	20.9	16.1	11.8	11.4	10.9
Children per woman	3.2	3.0	2.2	1.5	1.4	1.5
Marriage rate (‰)	7.8	9.4	7.4	7.3	6.6	6.2
Mortality rate under 1 year (‰)	77.5	55.5	24.3	11.0	6.4	5.0
Mortality rate (‰)	10.7	10.8	9.7	10.4	10.5	10.2
% Population over 65 years	8.0	9.7	11.4	13.6	15.1	16.4

Source: INE – Instituto Nacional de Estatística [National Institute of Statistics]

Having traditionally been the major care providers, families now find themselves faced with complex problems related to a growing dependent population (the elderly, for example) and, given the increase in female participation in the labour market, fewer resources for care provision. This growing inability to provide care has to do with changes in the morphological pattern of the family, and with its relationship to the labour market and other institutions of care provision, such as the state and the market.

Although it has never achieved the welfare provision levels of other European countries, Portugal has, in recent years, adopted some of the restrictive measures that characterise the current phase of evolution of the welfare state in those countries (Hespanha 1999). These measures include: privatisation of state social services; private management of public services; devolution to civil society (or de-institutionalisation) of state welfare provision; shared accountability of citizens in social spending; and revitalisation of civil society support systems. It is "as if Portugal were going through a welfare state crisis, without ever having had [a welfare state]" (Santos 1993, 45).

The key issue is not only the importance of the family's contribution to the protection of individuals, but also the specific relations that exist between the welfare society and the welfare state, as well as between the welfare state and the market. This "state/family/market" link implies that the crisis in the system of social welfare inevitably has an impact on the other elements in the triad. The weakening of the welfare state may also bring about a similar process in the welfare society. As Claude Martin states, this may be where the southern European specificity is to be found: in fact, the development of social welfare systems took place in a period of economic recession, thereby jeopardizing their complete development, while the family was undergoing a process of change linked to the transformation of the labour market, a change which involved a profound reformulation of values related to the domestic sphere (Martin 1996).

Women, Welfare State and Welfare Society

The social well-being produced by the welfare society has heavy costs for women. Given the traditional division of labour that prevails in Portuguese families, women assume nearly all of the responsibility for domestic work and care for the dependent (children, the elderly, disabled people). It is important to stress that when we speak about the Portuguese welfare society and the importance of family social networks in the social provision of well-being, we are talking about the work, the daily life, the effort and the commitment of women.

Nowadays, new challenges have been introduced into the situation described above. Tradition and modernity co-exist today in Portuguese families, modifying the capacities of the welfare society and the status of women in the family and in society. On the one hand, family obligations, especially intergenerational obligations, still have an important role in defining family relations and gender relations within the family.[1] From this point of view, women continue to assume the traditional role of caregiver. On the other hand, women are increasingly entering the labour market and losing their ability to respond to all of the informal care demands that are expected of them.

As we can see in Table 2, Portugal has one of the highest female activity rates within the European Union. If we look at the activity rate of women aged 20 to 44, with children between 0 and 5 years old, we can see the specificity of the Portuguese case. What I will try to show is that in Portugal, the state has largely abandoned women on the issue of childrearing. Policy measures to support working mothers have fallen into "the trap of believing in formal equality in a society without any real equality" (Ferreira 1998, 176). Family policies take legally established gender equality for granted, overlooking the fact that in real life women and men have different responsibilities within the domestic sphere. In doing this, they have not only *not* integrated the promotion of equality, but have also contributed, in some cases, to reinforcing inequalities and traditional social practices within families.[2]

Table 2: Activity rate of women (20–44 years) in EU countries (1998)

Country	Without children	Children 0–5 years
Austria	85	68
Belgium	77	66
France	72	56
Germany	83	49
Greece	60	48
Ireland	81	46
Italy	68	45
Luxembourg	84	49
Netherlands	86	60
Portugal	**83**	**72**
Spain	67	40
United Kingdom	87	53

Source: CIDM (2001)

Looking at Jane Lewis' model of patterns of male and female paid work (Lewis 2001), we can classify Portugal within Model 5, the Dual-Career Model (see Table 3). This is sometimes forgotten when Portugal is classified as a "fourth model" or a "southern model" of welfare along with Greece, Spain and Italy (Ferrera 1996), all countries where the activity rate of women with small children is much lower. Looking at the right column of table 3, concerning arrangements for care, the following questions arise: Who supplies the care work in Portugal? What is the role of the state? What should the role of the state be?

Table 3: Lewis' model of patterns of male and female paid work and arrangements for care

1. Male-Breadwinner Model	
Male FT earner	Female FT caregiver
2. Dual-Breadwinner Model 1	
Male FT earner, female short PT earner	Care supplied mainly by female earner and kin
3. Dual-Breadwinner Model 2	
Male FT earner, female long PT earner	Care supplied mainly by kin, and state/ voluntary sector/market
4. Dual-Breadwinner Model 3	
Male PT earner, female PT earner	Care supplied by male and female earners
5. Dual-Career Model	
Male FT earner, female FT earner	Care supplied mainly by the market and kin/ state/voluntary sector
6. Single-Earner (Lone Mother Family) Model	
Female earner FT or PT, or FT mother reliant on state benefits	Care supplied either by the mother or by the mother, kin and the state

FT=full-time; PT= part-time   *Source: Lewis (2001, 157)*

Support for working mothers has been viewed in Portugal from the point of view of family policy, since social policy is still influenced by a strong "familism". The family is the central target of discourse in the social field, and continues to be the main frame of reference when speaking about social policies. This fact is somewhat surprising if we compare the situation of Portugal with that of neighbouring Spain, where the former dictatorship also fed on a strong familist ideology. Celia Valiente (1996), a Spanish sociologist who has studied these issues, shows that the weak investment in this area in her country is due to a clear break with the Franco regime legacy as regards family policy, which was strongly pro-natalist and anti-feminist. Thus, in Spain, social transfers have deteriorated and the investment in the area is practically non-existent, but these features of state intervention correspond to a position taken by the democratic regime, which has made a break with the past and refuses to establish a political program on this matter.

In Portugal, the situation is quite different. There was never a break with the familist ideology of the past. On the contrary, it has persisted in the discourse of public policies, and continues to be at the centre of the social discourse of both the government and the opposition, of the Right and the Left (at least that version of the Left which has been in power until now).

What are the characteristics of state action in this domain? An analysis of the political and legal discourses since the revolution of 1974[3] reveals several contradictions between political discourse, government practices, legislative action, and the social effects of policies. Some of these contradictions are certainly not exclusive to the Portuguese situation, but they have, in this country, a structuring character in the definition of the profile of the state system.

The first major contradiction is found between an explicit ideological commitment to the family and the subsidiary position that family policy occupies within the whole of the social policies. In almost all the programs of the 14 constitutional governments, we find a commitment to the "family question" that does not correspond to subsequent political action. The framework of state intervention has not had significant alterations since 1974. The legislation produced in the area of the family is scarce and primarily of a regulatory nature, issued by the government or the ministries (Portugal 1998). Social payments correspond to insignificant amounts,[4] and the infrastructures available for supporting families are frankly insufficient.[5]

We can only talk about the attempt to implement a true family policy during a short period of time. From 1980 to 1982, during the 6th, 7th, and 8th governments of the Democratic Alliance (a centre-right coalition), we find, in addition to a strongly familist discourse in government programs, some changes in the governmental structure that tried to respond more efficiently to the family question. In 1980, the State Office of the Family (Secretaria de Estado da Família) and the Interministerial Commission of the Family (Comissão Interministerial da Família) were established (Law 202/80), and in 1982 the Organic Structure of the Ministry of Social Affairs for Family Affairs (Estrutura Orgânica do Ministério dos Assuntos Sociais para os Assuntos da Família) was created. The latter included the Interministerial Commission of the Family, the Advisory Council of Family Affairs (Conselho Consultivo dos Assuntos da Família), the Cabinet of Studies and Projects for Family Affairs (Gabinete de Estudos e Projectos dos Assuntos da Família) and the General Directorate of the Family (Direcção-Geral da Família).

However, the practical results of these changes, expressed both in the political discourse of government programs and in some of the legislative measures adopted during this period, remained far behind the initial expectations and were not subsequently developed. In 1983, the State Office of the Family was abolished; the Interministerial Commission and the Advisory Council were never fully operational, although there were several attempts to reactivate them (the last dating from 1988) without any visible results. The General Directorate of the Family, which underwent its final remodelling in 1993, was the only one which survived until the recent socialist governments, and functioned only as an advisory organ, which centralized and produced information about the family, but had no powers of coordination or supervision of policies. After 1982, there was a clear retreat from the idea of a family policy, which became mainly the object of theoretical study and fragmentary legislative production.

The two most recent socialist governments (in power from 1995 to 2001) once again adopted the familist discourse in their programs, and they also revived some of the structures created between 1980 and 1982, by changing or abolishing them and substituting them with others. The structures that had been inoperative since the governments of the Democratic Alliance were substituted by the High Commissioner for the Questions of Equality and the Family (Alto-Comissário para as Questões da Igualdade e da Família) and by the National Council of the Family (Conselho Nacional da Família) in the first government and by the Ministry of Equality in the second one.

What was innovative in these socialist governments was the fact that, for the first time, family policies were expressly linked to equality policies. This was indeed different from what had been the prevailing discourse about family policy until then, but once again stated intentions were not followed by practical consequences.

In 1999, there was a fundamental piece of legislation on this issue, which had the objective of establishing a family policy: "The Plan for a Global Family Policy." This plan represents an attempt to formulate the foundations of a family policy. However, the way in which it is formulated allows us to anticipate that it will not easily lead to visible practical results. The text of the document does not leave space for much optimism. Its rhetoric is not much different from that of previous documents on the issue, namely those of the aforementioned Democratic Alliance governments, as well as previous Social Democrat Party governments, especially in the context of the commemorations of the International Year of the Family. The vagueness of the proposals made in the Plan, which do not establish priorities or concrete goals and measures to be implemented, leads us to view it as one more example of the profile of family policies since 1974: an area of strong investment in rhetoric, but of weak political action.

The current conservative government, from a new Democratic Alliance, has launched the "Lei de Bases da Família," a piece of legislation which is even weaker than the previous socialist government Plan. The text of this law serves mainly to convey an ideological discourse about what the family is and what it should be, and very little is established in terms of goals to be achieved by the state concerning a family policy.

This government has also replaced the different structures created by the socialist government with a single one, the National Coordinator for Family Affairs. The Coordinator is a woman who, when taking office in January 2003, said that her role was to defend the values of the traditional family and that we would never hear her speak about abortion, but only about the right to life.

Both political and legislative discourses on the family reveal an extremely conservative and traditional view, and the "Lei de Bases da Família" is perhaps the best example of this. In some areas, the political discourse is even profoundly moralist regarding what the family is and what it should be. In most texts on this issue, the family is defined in essentialist and naturalist terms, and very little attention is given to the current realities and changes in the family.

The actors involved in the design and application of family policies have very much contributed towards imprinting these characteristics on state action. An analysis of the different consultative and executive organizational structures that have been established over the years to define family policies shows that most of their protagonists have remained in office in spite of party changes. The analysis shows, on the one hand, the power of private institutions of social solidarity, and on the other, the fundamental importance of the Catholic Church, through the intervention of priests, as well as that of prominent figures from different sectors with close connections to the Church. I have already had occasion to assess the preponderant role of the Catholic Church in the definition of family policies in a case study on the commemorations of the International Year of the Family in Portugal

(Portugal 2001). My research showed that the primary force behind this event was the Church and not the state.

Finally, a last contradiction, although not exclusive to family policies, lies in the discrepancy between the legal framework and its actual application. Although our welfare state is based on universalistic principles, an analysis of state intervention in the area of maternity assistance reveals that there are large segments of the population that are excluded from state protection. The percentages of coverage are very low, both in terms of social payments and available infrastructures.

In 1991, out of all family allowances in the area of maternity, only child benefits had a rate of coverage above 75 percent. Birth grants reached exactly 75 percent of families, nursing allowances 64.5 percent, and maternity leave allowances only 53 percent (Portugal 1995). The socialist governments also introduced changes in this area, suppressing all these benefits and substituting them with a single allowance.[6] This measure introduced for the first time the logic of selectivity in social policies in Portugal, granting differentiated benefits according to family income.

Child Care in Portugal

In what is referred to as child care services, state intervention has also lagged far behind the political principles subscribed to by the different governments. Although the Portuguese Constitution establishes, in Article 67, "the creation of a national network for mother and child assistance, a system of crèches, and family-support infrastructures", the scarcity of facilities is emphasized by all the national and international reports on this question.[7]

Although the family support structures in the area of child care are, even today, considered insufficient, the ability of the existing services to respond to the care needs of children up to the age of six has grown significantly since 1974. This growth has been characterised by an enormous socio-legal and socio-pedagogic diversity (Conselho Nacional de Educação 1994). Child care services derive from several controlling bodies with varying administrative departments, different care duties, and different kinds of financing and organisation.

As regards control and ownership, services exist in both the public and private sectors. In the public sector, there are facilities run by both central government and local authority departments. The private sector includes charitable bodies, religious organisations, private institutions, companies, citizens' groups and parents' associations.

State obligations are met through two ministries whose functional organisations are quite different: the Ministry of Work and Social Security and the Ministry of Education. The latter has a centralised structure, whereas the Ministry of Work and Social Security, in its Social Security operations, is divided into Regional Centres (CRSS), which enjoy a high degree of autonomy.

Socio-pedagogic diversity can be added to socio-legal diversity, though the former results in part from the latter. In accordance with ministerial obligations, two different kinds of operations can be identified: the services run by the Ministry of Work and Social Security operate according to a welfare model, whereas in the Ministry of Education, the educational model prevails (Bairrão et al. 1990).

The lack of any integrated policy in this area and the prevalence of a compartmentalisation strategy of services has been, above all, prejudicial to the welfare of children up to three years of age. The issue of child care services for those up to school age encompasses two distinct questions: first, the question of looking after the child, which is to say, the need to provide safe supervision while the parents are at work ("taking care of the child"); second, the issue of pre-school education.

The three- to six-year age group was the one to gain from the establishment of a public pre-school education system following the 1974 Revolution,[8] and benefitted from discussions on the role and structure of the education system in Portugal. However, the needs of families in terms of care for children up to three years of age, for whom the question of supervision is superimposed on that of education, have been ignored by a succession of public policies. In 1997 the socialist government approved a law on pre-school education[9] which intended to implement a network of facilities that allowed a slight expansion of child care for children between the ages of three and six. However, the extent of formal provisions for children under three continued to receive practically no attention in the debate on public policies and priorities concerning day-care provision. By focusing on pre-school education for those over three years of age, child care has essentially been conceived from the point of view of the child's educational career, rather than from the point of view of promoting the conciliation of work and family life.

Contrary to the situation that prevails for three- to six-year olds, the state option for children under three years of age has consisted of diversifying the type of services, which has involved more flexible structures which require less investment, and are thus more profitable in economic terms. Thus, the 1980s saw an increase in the use of mini-crèches, nannies and family crèches. Although mini-crèches have not thus far enjoyed large-scale development (in 1997, there were only three), nannies and family crèches have been the only child care services to really expand for this age group. By 1997, there were 596 registered nannies, caring for 2300 children.

Two main features of the current state of official support of child care for children under three stand out: on the one hand, there is an attempt to find cheaper answers, and this has taken the form of legal regulation of models and solutions in the informal sector, such as nannies and family crèches; on the other, there is an increasing tendency to resort to private enterprise, both for-profit and non-profit, in order to establish a system of facilities in this area.

State services provide very few children with a formal mode of supervision. The most important providers of services in this area are the "Instituições Privadas de Solidaridade Social" (Private Institutions for Social Solidarity) (IPSS). It is these institutions that bear the brunt of responsibility for child care in our country[10].

State intervention in the sphere of child supervision services essentially consists of Social Action, responsible both for licensing and financing nannies and for funding the IPSS, the sole dynamic sectors in this area. There is no public policy that guarantees the rights of families to child care. Instead of assuming the universalistic principles proclaimed in the Constitution, the state has assumed a subsidiary role, increasingly opening the field to private enterprise.

In the sphere of child care there is, therefore, a welfare model which, far from offering an adequate response to the needs of most families, merely takes care of a minority and resolves only certain specific situations. The absence of state intervention means even worse problems for those people who have no access to the child care market, where prices are too high for most Portuguese families.

In short, the options available to families in terms of child care facilities are very limited. Public policies present such a deficient material context – in terms of both funding and infrastructure – that families' choices are extremely limited: given the paucity of valid alternatives, they have to make use, above all, of their own resources.

Some of the results of a survey that I carried out in the Coimbra district, in 1993, about aid to families that had had their first child,[11] revealed the importance of family networks in child care and the absence of state response to family needs. The survey showed that 80 children from the sample (35 percent of the total) were cared for by the mother; 60 (27 percent) were looked after by a family member; 44 (20 percent) were supervised by a nanny, and 33 (15 percent) were in a crèche. Only six children (three percent) were cared for by a domestic employee. This demonstrates that informal contexts for child supervision predominate – only 15 percent of the total were cared for by a formal child care service. The importance of the family model, however, is emphasised by the fact that approximately 63 percent of the infants are in the exclusive care of the mother or another family member (Portugal 1998).

The data from the survey and from the interviews that I carried out more recently[12] reveal the same conclusions: on the one hand, child supervision is essentially a family responsibility, and, on the other hand, families need the help of their relatives and friends on a daily basis in order to meet their child care needs.

One interesting feature of the family supervision model is the fact that, to a large extent, it relies on more than one person for care of the child. Families whose child is in the care of the mother often receive help from at least one member of their family. The task of child supervision is overwhelmingly shared by the maternal or paternal grandmother, but there are also mothers who received support from their sisters, sisters-in-law, aunts and cousins. When the child is in the care of a relative, the same pattern of sharing responsibility occurs: when the child is looked after by a relative, she usually has additional help from another member of the family network.

The multiplicity of agents involved in child care exposes some interesting issues: first, there is the mobilisation of the social network of relatives in response to the problem; then we have the polarising role of women: where there is the capacity to respond to the needs of families, this situation is due entirely to their action; finally, and this is largely a result of these other issues, there is an enormous fragility which this family mechanism exhibits in the face of formal solutions.

Supervision shared between different relatives makes each one an indispensable link in the chain and, therefore, the system is highly susceptible to the unexpected. Normally the responsibility for caring is divided up into distinct periods of the day, thus enabling the women involved, for instance, to engage in paid activity. Should anything unforeseen occur, such as illness, the entire system may collapse. The only reason why this does not happen more frequently seems to be that there is always some female relative who "can lend a hand". However, as these female hands are increasingly integrated into the labour market, they will become correspondingly less available.

These facts are important, therefore, in the discussion of what Wellman calls the "political economics of the community" (Wellman 1985, 70), or, the place of personal networks in systems of production and social reproduction. Women have been used, to a great extent, as a "reserve army" for the reproduction of families, supplying low-cost services of high quality and great flexibility. The utilisation of this army benefits the family and also contributes a great deal to other spheres which generate well-being, particularly the state sector, which is thus relieved of its responsibilities.

Final Comments

The empirical research studies that I conducted demonstrate the vitality of family bonds, and, in a larger sense, of the welfare society vis-à-vis the insufficiency of state assistance. However, they also reveal a series of problems in relations between the family and the state, as I suggested at the beginning.

First, the data emphasize a question originally formulated by Boaventura de Sousa Santos in his characterization of the welfare society, a problem equally emphasized by other authors (Hespanha and Alves 1995; Nunes 1995): the non-viability of the substitution of action by the welfare state with the contributions of the welfare society.

The application of public policies is based on respect for citizenship and social rights. The welfare state is founded on principles of egalitarianism, its objective being to reduce the inequalities created by the market. The welfare society, on the other hand, circulates goods and services based on definitions of moral duty constructed in the spaces of inter-knowledge. Its weakness as a mode of organizing solidarity becomes apparent when we consider those individuals who are excluded from those spaces (Nunes 1995).

In the case of child care, the empirical research has shown that the production of social well-being within an unequal socio-economic structure reproduces inequality: the family resources of underprivileged families are limited when compared to those of better-off families. Occurring in an unequal class structure, the action of family networks doesn't change the life conditions of the families, and thus reproduces social inequality.

However, the action of the state system, if it is efficient, can in some ways counteract this situation. Both at the level of social payments and at the level of provision of infrastructure, state action can be fundamental in meeting some of the needs of underprivileged families. In spite of the insignificant amounts of Portuguese family benefits, 60 percent of the families interviewed in the 1993 survey considered these benefits "important" or "very important" in confronting the expense of child care.

Another problem revealed by the empirical research is the scarcity of means in the welfare society. In the case of child care, the elements involved are exclusively women – it is they who continue to bear most of the responsibility for "raising" children and "taking care" of them. But with growing numbers of women entering the labour market, the number of people on whom families can count to answer their child care needs will become increasingly smaller.

Thus, families face a double scarcity of resources: inadequate state provision and fewer alternatives within their social network. The growing inability of the welfare society to respond to the needs of families is all the more problematic since all the surveys conducted until now reveal that families clearly prefer informal models of child care, in which the family itself has a predominant role.[13]

The key question concerns the profile of state intervention in child care. Should we expect the state to assume its constitutional obligations when the family itself is willing to exempt it from them?

The state has a strong tendency to abandon certain sectors of social policy in moments of crisis: the argument of self-sufficiency is used to justify the passivity of the state (Hespanha 1995). The point that should be emphasized is that the state is not only a *provider* of welfare, but also a legitimate *regulator* of societal values and activities (Mishra 1990). Minimizing the role of the state in the first case is very different from its abdication in the second.

Translated by Teresa Tavares and John Mock

Notes

1. During 2001, I carried out 60 in-depth-interviews with women and men, from different socio-economic backgrounds, aged 24-34 years. The interviews show the weight these obligations still hold over the younger generations. These families depend a great deal on the help of their parents in order to cope with their daily life, and they feel a strong obligation towards reciprocity.
2. The Law of Protection to Maternity and Paternity is an example of this tendency.
3. This analysis was based on 1) the programs of the 13 constitutional governments in power since 1974 and 2) the legislation produced within a broad definition of "family policy" between 1974 and 2000.
4. Until 1997, family benefits included the "Abono de família", the main family benefit provided to each child until he/she leaves the school system (€13.47 in 1996), the birth grant (€118.96), the marriage grant (€98.91), and the nursing allowance, a monthly benefit covering children up to ten months (€21.90). In 1998, all these benefits were replaced by one single allowance, the "Subsídio familiar a crianças e jovens" (Family allowance for children and youth) whose maximum (for families with low income and more than 2 children) is €113,65 during the first year and €40,15 thereafter.
5. Every report published up to now, whether national or international, has emphasised the inadequacy of equipment and services in Portugal. See Bairrão et al. (1990), Conselho Nacional de Educação (1994), Comission des Communautés Européenes (1998).
6. Cf. footnote 4 above.
7. The latest data from the European Commission, from 2000, show that the access to formal child care services is 75 percent for 3 to 6 year olds and only 12% for children under 3 (http://europa. eu.int/comm/employment_social/equ_opp/statistics/childcare).
8. The public pre-school education system was created in the 1978/79 academic year with the establishment of 142 kindergartens which catered to approximately 2900 children (Ramirez et al. 1988, 48).

9   Law no. 5/97, 10 February, "Lei Quadro da Educação Pré-Escolar".
10 In 1993, IPSS were responsible for 81 percent of the formal child care services in Portugal. With the recent expansion of the network for children over three, this responsibility is now certainly greater.
11 This survey was made in November 1993. Two hundred and twenty-three families whose first child was born between January and June 1993 were questioned. Their children were thus between 4 and 11 months old at the time of the survey. One sample per locale, associated with the health centres in the district of Coimbra, was used, and only the mothers were questioned (self-administered questionnaires).
12 Cf. footnote 1 above.
13 In the 1993 survey, 94 of the women that did not take care of their children stated that they would prefer another solution than the one at their disposal. 51 percent of these women said that such a solution would be "to stay at home and look after him/her" (Portugal 1998). All the other studies carried out on this matter reveal the same results. Especially when speaking of children under three, Portuguese families clearly prefer family supervision (CAIF 1993; Torres and Silva 1998). Other studies have shown similar results regarding the care of the elderly (Hespanha and Ferros Hespanha 1995).

References

Andreotti, Alberta, et al. 2001. Does a Southern European Model Exist? *Journal of European Area Studies*, vol. 9, nº1: 43–62.

Bairrão, Joaquim, et al. 1990. *Perfil Nacional dos Cuidados Prestados às Crianças com Idade Inferior a Seis Anos*. Lisboa: Fundação Calouste Gulbenkian.

CAIF. 1993. *Relatório. Situação Actual da Família Portuguesa (Report. The Portuguese Family Today)*.

Carreira, Henrique Medina. 1996. *As Políticas Sociais em Portugal*. Lisboa: Gradiva.

CIDM. 2001. *Portugal. Situação das Mulheres 2001*. Lisboa: CIDM.

Comission des Communautés Européennes. 1998. *Conciliation de la vie professionelle et familiale en Europe*.

Conselho Nacional de Educação. 1994. *Projecto de Parecer sobre a Educação Pré-Escolar em Portugal*.

Ferreira, Virgínia. 1998. Engendering Portugal: Social Change, State Politics and Women's Mobilization. In António Costa Pinto (ed.) *Modern Portugal*. Palo Alto, CA: Sposs.

Ferreira, Vírginia, Teresa Tavares, and Sílvia Portugal (eds.). 1998. *Shifting Bonds, Shifting Bounds. Women, Mobility and Citizenship in Europe*. Oeiras: Celta.

Ferrera, Maurizio. 1996. The 'Southern Model' of Welfare in Social Europe. *Journal of European Social Policy*, 6 (1): 17–37.

Hespanha, Pedro. 1995. Vers une société providence simultanément pré- et post-moderne. L'état des solidarités intergénérationnelles au Portugal. In Claudine Attias-Donfut (ed.) *Les Solidarités entre Générations. Vieillesse, Familles, État*. Éditions Nathan.

Hespanha, Pedro. 1999. Em torno do papel providencial da sociedade civil portuguesa. *Cadernos de Política Social*, 1: 15–42.

Hespanha, Pedro, and Ana Isabel Alves. 1995. A construção da habitação em meio rural: um domínio da sociedade-providência. *Revista Crítica de Ciências Sociais*, nº42: 125–152.

Hespanha, Pedro, Claudino Ferreira, and Sílvia Portugal. 1997. The Welfare Society and the Welfare State. The Portuguese Experience. In Maurice Roche and Rik van Berkel (eds.) *European Citizenship and Social Exclusion*: 169–183. Aldershot: Ashgate.

Hespanha, Pedro, and Maria José Ferros Hespanha. 1995. The Welfare-Family in a Changing Context. On Social Modes of Provision of Elderly Care in Portugal. Paper presented at *The European General Practice Research Workshop*, Oporto, May 1995.

Lewis, Jane. 2001. The Decline of the Male Breadwinner Model: Implications for Work and Care. *Social Politics*, vol. 8, nº2: 152–169.

Martin, Claude. 1996. Social Welfare and the Family in Southern Europe. *South European Society & Politics*, vol. 1, nº3: 23–41.

Mishra, Ramesh. 1990. *The Welfare State in Capitalist Society. Policies of Retrenchment and Maintenance in Europe, North America and Australia*. Harvester: Wheatsheaf.

Mozzicafreddo, Juan. 1992. O Estado-Providência em Portugal: estratégias contra-ditórias. *Sociologia – Problemas e Práticas*, nº12: 57–89.

Nunes, João Arriscado. 1995. 'Com mal ou com bem, aos teus te atém': as solidariedades primárias e os limites da Sociedade-Providência. *Revista Crítica de Ciências Sociais*, nº42: 5–25.

Portugal, Sílvia. 1995. As mãos que embalam o berço: um estudo sobre redes informais de apoio à maternidade. *Revista Crítica de Ciênciais Sociais*, nº42: 155–178.

Portugal, Sílvia. 1998. Women, Child Care and Social Networks. In Vírginia Ferreira and Teresa Tavares (eds.) *Shifting Bonds, Shifting Bounds. Women, Mobility and Citizenship in Europe*: 345–355. Oeiras: Celta.

Portugal, Sílvia. 2001. Os trajectos da globalização das políticas sociais. Da retórica global às práticas locais no Ano Internacional da Família. In Pedro Hespanha and Graça Carapinheiro (eds.) *Risco Social e Incerteza. Pode o estado social recuar mais?* Porto: Afrontamento.

Roche, Maurice, and Rik van Berkel (eds.). 1997. *European Citizenship and Social Exclusion*. Aldershot: Ashgate.

Santos, Boaventura de Sousa. 1993. O Estado, as relações salariais e o bem-estar social na semi-periferia: o caso português. In *Portugal: um Retrato Singular*. Porto: Afrontamento.

Torres, Anália, and Francisco Vieira da Silva. 1998. Guarda das crianças e divisão do trabalho entre homens e mulheres. *Sociologia. Problemas e Práticas*, nº28.

Valiente, Celia.1996. The Rejection of Authoritarian Policy Legacies: Family Policy in Spain (1975–1995). *South European Society & Politics*, 1 (1): 95–114.

Wellman, Barry. 1985. Studying Personal Communities. In Peter V. Marsden and Nan Lin (eds.) *Social Structure and Network Analysis*. Beverly Hills: Sage.

Virgínia Ferreira

The Politics of Reproduction in Post-1974 Portugal

Introduction

One of the major changes of the last three decades is the increasing integration of mothers into the labour force. Nevertheless, empirical evidence points to the fact that both pregnancy and motherhood are still factors of discrimination against women as workers. A female candidate for a job in her twenties or thirties is always seen as a potential mother by the employer, which means, in his mind, lower productivity, high absenteeism and lack of commitment to the job. This image is irremediably (so it seems) associated with women workers throughout their child-bearing years (more or less between 15–50).

In Portugal, which has one of the highest rates of temporary work (over 20 percent) in the European Union context, employers often request that prospective female employees not get pregnant during the duration of the contract, and there have been some dismissals of pregnant women. This is of course against the law, but employers argue that in these cases, the dismissal may be considered fair because the employee did not fulfil all the contractual terms. Unfortunately, we can find similar examples in other European countries.

Pregnancy and motherhood can thus be considered as the last and most difficult components to be overcome in the stereotyping that discriminates against women as workers. Thus, it is very important to choose the right strategy to claim women's rights in the workplace. The strategy employed will have repercussions on social ideology and ways of living, since the politics of reproduction is a central vector in the determination of the level of human well-being. Being a multidimensional sphere, the politics of reproduction may be analysed from multiple perspectives and may activate multiple knowledge domains. I chose to approach the issue from the perspective of the institutional and state framework. Thus, in this paper, I will make an institutional analysis of the main strategies and actors involved in the design and enforcement of the protection of motherhood in the workplace in Portugal. I will, in the first place, briefly discuss the relationship between social rights and political and civil rights, as some feminist writers have problematized it. Secondly, I will analyse three strategies that women have deployed to expand social rights, especially the right to work: the strategy of equality, the strategy of workers' rights and the strategy of health and security at work. Finally, I will discuss the most relevant aspects of the controversy about abortion, as an illustration of the politics of reproduction in Portugal.

Strategies to Improve Women's Position in the Workplace

Let us see one possible typology of these strategies and look for the potential consequences of each one of the types considered. I will follow the typology presented by Joanne Conaghan (1993) in her article "Pregnancy and the Workplace: A Question of Strategy?" Although her typology was designed only for pregnancy, I think that the controversies about reproduction, in general, follow similar lines. According to this author, there are three strategies that feminists have employed in order to improve the position of pregnant workers: the Equality Strategy, the Workers' Rights Strategy and the Health and Safety Strategy.

The equality strategy

It is impossible to define, in a consensual way, what equality between women and men means, when it refers to the situation of pregnancy in the workplace. The controversy is about whether or not pregnancy should be accorded 'special' consideration in the workplace or whether it should be treated like other short-term 'disabilities'. Some employers argue that pregnancy protection is inconsistent with the rule of equality before the law, because it treats certain employees (pregnant workers) preferentially on the basis of sex. Feminist groups are usually divided about this issue: some are for and others against protective legal provisions. Those who are against avoid emphasizing the unique experience of pregnancy and motherhood, fearing that this will reinforce stereotypical notions of women's 'natural' role as mothers. In this line of thinking, pregnancy should be viewed as a short-term disability and feminists should campaign for better disability provisions for all workers (Conaghan 1993, 75).

Advocates of 'special' treatment, by contrast, insist that pregnancy should be recognized as a unique and enabling condition requiring especially tailored policies. Treating it like an illness will not lead to the recognition of the social value of pregnancy and childbearing.

The critics of both the legal equality and special treatment positions point out that they postulate the same male norm. As Joanne Conaghan stresses, depending on how difference is defined, the concept of equality is perfectly consistent with both positions. If we consider pregnancy in terms of its immediate financial and administrative consequences in the workplace, then it is arguably 'similar' to other disabilities. But we have to consider it differently if we take into account the fact that the majority of cases of 'similar' disabilities are not voluntary, whereas pregnancy, most of the time, is.

The workers' rights strategy

Under this strategy, the issue is viewed in terms of practical needs – job security and better childcare provision. In part, this is an expression of the traditional liberal aspiration to maximize freedom of choice – women wish to be able to choose to have children without compromising their economic independence. But, more realistically, it reflects a desire, common to all workers, to seek some measure of legal protection through the introduction of statutory rights.

The health and safety strategy

The most fruitful strategy currently employed in Portugal to improve maternity provisions invokes health and safety reasons for expanding the legal protection of pregnant workers. In the context of European law, the Framework Health and Safety Directive of 1989 provides a set of "measures to encourage improvements in the safety and health at work of pregnant workers and workers who have recently given birth or who are breastfeeding" (Preamble). These measures include: (1) protection of pregnant and breastfeeding women against exposure to harmful agents and processes, including, where necessary, the adjustment of working conditions; (2) time off for pregnant/nursing mothers; (3) A substantial period of paid maternity leave (at least 14 weeks); (4) prohibition of dismissal on pregnancy-related grounds.

In the context of European law and politics it may make more sense to rely on the arguments of health and safety, no matter how oddly misplaced that can sound, rather than to make the case in terms of equal opportunities or workers' rights. So, the aim is "to guarantee workers [...] the exercise of their health and safety protection rights" (Pregnancy Directive, Art. 11).

As Conaghan (1993) acknowledges, the most severe objections to this strategy have come from the feminist perspective: 1) It reinforces the association of pregnancy with ill-health, although maternity is a very natural and healthy condition; 2) It does not avoid the pitfalls of protective labour legislation, and legitimates social and legal practices which exclude and dis-empower women as the weaker sex; 3) It confuses health and safety during pregnancy with the health of the foetus, which leads to the legal construction of the foetus as 'a locus of rights', thus seriously threatening women's physical autonomy.

The Political Context in Post-1974 Portugal

As I argued elsewhere (Ferreira 1998a), after the 1974 Revolution, the existence of large women's organizations connected to political parties, especially Communist parties, had a major influence on the strategies adopted in arguing for women's rights in Portugal, as it did in other Southern European countries that came out of dictatorial regimes during the 1970s. The position adopted was typical of the traditional left, which can inspire women to demonstrate against the working classes' poor standard of living, considered in the abstract, but cannot inspire them to demonstrate against the rape of their next-door neighbour. In line with this position, when urged to demand the decriminalisation of abortion, the largest organization of women, affiliated with the Communist Party, answered: "Abortion will not help to free the country." That is probably one of the reasons why abortion is still prohibited in Portugal.

In any case, feminism has exerted a strong, although diffuse, influence on the institutions of modernised Portugal, especially the media and the political parties. This is so much the case that if you want to see consensus spreading among political opponents, you only have to propose to them a debate on any women-related issue, with the only exception of abortion. Then, you will see that everyone agrees with one another, and the air will immediately clear up. That is what we can call "diffuse feminism."

In this context, it would not be exaggerating to assert that, all of a sudden, as a perverse effect of the Revolution, we got a "woman-friendly state" apparatus, even if we did not have the political culture and the social and political history of the Scandinavian welfare states, wherein this expression was initially created by Helga Hernes. In a country so heavily marked by traditional and rural culture, it is hard to understand how that could ever be possible. I think that, in the case of Portugal, more than any other Southern European country, with the possible exception of Greece, the achieved legal equality between women and men was seen as an inexorable part of modernisation, and perhaps only secondarily as a part of democratisation. Above all, it was one of those negotiable issues that served to prevent, at any price, the emergence of a proletarian political regime.

Two years after the Revolution, the new Constitution ratified the *acquis révolutionnaire*. There was a revolutionary Constitution, which asserted the construction of socialism as the main purpose of our political regime. It was then relatively easy to introduce several changes that enacted women's most important legal rights, with the generalisation of the legal equality principle as one of the major changes of the new legal order.

The subsequent revision of the main legal codes (criminal law, civil law, et cetera) did incorporate these changes. Thus, as far as the family is concerned, we can mention the following: the extension of divorce to all marriages (including religious), the abolition of the status of household head; the legal equality between husbands and wives, and between fathers and mothers; the abolition of the category of illegitimate children; and the legal recognition of common-law marriages.

Feminism was rejected, but some of its ideas were co-opted and watered down by the discourse of modernisation and democratisation. For this reason, a proposal to include a separate article on the protection against sex-based discrimination in the Constitution was defeated. The right of both sexes to equal legal treatment is mentioned along with other conditions: race, ethnicity, religion, political and ideological ideas, education, and economic and social situation. This is mentioned by Lia Viegas (1977) in her book about Portuguese women and the new Constitution, but as far as I know, it never came to be an object of public debate.

After an initial period of greater political radicalisation, which came to a close by the end of 1975, the Socialist Party become the dominant political force, and then feminist ideas became part of the official ideology. This had the effect of pushing the influential Communist Party (with almost 20 percent of the votes in the 1979 legislative elections) to an active opposition, which led to women's mobilisation around the big struggles of the party – the defence of nationalisations, land reform, trade union unity, and workers' rights in general. Therefore, there was no philosophical or ideological dissent about the legislation that was being enacted on issues relevant to women.

It is symptomatic that the great cleavages between the different feminist perspectives never developed as they did in other countries. They came out during discussions around specific problems in settings where it was possible to gather people from every tendency (lesbian, socialist, radical, and so on), but, as these tendencies were not publicly assumed, they ended up looking like personal quarrels. The same process could be observed in Greece, as Eléni Varikas remarked, in spite of the fact that there was in this country much more feminist mobilisation than in Portugal (Varikas 1985).

It seems, therefore, that legal equality between women and men in Portugal was not the result of any specific strategy or struggle by feminist women's groups. The legal changes emerged as a component of the country's modernisation and democratisation, as an achievement of the civil and political rights due to all individuals, as an achievement of the full citizenship so long denied and crushed by the dictatorial regime. That is why all these changes took place very smoothly, with no opposition, with the only exception, again, of abortion: the proposal to legalise abortion, in 1984, mobilised both conservative sectors (especially the Catholic Church) and female supporters of a pro-choice politics.[1] In short, the legal equality between women and men has been set up without the need to justify it. There were no arguments about sexual difference or sexual equality. It was as if the progressive sector said to itself, "this is the latest fashion in the more developed countries, they themselves are now trying to change their laws in this direction, and as we are now remodelling the whole legal framework, we can do even better than they." And it was as if the conservative sector shrugged its shoulders and thought, "Who cares? *De jure* equality will not profoundly change *de facto* inequality."

Another relevant aspect of the legal-institutional apparatus of the post-revolutionary period is the way in which the State conditioned the pattern of women's insertion into economic activity outside the household by adopting a universalistic conception of citizenship. Here also, similar to what Jane Jenson (1986) discusses in the case of France, the concept of citizenship includes the right to work. Anglophone societies have a more particular understanding of citizenship insofar as the concept splits into two different spheres: one for the male family providers and another for the female agents of reproduction.

The legislation coming from such contrasting politico-juridical frameworks is very different. The first type is universalistic, and creates mechanisms for substituting women's presence in the home, while the second type is separatist, and privileges the transfer of money that women are supposed to manage in the home. We should not, however, think that the practices actually contrast as much as they appear to in the previous statements, since in both types of society there is segregation in employment. Nonetheless, there do exist fundamental tendencies that ground and justify the dichotomy, and we cannot forget that political discourses end up operating powerfully at the level of social expectations. The reflections of different policies are mirrored, for example, in the differences in the prevalence of part-time work among women.

The State greatly reinforced its intervention both at the administrative level and in the sphere of social reproduction (health and education, principally) in the post-1974 Revolution period, the moment from which it makes sense to characterise the juridical-institutional framework in Portugal in terms of universalistic citizenship. The new codes of Civil, Penal and Family Law developed after the 1974 Revolution were the most advanced of the time and introduced fundamental legal changes without women being specially mobilised to claim them or men to oppose them. In a certain way, we can consider that the State itself seems to have found an easy (and politically inexpensive) field to introduce what could have been viewed as a genuinely radical transformation.

Discursive Strategies to Protect Maternity

As we can see, the rhetoric used by the State to reform the legal order has varied over the last thirty years. References to the reparation of historical injustices suffered by women and to the need to harmonize institutions with international norms disappeared with the end of the revolutionary crisis (1974–1976). During this period, the universalistic principle of equality was opposed to the rights of workers, as witnessed in the debates in the Constituent Assembly. The Portuguese Communist Party was in favour of an article on women's rights based on the following premises: "(1) Women have the same rights and duties as men and therefore cannot be the object of discrimination in any sphere of economic, cultural or political life; (2) The basis for the equality of rights and duties of women is the right to work and to an equal wage for equal work." The Communists defended this article according to the discourse of workers' rights. It was rejected by the Socialist and the Social Democratic parties on the basis of universal rights logic (Ferreira 1998a). The article that consecrates legal equality thus cites sex alongside race, political and religious creeds, and social class. Ordinary legislation, however, has made use of the logic of workers' rights. The granting of maternity leave is one such example: according to the preamble to Decree Law 112/76, of February 7, it was based on the need to "improve the living conditions of the less favoured."

In Portugal, in 1979, a number of rights for pregnant workers were achieved, including the right not to be unfairly dismissed on grounds of pregnancy, and limited rights to maternity pay and leave (Decree Law n.º 392/79, of September 20). This set of maternity rights derived from the status of women as workers. Based on a concept of 'work' and 'worker' that is stereotypically male, the legal provisions fail to capture the varied biographies of women's working lives. The qualifications for full entitlement to maternity rights exemplify this well. To qualify for maternity pay, leave and reinstatement, a woman must be an employee, that is, engaged in a contract of service, and not a contract for services, for at least six months. Inevitably, these provisions ensure the exclusion of self-employed women, women working casually, women on temporary contracts (23 percent in 2001) or with interrupted work patterns. Clearly then, the concept of work, upon which maternity provisions are based, does not accommodate the wide and varied working patterns of women.

In part, the limitations inherent in the provisions reflect their genesis as a response to labour changes rather than working women's needs. Because the maternity provisions reinforce an existing tendency to conceive of home and work as separate and independent realms, because they do not challenge the prevailing view that childcare is the responsibility of mothers rather than fathers, the province of the family rather than the workplace, they reinforce the very ideologies they purport to challenge.

The 1970s were favourable to an ideology of workers' rights, but the 1980s were not. The current tendency to deregulate the labour market renders existing maternity provisions and reform efforts vulnerable. Thus, the workers' rights strategy, while bringing limited benefits in the 1970s, was of little use in the changed political and economic climate of the 1990s.

After 1984, when the law protecting maternity and paternity went into effect, legal change was based solely on the argument that constitutional principles establishing citizens' equal rights before the law had to be made a reality. This has given rise to a number of legislative initiatives. The most common are those that deprive women of previously enshrined "special protection." Some examples of this are the lifting of restrictions on night work (except during pregnancy and maternity) and the levelling of the age of retirement. Until 1993, women were entitled to retire at 62 years of age and men at 65. Today, the retirement age for both is 65. The government declared itself in favour of equality and argued that "this differentiation in terms of retirement age was all wrong." Enmeshed in the web of the rhetoric of equality, the trade unions and women's organizations hardly reacted to this measure, despite the climate of job insecurity and redundancies.

This line of argumentation is also frequently reinforced by the assumption that men equally share the burden of domestic and family responsibilities. This is apparent in Art. 68 of the Constitution (1/89, of July 8) which reads "(1) Fathers and mothers have the right to social and State protection when carrying out their irreplaceable task of childrearing and education, being ensured job guarantees as well as the conditions for participation in the civic life of the nation; (2) Maternity and paternity are socially eminent values; (3) Women workers have a right to special protection during and after pregnancy, including leave from work for an adequate period of time without loss of wages and benefits." The 1976 Constitution, however, only mentioned the irreplaceable childrearing role played by women and the socially eminent value of motherhood. The Constitutional revision of 1982 thus placed maternity and paternity on an equal footing, consequently attributing the same weight to the obstacles to economic and civic participation encountered by mothers and fathers. Clearly, only a small minority of men participate in childrearing activities or domestic tasks (Ferreira 1998b). Formal equality is not complemented by family support structures and effectively aggravates material inequalities between the sexes (see the chapter by Sílvia Portugal).

A brief description of the legal rhetoric on social relations between the sexes allows us to conclude that the "defence of the rights of women workers" was dominant in the ten-year period between 1974 and 1984, when the law protecting maternity and paternity was passed. Thereafter, the rhetoric of "equality between the sexes" became dominant. Legislators worked on the assumption that equality between men and women either already existed or would soon become a reality in the economic and family spheres.

During the 1990s, the discourses on the protection of maternity were either based on the strategy of equality (as in the example given above about the levelling of the retirement age for both sexes), or on the strategy of health and safety at work. This strategy has some advantages and disadvantages, as we've seen. One of the advantages is that it depoliticises the question of reproductive rights, turning it into a matter of the well-being and health of the community. In a certain way, it was this logic that led to the increasing acceptance of the discourses that demand the sharing of care for family members by women and men. Thus, the most salient topics of the discourses produced, especially after the second half of the 1990s, were the conciliation of work and family for both sexes and fathers' new rights associated with paternity (a five-day fully-paid paternity leave after the birth of a child, and a fifteen-day fully-paid parental leave immediately after the end of the mother's maternity leave).

This discourse assumes that maternity is not the exclusive problem of women and, in a way, socializes it. At the same time, it adds new facets to the problem as rose out of the debate about paternity leave and the adoption of grandmother leaves (for adolescent mothers, in this last case): it undermines women's autonomy in what concerns the fulfilment of their reproductive rights. These risks are particularly evident in the case of abortion, which I discuss below, since I believe this is a paradigmatic issue in any politics of reproduction.

The Abortion Question

I situate the turning point of the abandonment of the discursive strategy of workers' rights in 1984, because it was then that a mitigated version of the decriminalisation of abortion was enacted. In fact, we could say that the law protecting maternity and paternity was a kind of excuse for passing the law on abortion. This law passed also in 1984 (Law no. 6/84, of May 11), within the same package, and it provides for abortion in cases of deformity, rape, and health risks for the mother (including psychological health).[2] This law could be positive if the medical profession were willing to apply it or if the State had created the necessary clinical infrastructure for its application. Neither of the two has occurred, and thus few women have had legal abortions in Portugal. A survey conducted by the Association for Family Planning (APF) in 1991 showed that, of the 52 hospitals surveyed, only 17 practised abortions. Of the ten central hospitals, only five practised abortions. Since the law came into force in 1990, only 397 legal abortions have been performed. Thus, the overwhelming majority of abortions are performed illegally.[3]

The controversy about the decriminalisation of abortion is an excellent point for observing the politics of reproduction in every society. The 1984 law was proposed by the Socialist Party (PS) and designed to defeat a more liberal proposal that had been presented to Parliament two years before by the Communist Party (PCP). Although the PCP eventually recognised the importance of abortion as a conditioning factor in the lives of Portuguese women, due to its continued emphasis on the elimination of social rather than sexual inequalities, the discourse it produced during the public hearings completely obscured the fact that women, as a social group, are especially implicated in the issue of abortion (Reinhold 1988). In presenting the bill to Parliament, the PCP asserted that it concerned "citizens," "couples," "parents," "children," "democracy," "Portugal," and "all of us." The decriminalisation of abortion was, then, not a "women's issue" or a "matter of women's rights." The PCP argued that three principal aspects were at stake: the fact that the law was not being enforced; the fact that deaths were occurring as a result of illegal practices; and the fact that it was a question of class, since the victims were mostly women workers and poor women. Thus, the bill identified only a specific group of women (women workers and poor women), and defined the question as a social issue rather than a gender issue.

This way of viewing the problem is very different from what can be seen in other countries, where the liberal tradition of individual rights is much more deeply established. In these countries, the abortion issue is usually viewed as a conflict of interests between the right of women to choose whether to have a child and the foetus's right to life. In Portugal, this perspective came to the fore during the second debate on the bills presented by the PCP and the PS in 1984, which eventually led to the passing of the bill presented by the latter party. In this second debate, the question was more patently posed in terms of individual rights – the rights of women, on the one hand, and rights of the foetus, on the other.

What happened between 1982 and 1984 to justify this change in the discourse? What happened was precisely a strong mobilisation of women's groups, which, under the coordination of CNAC (National Campaign for the Right to Abortion and Contraception), organized meetings, debates and demonstrations throughout the country in order to generate a favourable public opinion concerning the decriminalisation of abortion and the free access to contraception, which had been banned for women under 18 in 1980. The mobilisation was so successful that some authors argue that there was an actual feminist movement in Portugal during this period (Magalhães 1998). This explains why, at the time of the second parliamentary debate, the national press, according to a study I conducted then with Graça Abranches, carried a significant number of pieces with the views of the Catholic Church, defending the right to life as an absolute value. The press also stressed discourses inspired by religious morality (on the part of the opponents of decriminalisation) and by scientific reason (on the part of the defenders of decriminalisation). The legal-social arguments that had been dominant during the first debate now took second place. However, it should be stressed that, in both periods, the press articles that we analysed (over 900) gave visibility mostly to the discourses of men and political parties (Abranches and Ferreira 1986, 482).

The debate has been more polemical in countries where questions are posed in terms of individual rights. Pro-choice advocates frame the issue in terms of individual responsibility and freedom. Pro-life advocates invoke equal opportunities for all, no matter how vulnerable. In the United Kingdom, for example, the reason why the discussion about abortion did not reach the stridency it did in the U.S.A. is that there is a greater indifference regarding religion and there are no fundamentalist groups organized against abortion. Furthermore, the legal tradition of each country also influences the terms of the debate. The Portuguese legal tradition is fundamentally based on legislation designed by Parliament, which makes it more resistant to change, rather than on jurisprudence, as in the U.S.A., where a Supreme Court decision can eventually be overturned by another, thus making legal instability an inherent part of the system.

A concern for health and safety during pregnancy encompasses the health of the foetus as well as the mother. The emerging legal construction of the foetus as 'a locus of rights' seriously threatens women's physical autonomy; in the field of paid work, concern for the foetus has often justified the imposition of restrictions on women in the form of foetal protection policies. This is already visible in some formulations about woman/child health protection, made possible by the new ultrasound and related technologies. If we look carefully at Lennart Nilsson's famous photos of foetuses, published in 1965 in *Life* magazine, we will notice that the foetus floats in a non-identifiable 'environment'. The photos with a black background suggest a foetus that develops from the resources at its disposal, and it seems to be lighted from behind. It is an inert foetus, floating and disembodied, thus reproducing the old myth of man's self-creation. A myth in which woman is merely the keeper of the seed a man planted in her. The new invasive technologies of medical surveillance give us an image of the foetus that is very similar to Nilsson's photos. By making the female body transparent, they erase the mother as a subject, and in her place the foetus emerges as a super-subject. Thus, the same woman whom no court would compel to subject herself to a blood transfusion to save a life, becomes, when pregnant, legally and clinically seen as a mere system of support for the foetus's life (Bordo 1993). There are doctors who see the foetus as their real patient, and jurists who believe they should demand from the State the protection of the rights of the foetus, even at the cost of the rights of the pregnant woman. In the ongoing constitutional revision during the current legislature (2002–2004), there is a proposal under discussion, presented by the conservative party in power, the Social Democratic Party, that proposes to establish in the Constitution the State's duty to protect life. The clear aim of this proposal is to establish the foetus as a subject of rights. The argument of the defence of the weakest link is used in the justification of this proposal, and has also been used in the ongoing discussion in Parliament in relation to the regulation of recourse to medically assisted reproduction techniques. Following the guidelines recommended in the last decade by the National Council of Ethics for the Life Sciences, the proposed regulation expressly excludes cloning, the genetic manipulation of embryos, the utilization of "surrogate mothers," the transaction of donated biological materials, and the creation of surplus embryos solely for scientific aims, and it limits the recourse to medically-assisted procreation by heterosexual couples.

Conclusion

In Portugal, the extremely rigid and conventional pattern of gender relations, associated with other aspects of Portuguese society, has not allowed the emergence of significant women's movements. Thus, the politics of reproduction has emerged as a derivative issue, a kind of second thought, and it has not taken a prominent place among the substantive policies of the State, unlike the rhetoric about the "family" and its well-being, which is indispensable in any political discourse.

Thus, the sphere of production has imposed the dynamics of reproduction. This is why Portuguese women have one of the lowest rates of fertility, along with one of the highest rates of economic activity, within the European context. It can therefore be said that while the legal order established in the 1970s is based on a universalistic concept of citizenship, it effectively reinforces unequal and unfair social practices by considering men and women equal producers and reproducers.

As we have seen, at the present stage, symbols, discourses and laws continue to promote the traditional image of the mother. Thus, although we should keep an open mind in relation to the health and safety strategy of the pregnancy issue, we should not lose sight of the distinction between the measures that are predominantly working-mother-focused and those that are exclusively foetus-centred. At the same time, I think it is strategically important to continue to develop the potential of this strategy in what concerns the expansion of the rights and obligations associated with fatherhood.

Notes

1   It is interesting to note that the debate was dominated by religious and moral discourses. The political discourse on abortion was more clearly produced by advocates of abortion decriminalisation on the occasion of the 1998 referendum, in which the "no" vote won by a thin margin (51%).

2   Presented to Parliament by the Socialist Party, Law no. 6/84, of May 11, legalizes the voluntary interruption of pregnancy (VIP) in certain situations. It establishes prison sentences of 2 to 8 years for those who perform or help to perform abortions, except in the following cases: risk of death or irreversible damage to the physical and mental health of the pregnant woman; risk of severe illness or foetus malformation (until the 16th week of pregnancy in both cases); and rape (until the 12th week). Parental permission is required in the case of minors. In any of these situations, the opinion of two doctors is necessary, and whoever initiates the VIP process cannot perform it. The law also establishes a three-day period of reflection.

One of the main keys to understanding why in Portugal such a restrictive law on abortion decriminalisation has not been enforced is that those who have been in power since the law was passed have publicly declared their opposition to abortion – first the Social-Democrat Aníbal Cavaco Silva, who was Prime Minister from 1985 to 1995, and then the Socialist António Guterres, who was Prime Minister from 1995 to 2001.

Being against abortion, what did both do? Did they change the law? Did they tighten the surveillance and repression on the illegal abortion network? Did they punish the women who turned up at public hospitals with complications from badly-performed abortions? Did they prohibit doctors from treating those women, or did they compel doctors to denounce them? These are obviously rhetorical questions. The former Prime Ministers did absolutely nothing. They let things run their course. They neither regulated the law in order to provide for its effective application, nor punished its violators. The tacit agreement established in our society is thus based on hypocrisy. Silence reigns as long as there are no deaths, no accusations. Hypocrisy, danger and risk thus shroud the practice of abortion in Portugal. Is it possible to anticipate any changes at this level? It is obvious that we can always look at the experience of other countries and learn from it. One thing is clear: this kind of tacit agreement runs the risk of disintegration if a period of populism sets in, a period when fighting crime is politically rewarding for certain politicians and political parties. Then, both abortionists and women who abort will experience persecution and imprisonment in order to "expiate their sins and the nation's sins."

3   In this study, the APF mentioned the following reasons for the small number of abortions: 1. Women's lack of information on legal provisions; 2. The deficient organization of official health services; 3. The limitations of the law itself as regards the possibility of performing abortions; 4. The doctors' right to claim conscientious objection.

Between 1984 and 1990, the Portuguese Judiciary Police received 222 complaints about the crime of abortion. According to some sources, in 1987, more than 1200 women were humiliatingly subjected to legal medical exams at the Institute of Legal Medicine because their names were registered in a notebook collected by the police at the house of a midwife under investigation for abortion. This was a totally arbitrary intervention, since such exams can only produce conclusive results within ten days of the abortion. At the end of 1990, the Consultative Committee of the Commission for Equality and Women's Rights approved a protest against this action by the police. As far as is known, no indictments resulted from these investigations. Recently, 17 women were indicted, but only as a pretext for accusing a nurse of several crimes associated with the abortion practice (namely, theft of medicines and prescriptions from the hospital where she worked). She was sentenced to eight years in prison.

References

Abranches, Graça, and Virgínia Ferreira. 1986. O Debate sobre o Aborto e a Ortopedia Discursiva da Sexualidade. *Análise Social* XXII: 92–93, 477–492.

Bordo, Susan. 1993. *Unbearable Weight: Feminism, Western Culture, and the Body.* Berkeley: University of California Press.

Conaghan, Joanne. 1993. Pregnancy and the Workplace, A Question of Strategy? *Journal of Law and Society* 20 (1): 71–92.

Ferreira, Virgínia. 1998a. Engendering Portugal, Social Change, State Politics and Women's Mobilisation. In António Costa Pinto (ed.) *Modern Portugal*: 162–188. Palo Alto, CA: Sposs (The Society for the Promotion of Science and Scholarship).

Ferreira, Virgínia. 1998b. Mulheres em Portugal, Situação e Paradoxos. In Leonel Moura and Maria Nobre Franco (eds.) *Pavilhão do Território*: 86–147. Lisboa: EXPO 98, Ministério do Planeamento e da Administração do Território. (Portuguese, Spanish and English versions).

Jenson, Jane. 1986. Gender and reproduction, or babies and the state. *Studies in Political Economy* 20: 9–46.

Magalhães, Maria José. 1998. *Movimento Feminista e Educação – Portugal: Décadas de 70 e 80.* Oeiras: Celta.

Reinhold, Susan. 1988. *Her Legitimate Mission: Debates on Abortion, Conflicting Visions of the World, and the Consolidation of Liberal Democracy in Post-Revolution Portugal.* Stanford University, mimeo.

Varikas, Eléni. 1985. Les femmes grecques face à la modernisation institutionnelle: Un Féminisme Difficile. *Les Temps Modernes* 473 (Déc.): 918–934.

Viegas, Lia. 1977. *A Constituição e a Condição da Mulher.* Lisboa: Diabril.

Linda Gordon

"Choice" versus "Right to Life:" Political Contestation About Reproductive Rights in the United States[1]

The slogan "reproductive rights" developed within the socialist-feminist stream of the women's liberation movement of the US in the early 1970s. The phrase was an alternative conceptualization of "birth control" or "population control," an alternative that took a more holistic view of what reproductive freedom might mean. The concept took shape in a campaign against coercive sterilization. Exposing and campaigning against the practice of coerced sterilization of poor women, particularly African Americans and American Indians and those who relied on public assistance, feminist reproduction control advocates advanced the program that the freedom to limit reproduction could not be real freedom without the complementary freedom to reproduce and to be able to raise one's children in decent conditions. Many feminist groups sought to create an overall women's policy program that included reproduction control, health care, child care. While there were many issues, theoretical and political, on which 1970s feminists did not agree, this reproductive rights program claimed virtual unanimity within the movement.

Unfortunately that movement declined in strength in the next decades, weakened primarily by a large conservative reaction – precisely the reaction that is today threatening world peace. I devote a large part of this paper to an analysis of the theory and practice of that reaction because through such an analysis, we can also get a better understanding of the historical significance of the campaign for reproductive rights.

The reproductive rights battle is intensifying rather than quieting down. As the US government has become increasingly controlled by Christian fundamentalists, who share, ironically, the same Manichean worldview as Islamic and Jewish fundamentalists, the war that we are expecting can only make the struggle for reproductive freedom harder. As many in the US have looked toward Europe to save us from a disastrous and sadistic imperial adventure, we also hope that saner polities might help temper the American drive toward fundamentalism. So allow me to say that in what follows, the stakes are higher even than reproduction control but affect the future of the world in its entirety.

This paper has the following sections: i) the feminist campaign for reproductive rights and its ideology; ii) the conservative campaign against abortion and its ideology; iii) the strategy and tactics of the "Right to Life movement;" iv) the recent – 1990s – foci of the Right-to-Life campaign; v) the current balance of the abortion fight; vi) the extension of the anti-abortion campaign to contraception; vii) the 1980s moral panic about teenage pregnancy; and, finally, viii) the attack on the welfare and regulatory state.

I.

Campaigns for reproduction control have been a central aspect of industrialization, urbanization, modernity, or whatever similar label we are comfortable with. In the US, there have been controversies about reproduction control for more than 150 years. But nothing prepared us for the centrality of this struggle to US and global politics at the turn of the 21st century. The major reason for the heightened passion about reproduction issues is that they seemed to express the core aims of the women's liberation movement, and for this reason became the major focus of the backlash against feminism. Birth-control politics has become an arena for conflict between liberal and conservative ideas about family, personal freedom, state intervention, religion in politics, sexual morality, and social welfare – even, perhaps, about war and peace.

For this reason, reproduction-control issues disproportionately influenced the women's movement, and not always for the good. Many other issues lost priority as feminists had to respond to the powerful political backlash against reproductive rights and the result was, in part, the narrowing of the appeal and the base of the movement. It was, you could say, our own fault, as we so badly underestimated the radicalism of what feminism meant in the 1970s and, therefore, the intensity and funding of the opposition.

My general argument here is that the political contestation over these issues has been preeminently a contest of meanings, a competition for how reproduction control should be understood. This competition has never been so polarized. The various alternative historical meanings of reproduction control – women's rights, individual freedom, family planning, population control, eugenics – were narrowed to two major interpretations: a liberal vision in which birth control is an individual right, a woman's right, essential to sex equality and sexual freedom; and a conservative vision in which reproduction control is a modern convenience that must be closely restricted lest it become destructive of social cohesion and sex/family morality.

The legalization of abortion in the early 1970s represented a major gain for feminism. But it rested on an earlier compromise that was to return and haunt us. In the 1870s, it was not common to distinguish abortion from contraception; both techniques of reproduction control were banned. In the early 20th century feminists crafted a compromise: by separating abortion from contraception, they were able to legalize the latter while accepting the continuing prohibition of abortion. Thus in the 1970s, antifeminists were able to make the argument that abortion was a unique evil. This was important at a time when the women's movement was at its peak and an assault on reproductive rights altogether might have been extremely unpopular.

The women's movement, on the other hand, did not advance abortion as a simple family-planning method. Rather the movement called for women's autonomous control of their reproduction, signaled by the slogan "control over our own bodies," once again marking their claim for reproductive rights with a critique of male domination and a demand for women's liberation. This wave of birth-control agitation rested on a more grassroots and comprehensive feminist program than had the previous wave: a program that invented a new word – "sexism" – condemned practices once not even reprehensible, and invented an analysis that challenged not only sex inequality but gender itself, including the view that motherhood had to be women's primary identity.

This feminist radicalism set in motion a dialectic of influence and counter-influence. The conservative response identified abortion and unlimited access to contraception with sexual permissiveness and subversion of "tradition," the family, "morality," and the word of God. Like previous antifeminist reactions, this one was by no means simply a men's movement, but equally a movement of women who did not see their own interests in the dominant feminist imagery, and even saw feminism as antagonistic to women's interests. In the 1970s, a new conservatism focused far more on these social/sexual issues and less on economic ones than had earlier conservative responses, and made birth-control issues, particularly abortion, far more prominent in the conservative political agenda. This new conservatism was deeply shaped by fundamentalist Christianity.

In response to the conservative attacks and the (inevitable) weakening of the feminist movement in the 1980s, the campaign for reproductive rights tried to hide its feminist identity. This compromise initially enabled a liberal coalition of feminist, family planning, and population-control organizations, in favor of abortion and contraceptive rights. By retreating from emphasis on gender equality, and by reliance on the individual's right to privacy and "choice," the reproduction control movement repudiated the concept of abortion rights as a *social* right, part of a larger group of reproductive rights which included a right to medical care, child care and welfare support. Abortion came increasingly to seem an issue most urgent for prosperous, even professional women. Although abortion rights are favored by a considerable majority of Americans, the activist groups actually shrank in size, leaving them less well positioned to resist the onslaught of fundamentalism.

In the US, abortion became intensely controversial only *after* it was legalized; previously, illegal abortions were common and not widely stigmatized. This fact has produced the suggestion that abortion was legalized "prematurely" – that is, before public opinion was fully supportive of the reform – or wrongly, defying majority sentiment. The evidence does not support these conclusions. Abortion was not legalized by the Supreme Court in the *Roe v. Wade* decision of 1973. In fact, seventeen states had legalized or decriminalized it beforehand, often in response to active feminist reform campaigns, and this kind of local change conditioned the high court's decision that state statutes universally prohibiting abortion should not stand. Abortion was widely practiced and provoked little fervor in these years.

A better explanation of the escalation of anti-abortion feeling was that abortion had changed its meaning through its reinterpretation by the revived women's movement. One might speculate that had there not been a feminist movement, abortion might have been decriminalized with less opposition – and one might equally speculate that had abortion remained illegal the opposition to other aspects of the feminist program would have been the more intense. What did happen was the spread of a feminist understanding of abortion as a right of self-determination to which all women were entitled, replacing the previously dominant view of abortion as, alternatively, a form of medical treatment or an unpleasant and risky but often necessary private solution to a common problem. Abortion was a widely practiced birth-control method, available and legitimized in most societies even when illegal. It is only since the birth of the Right to Life movement that a substantial group of women report feeling agonies of guilt in deciding upon abortion. The morality of abortion, often presented today as a basic, metaphysical, timeless, and universal question, has in fact been changed by historical experience and possibility.

One impact of the 1973 *Roe v. Wade* decision was reconfirmation of medical control of abortion. The Court situated women's rights to abortion in a right to privacy, but not an absolute right; it was limited by the doctor's discretion throughout, and by the state's "justifiable interest" in the health of the pregnant woman and in "preserving the potentiality of human life" in later pregnancy. To adjudicate conflicts between women's desires and state interests, the Court placed "the right of the physician to administer medical treatment according to his professional judgment" and categorized abortion as a medical decision. Making physicians into agents of the state opened a door to several anti-abortion tactics, as I will discuss below.

Using the spirit and argumentation of the "privacy" defense of abortion rights, the dominant pro-abortion-rights lobby fixed on "choice" as its slogan. This language called upon the emotional and political power of the idea of freedom – as in freedom of choice – in American political discourse. Moreover, the slogan "choice" evoked commitments to civil liberties and women's autonomous decision-making and de-emphasized abortion itself. But it also revealed and reinforced some of the limitations of the pro-abortion-rights case: the abstract right to privacy suggested that a procedure legalized was actually accessible, by trivializing the effects of non-legal barriers to reproductive self-determination, notably poverty. The "choice" slogan could have accompanied a campaign that highlighted access to all reproductive options, but in fact the movement's most visible emphasis was on legal barriers (a legacy of civil rights). Moreover, the emphasis was on individual rights, and implicitly denied the validity of any social regulation of reproduction. The notion of a reproduction policy that could work to promote other social goods – for example, the eradication of infant mortality, or the improvement of sexual relations – was de-emphasized in favor of arguments based on individual liberty and privacy (quoted in Pollack Petchesky 1984, 291).

II.

Just as the *Roe v. Wade* decision was based on a new, abstract, and allegedly gender-neutral right – privacy – so the anti-abortion movement introduced a new, allegedly ungendered argument: the rights of the fetus. There were other anti-abortion themes, such as women's "selfishness" and "frivolity" in rejecting maternity (a theme familiar from the nineteenth century campaign). But the fetal-rights argument was to become steadily more prominent, not only legally but also in the popular consciousness. It transformed abortion from a traditional form of reproduction control into murder.

Only in seeing Right-to-Life ideology as saturated with anti-feminism does its strength become understandable. Abortion came to represent a multi-dimensional attack on the "traditional" family and gender system. One dimension was, of course, sexuality: A reproduction-control method potentially controlled exclusively by women, abortion could allow women non-marital and multiple sexual partners without the restraint of possible childbearing. Indeed, the anti-abortion discourse has a pungently punitive aroma, often appearing in the notion that those who would enjoy sexual pleasure must be ready to accept their punishment. Despite lip service to sex equality, most anti-abortionists believe that women must accept as inevitable a direct path from sexual intercourse to motherhood.

This prudery, in the Victorian mode, ordains not only a double standard for men and women but also the hypocrisy of many leaders. The sex scandals involving several fundamentalist Christian ministers, and their survival as leaders nevertheless, remind us that the Christian sin-and-redemption narrative remain more powerful in religious discourse than simpler stories of consistent virtue (Harding 2000). But the hypocrisy does not mean that anxiety about abortion is inauthentic; the longing for a stable gender system and for sexual constraints on women expresses a drive to reduce sexual anxiety and gender uncertainty.

Another dimension of the anxiety provoked by legal abortion involves mothers' wage-earning work. Here anti-abortion protestors express a material tension experienced by all but the wealthiest parents. The protracted refusal of US domestic policy to recognize the economic necessity of employment by so many mothers has deprived them of basic provisions to make their double job possible – such as a living wage and livable benefits, affordable day care, affordable housing, medical insurance, parental leave, sick leave when they or their children are ill, and flexible schedules. Behind this failure lies a weakened but still breathing loyalty to the family wage, that is, to the standard that husbands/fathers should single-handedly earn enough to support non-earning wives/mothers and children. This family-wage standard has *never* been possible for the majority of Americans, now less than ever. In their fantasy nostalgia for the family wage, anti-abortionists search for blame, ignoring structural economic change and defining a wilful, evil feminism as the guilty party. In that story there is a wicked siren who lures women from their fulfilling maternal destinies into the job market. In fact, feminism is but a small factor among the reasons, overwhelmingly economic, that women work for wages.

Closely related to the fear that feminism pulls women out of their homes is an anxiety about the loss of motherhood – a loss not only to children but to marriage and the society as a whole. The "family values" of the late-twentieth-century social conservatives involved the construction of yet another fictive "nostalgia," for a mother who was ever comforting, providing, self-sacrificing – the fantasy of a perfect mother. Motherhood became an expression of longing for a caring relationship in which one is an individual rather than one of a mass. After all, being mothered is for most people their earliest experience of being treated as subject, not object. Abortion became for its opponents a powerful anti-motherhood symbol, and indeed, the antithesis of motherliness. The redefinition of the fetus as a preborn child makes abortion into killing babies, thus positioning aborting women as murderers of their own children.

So focusing on the fetus played an essential role in this discourse. The first campaigns against abortion, in the mid-nineteenth century, focused primarily on women's rights, attacking the selfishness of those who would evade their maternal calling, and only secondarily on the "dysgenic" implications of "race suicide"; the status of the fetus was a minor theme and these anti-abortionists did not attribute legal rights or personhood to the fetus.[2] But women's lives had changed so greatly by the 1970s that no campaign directly attacking women's option to delay or limit childbearing could have become mainstream. By shifting the focus away from women, women's rights, and reproduction control, however, to the fetus and even the embryo and their postulated rights, the anti-abortion movement was able to create an anti-abortion discourse sufficiently compatible with the late-twentieth-century gender system to garner widespread support (Pollack Petchesky 1987).

Underlying all this discourse is religiosity – most anti-abortion advocates are not just church-goers but personally involved in a relation with God. Many have been "born again," i.e. they have experienced a rebirth of Christian devotion in their own lives, and they deeply resent secular culture, with its tolerance for religious difference. (Many find it difficult to mask their belief that non-Christian religions are, at best, inferior.) Many consider women's expanded public-sphere activity and withdrawal from domesticity to be one of the aspects of secularism they most detest, but it is not the only aspect. The movement decries the separation of church and state, the teaching of (secular) science and social science, the legal and moral discourse of individual rights, the decline of parental authority, the tolerance of homosexuality (Cavanaugh 1986). This hostility to secularism also expresses a conservative populist class politics: like the Ku Klux Klan of the 1920s, they associate secularism with liberal elites. But there are other religious positions that are considerably more complex and less conservative. African-American and Mexican-American religious people, for example, often consider abortion a major sin without such hostility to other aspects of secular culture.

Anti-abortion attitudes have also been complicated by racial and imperial concerns. Birth-control and population-control advocates at times focused on reproduction limitation so as to evade demands for fundamental structural change – such as, for example, land reform – in order to ameliorate poverty and inequality. Yet contemporary anti-abortion advocates are often the same people who defended segregation and cheered the dogs and water hoses directed against civil-rights activists. Male church and nationalist leaders have been historically anti-abortion (and often anti-contraception as well). But as population control gave way to a woman-centered reproduction-control agenda, as black feminism developed, and as anti-abortion activism grew more strongly associated with the political Right, black positions fluctuated. As one socially conservative minister wrote about abortion demonstrators,

> I have never heard any of them say that they should have blocked the entrances to the jails where we were beaten and tortured ... over the past few years there have been only a few Southern, white, evangelical Christians who

have asked our forgiveness and extended a hand in reconciliation. On the contrary, for every step we take in their direction, it seems that most take another step toward the suburbs (Perkins 1989, 22).

Some leaders shifted their views because of pressure from below. Congressman Floyd Flake of New York, for example, gave up his opposition to public funding for abortion after his polls showed his constituents to be mainly pro-abortion rights (Blacks 1989).

African-American women in particular were generally pro-choice in the 1970s and 1980s and increasingly public about their views but, as on so many other issues, women of color often felt alienated from the mainstream abortion-rights movement. This was not only because the movement was overwhelmingly white – many black activists have a history of working actively with whites on issues of mutual concern – but, perhaps more importantly, because the movement has been white and middle-class in its priorities. Its single-minded focus on abortion rights does not meet the needs of women who are poor and/or discriminated against, who have equally strong needs for contraception funding, prenatal care, and pediatric care, for example (Ross 1998, 161-207). As Loretta Ross said of the pro-choice movement, speaking for the Women of Color Program of NOW, "Until you can hook up infant mortality and sterilization abuse, you're going to have ambivalence because it doesn't reach the issues that are immediate for us." (Quoted in Dionne Jr. 1989, 28)

The anti-abortion movement is thus an unstable coalition with internal political differences. Nevertheless, national Right-wing funding and leadership have been dominant, and women-centered rank-and-file sentiment has not been able to shift the overall political meanings and impact of anti-abortionism away from social and sexual conservatism. Liberal Right-to-Lifers have not been able to challenge conservative opposition to sex education, to easier access to contraception, to insurance funding of contraception, to emergency contraception, and to a safety net for poor children.

III.

Given its generous funding base, the Right to Life movement has been able to conduct an expensive professional publicity campaign, using billboards, print and TV advertisements, websites, counterfeit "cemeteries" for fetuses, counterfeit abortion services, with national and local paid leadership. In the late 1980s, anti-abortion advocates developed fake abortion clinics that offered neither abortion services nor open-minded counseling but rather presented clients with gruesome slide shows and misinformation about the allegedly great dangers of abortions. By 1988, there were an estimated 800 to 2000 fake abortion clinics in operation, involving an estimated 480,000 consumers.[3] Anti-abortionists began to operate homes for unwed mothers, attempting to revive institutions that had become largely extinct (Gross 1989, 1, 13).

Nevertheless, Right to Life was also a mass participatory movement. Its members picketed and obstructed abortion clinics, demonstrated at the homes of abortion providers or abortion-rights spokespeople, and protested abortion-rights candidates and events. They sat down at clinics, even chained themselves to fences, requiring police to carry them off. They picketed and obstructed abortion clinics – during 1985 alone, 80 per cent of clinics were affected – inflicting embarrassment and anguish on abortion clients, turning some away, and deterring others who could not face the persecution. Clinics were harassed in many other ways: picketing homes of staff members, tracing patients' license plates, jamming telephone lines, vandalism, mass scheduling of fake appointments. Right to Life movement members entered clinics posing as patients in order to condemn abortion to other patients.

In the 1980s, the Right to Life movement spawned violent offspring who employed arson, bombs, and guns as well as rhetoric. In 1984, there were 161 acts of violence against clinics and twenty-one death threats; in 1985 and 1986 there were approximately 400 cases a year of harassment or violence against clinics (Antiabortion 1985; Donovan 1985, 5–9; Boardman, 3). Comparing abortion to murder, even (frequently) to the Holocaust (Neustadter 1990, 76-83), some anti-abortionists took the next step, and justified assassinating abortion providers. (Killing one to save the lives of many, they said.) The American Coalition of Life Activists distributed "wanted" posters targeting specific abortion providers.[4] Soon after came the "Nuremberg Files" website:[5] Extending the holocaust metaphor to label abortionists as guilty of crimes against humanity, computer programmer Neal Horsley established the site in 1995, attempting, in his words, "to record the name of every person working in the baby slaughter business …" The site lists names in six categories – baby butchers, clinic owners and workers, pro-abortion-rights judges (called "shysters"), politicians ("mouthpieces"), law enforcement workers ("their bloodhounds"), and "Miscellaneous Spouses & Other Blood Flunkies." Names of those murdered are visibly crossed out. Visitors to the website are asked to provide more names and detailed personal information about each, including addresses and phones, photos, photos of cars, houses and friends, and civil suit records including divorce files.[6] From 1977 through 2000, anti-abortionists committed seven murders (three doctors, two clinic employees, one clinic escort, and one security guard), 17 attempted murders, 40 bombings and 163 arson attacks (causing $8.5 million damage since 1990), 80 attempted bomb or arson attacks, and 369 invasions of clinics. The acts of vandalism, assaults, and threats number in the thousands, although the overwhelmingly negative public response has reduced the incidence of the worst violence.

The leading Right to Life strategy has remained legal, however. For much of the 1970s, 1980s and 1990s, the movement pressured state and federal legislatures to ensnare abortions in a thicket of regulations and prohibitions. In the 1980s, these requirements included, for example, a waiting period between the request and the performance of an abortion; birth and death certificates for fetuses; providing the patient with a description of the fetus and its physiological characteristics; "informing" the patient that "the unborn child is a human life"; limiting abortions to hospitals (thereby raising the cost); using extraordinary measures (such as enforced cesarean sections) to get aborted fetuses to survive; requiring permission from minors' parents and/or women's husbands. In the 1990s, further restrictions were added: post-viability abortions require the consent of a second physician; the physician must determine gestational age, weight, and lung maturity before abortion; birth-control clinics receiving public funding may not inform women of their legal right to an abortion; detailed information about abortionists and patients must be reported publicly.[7]

Contributing to legal victories for abortion rights was the fact that, in contrast to the nineteenth- and early-twentieth-century situation, mainstream physicians and the women's movement were usually in the same camp. In the *Thornburgh* case, for example, an *amicus* brief by the American Medical Association, the American College of Obstetricians and Gynecologists, the American Academy of Pediatrics, and the Nurses Association of the Obstetrical College, and another by the American Public Health Association, asserted that the "information" required to be given to abortion clients was inaccurate. The medicalization of birth control had strengthened, at least in the short run, the legal pro-choice case.

But conservative court appointments during the Reagan years shifted the balance of decisions. The greatest defeat for the pro-choice side came in several decisions between 1977 and 1980 upholding state laws and the federal "Hyde amendments" prohibiting use of public funds for abortion except in cases of extreme danger to a woman's life.[8] Prior to 1977, approximately 295,000 women per year had abortions paid for through Medicaid. Following the funding cutoff, 80 per cent of poor women desiring an abortion either scraped together the money at great cost to themselves or their families, or resorted to unsafe nonmedical or self-induced abortions; 20 per cent gave birth.[9] The result has been to create a dual health care system with respect to reproduction, in which government effectively deprived poor women of choice, placing a tax on abortion and offering financial incentives to carry pregnancies to term or to accept sterilization. This is a policy consistent, of course, with 1980s conservative economics and judicial thought, returning to a classical liberal view of freedom in which blindness to the material obstacles to choice results in a double standard of justice. The Reagan administration attempted to interfere with private organizations offering reproductive choice by attaching restrictions to the use of Title X – federal funds for family planning and research in reproduction and contraceptive development – by clinics that provide sex education and abortion counseling.

By the late 1980s, the Supreme Court's balance had shifted, notably in the *Webster* and *Casey* decisions. In these decisions, only a minority of Supreme Court justices voted to reaffirm *Roe v. Wade* and in the latter decision, the Court promulgated a lower standard of scrutiny of state restrictions on abortion.[10] Appointments by Bush II are likely to continue this trend, and possibly even overturn *Roe v. Wade*.

IV.

Among important recent themes in anti-abortion litigation is so-called "partial birth" abortion. This term, coined by the anti-abortion camp and not recognized by the medical profession, is intentionally ambiguous. Proponents of the ban on partial-birth abortion allege that they are targeting only late-term abortions in which the fetus is partially extracted from the uterus and then killed while still in the birth canal. But all human tissue taken from a living person is itself living. So a "living" embryo or fetus enters the birth canal in many early abortions – which means that, according to the Centers for Disease Control, 99 percent of all abortion procedures could fall under such a ban. The fact is that fewer than 0.01 percent of abortions are performed during the third trimester and these are usually precipitated by medical emergencies involving risks to the pregnant woman's health, severe damage to the fetus, or psychological denial of the pregnancy until too late for a typical abortion, a problem most common among poor teenagers with high levels of sexual ignorance and shame.

Even the conservative Supreme Court was forced to overturn "partial-birth" bans, in *Stenberg v. Carhart* in June 2000. Although 31 states had passed laws against "partial-birth" abortion, the Court ruled against them on several grounds: that their deliberately vague terminology left physicians without clarity as to what specific procedures were allowed – not to mention the disturbing precedent of allowing legislatures to dictate medical practice; that they fail to include an exception to preserve the health of the woman; that they impose an undue burden on a woman's ability to choose an abortion; and that they prevent women seeking abortions from benefiting from the medical procedure their doctors believe is best in the particular case.[11] As I write, the US Congress has passed such a ban; it is being immediately challenged in the courts and the outcome is uncertain.

The story of the abortion drug, mifepristone, once called RU-486, demonstrates the power of the anti-abortion forces but also, possibly, their ultimate defeat by the widespread need for reproduction control. More than twenty years ago the Roussel Uclaf pharmaceutical laboratories synthesized a drug that blocks progesterone, a hormone needed to sustain pregnancy. By 1983, European trials of the drug having been successful, the Population Council began testing it in the United States. A 1988 conflict in France illustrated how the issue might have been resolved in the US with different political leadership: the French Ministry of Health approved the drug, then anti-abortion protests led Roussel Uclaf to suspend marketing it, but the minister of health ordered it back on the market, calling it the "moral property of women." In the US, unfortunately, this remarkable notion – that birth control is women's moral property – was neither appropriated by political leaders nor developed by intellectuals.

Soon afterwards most European countries approved mifepristone.[12] The Clinton administration directed the Department of Health and Human Services to support development of the drug and Roussel Uclaf donated its US rights to the Population Council. But anti-abortionists were able to delay approval through a variety of tactics. After a decade of delay, the Food and Drug Administration approved the drug in September 2000, but immediately thereafter, Bush II's ascent to the presidency gave anti-abortionists renewed hope. They have tried to restrict the drug by introducing bills in at least twelve states and the US Congress that would make it illegal to prescribe or use or provide public funds for mifepristone.

Meanwhile, in 2001, another abortion-related controversy, over stem cell research, grabbed the headlines and presented an explosive dilemma for President Bush. The conflict illustrates how anti-abortion passion reaches beyond the boundaries of reproduction control itself. The purpose of stem cell research – treating or even curing currently incurable disease – is surely approved by everyone. But the most useful and easily accessible stem cells come from embryos. The cells that make up very early embryos are not yet specialized, and can develop into any of the 220 cell types that make up a human body. (Adults also have stem cells, but they multiply more slowly and may not be undifferentiated enough to be useful.) And that is what makes them valuable – in theory, they can multiply endlessly and be transplanted into a patient and coaxed to replace damaged tissue of various kinds. This procedure has been successful in rats and mice, and researchers are confident that in the near future it will work for humans too.

The best source of embryonic stem cells is not abortion clinics but fertility clinics, specifically, the "extra" embryos left over from laboratory fertilization attempts. Typically, once a successful pregnancy and birth is created, these extras are discarded. Hard-line anti-abortionists take the position that any use that requires destroying embryos is murder, and harvesting stem cells destroys the embryos. These fundamentalist views seem uncompromisable because followers have become invested in the kind of all-or-nothing purity that so often accompanies faith-based ideologies. Other anti-abortion leaders and loyalists have drawn a line between lab-created embryos (acceptable) and what is removed in an abortion (unacceptable). They speak of friends and relatives with incurable diseases. And they are perhaps sensitive to public opinion polls that run 3-to-1 in favor of stem-cell research. This compromise by anti-abortionists suggests that, when sex and gender are not at issue, their commitment to preserving all unborn life may be considerably less passionate. President Bush, having won office through a coalition of Christian-Coalition social conservatives with more secular economic conservatives, ordered in August 2001 that federal funds might be appropriated for research using already-created stem cells but not for research that required creating new ones. Tilted to avoid alienating social conservatives, his ruling is unlikely to satisfy those who favor a robust research program and those who long for better cures for Alzheimer's, juvenile diabetes, Parkinson's and other diseases. Moreover, nothing will stop privately funded research, and the absence of federal funding will make the research less well supervised and will surely speed the development of a market in body parts and physiological elements.

V.

Which side is winning the abortion conflict? It depends on what evidence is used. In the 1990s, abortion rates fell from 26 per 1000 to 23 per 1000 among women aged 15 to 44 (Henshaw 1998). But what caused the decline? Anti-abortion groups hail it as a victory, attributing it to popular moral revulsion against abortion and more abstinence, at least among the unmarried. Pro-abortion-rights groups evaluate the decline as reflecting some gains and some losses. To the degree that the decline results from better contraceptive use and less sex among young teenagers, it is a good thing. To the degree that it reflects women's loss of access to abortion, the decline is not a good thing.

The Right-to-Life movement won a major victory in shifting the meaning of abortion in its favor. The very concept of a "Right to Life," the focus on the rights of the unborn, the gory pictures, and the moral damnation of aborting women have enveloped abortion in shame and loathing even among many of those who support abortion rights. The notion of abortion as murder has created a great deal of guilt. No doubt many abortions were thereby prevented, but there has also been some resistance to this shame. Right-to-life advocates have tried to create an official, abortion-induced pathology: the so-called post-abortion trauma syndrome. The National Right to Life Committee and its ally, the American Rights Coalition, encouraged women who have had abortions to sue their doctors for malpractice suits and offered the services of lawyers to that end. This strategy aimed both to intensify trauma about abortion and to intensify the degree of trauma associated with abortion in public opinion. The strategy also sought to raise the cost of malpractice insurance in an attempt to put abortion clinics out of business. However, the right-to-lifers could not even convince anti-abortion Surgeon General C. Everett Koop to support their claim as to the existence of a post-abortion trauma syndrome, since hundreds of studies found no evidence of it. Studies found that depression was far more common after childbirth than after abortion, and the most common post-abortion emotional reaction is relief.[13]

In terms of "public opinion," often a volatile and malleable construction, the most interesting news is how little has changed. A stubborn majority of U.S. residents continue to oppose the criminalization of abortion.

Abortion opinion, however, is not a simple either/or matter. Most Americans do not support abortion in all circumstances: many are hostile to third-trimester abortions (which, in fact, constitute less than 0.01 per cent of all abortions); others oppose abortion for "frivolous" reasons. And poll responses, of course, always depend very much on what is asked. In 2001, Americans were deeply split, 52% identifying as pro-choice and 43% as pro-life.[14] If those polled are given four options, they divide in this way:
- Abortion should be legal in all cases – 21%
- Abortion should be legal in most cases – 38%
- Abortion should be illegal in most cases – 25%
- Abortion should be illegal in all cases – 14%[15]

Or, with a question designed to find a middle ground:
- A woman should be able to get an abortion if she decides she wants one no matter what the reason – 35%
- Abortion should only be legal in certain circumstances such as when a woman's health is endangered or when the pregnancy results from rape or incest – 50%
- Abortion should be illegal in all circumstances – 12%[16]

The polls offer some insight into correlations between beliefs about abortion and other issues. Opposition to abortion is correlated with religiosity (meaning, intensity of religious commitment) across all racial and ethnic groups, including African-Americans and Latino/as. Yet 37 percent of those who have abortions say religion is very important to them.[17] Latinas differ among themselves greatly on abortion: Puerto Rican women are quite positive about it, Chicanas less so. But the Church's views do not represent those of actual US Catholics who divide pro/con on abortion more or less like the public at large: 55 percent believe abortion should be generally legal, only 43 percent that it should be illegal in all or most cases.[18] African-Americans are less likely to approve of abortion than whites, but this differential is declining and blacks have become steadily more positive toward abortion over the last two decades. The black/white difference in part reflects class differences: more educated and more secular people support abortion more strongly. But black attitudes are also independently formed, by the legacy of racism in family-planning programs that we have seen, challenged by the traditions of independence and even feminism among black women. Moreover, despite somewhat more negative attitudes, adult black women are twice as likely to use abortion as whites.[19] By contrast, among teenagers, whites are more likely to use abortion, but this differential is almost entirely a function of class or socioeconomic status rather than race – the more prosperous, the more likely teenagers are to terminate pregnancies.

The greatest anti-abortion success has been in reducing women's access. A variety of efforts contributed to this change: violence, withdrawal of funding, lack of training for medical students, state restrictions, harassment and shaming. Costs are one of the greatest obstacles. The legalization of abortion at first produced a remarkable dip in price. Just as prohibition always raises the cost of that which is prohibited, so legalization reduces the cost: typical abortion costs in 1996 were only half the costs in 1973. The ban on public funding inflated the costs for those who most needed the help. Women with family incomes under $15,000 were twice as likely as the national average to seek abortions while those with incomes above $60,000 were half as likely (Henshaw and Kost 1996). As of April 2000, 34 states provided no medical insurance that covers abortion. Funding prohibitions also affect military employees, federal and many state and local employees, residents of the District of Columbia, members of the Peace Corps, prison inmates, Native Americans and many other groups whose medical insurance is, by one restriction or another, prevented from paying for abortions. Such defunding not only prevents access but causes delays – on average, women delay two to three weeks as they search for money to pay for abortions. These delays further increase the costs of abortion – doubled at 16 weeks pregnancy, tripled at 20 weeks – and, if the delay extends beyond the first trimester, make it harder to find an abortionist. 60 percent of Medicaid recipients suffer hardship from lack of public funding for abortion, while in states where Medicaid will pay, the abortion rate among covered women is 3.9 times higher. Where public funding is banned, approximately 20 percent more pregnancies are carried to term (37 percent more in a rather poor state, North Carolina). Among African-Americans, defunding accounted for half of the decrease in abortions.[20]

The number of abortion providers has shrunk considerably. Anti-abortion-rights campaigns succeeded in putting abortion applicants in a vice, squeezing them between, on the one hand, state laws requiring that abortions be performed only in hospitals and, on the other hand, campaigns pressuring hospitals not to provide abortions. In 1997, there were 600 fewer hospitals offering abortion services than in 1979 (Henshaw and Kost 1996).[21] This reduction was accomplished in part through pressure on hospital boards and in part through mergers by which Catholic hospitals swallowed others. Since 1990, a record number of secular community hospitals have merged with religious ones, and the Catholic hospitals are particularly restrictive. In 2000, Catholics provided 15 percent of all hospital care in the US, forbidding contraception as well as abortion services; 82 percent of these hospitals forbid emergency contraception even in cases of rape. In 91 percent of rural counties, Catholics run the only hospital, although in 95 percent of these counties, only a minority of residents are Catholic. Even medical schools caved in to anti-abortion intimidation, eliminating abortion training for students. In 1991, only twelve percent routinely included training, even for first-trimester procedures, 57 percent offered it as an elective, and 27 percent offered no training at all.[22]

VI.

Buoyed by its victories, the anti-abortion movement soon dared to attack the right to contraception. The more extreme, or more forthright, anti-abortion leaders openly condemn contraception because of their hostility to sexual activity. "I think contraception is disgusting – people using each other for pleasure,"[23] remarked Joseph Scheidler, head of the Pro-Life Action League. Or Father Paul Marx, President, Human Life International, developing the connection more thoughtfully: "You can't stop abortion without fighting contraception: it is the gateway to abortion. Not one of the 81 countries I've worked in has 'clean' contraception without abortion – not one. Once there's contraception – separating sexual activity from procreation and teaching people to use each other's bodies for selfish pleasure – abortion is always used as a backup."[24]

On the whole, the movement avoids general condemnation of contraception but tries to restrict access to it through funding and prohibitions directed particularly at young people. Make contraception too easily available, Right to Lifers argue, and it will license sex outside of marriage, especially among the young. They have the same objection to "emergency contraception," a high dosage of birth-control hormones that, if taken within 72 hours after intercourse, prevent pregnancy. During the Reagan and Bush I presidencies, Title X funding for contraception (in real dollars) fell by 72 percent and total public funding by 27 percent, while the costs of contraception were growing faster than inflation (Harrison and Rosenfield 1996, 227). New regulations to Title X proposed by the Reagan administration in 1987 and 1988 not only prohibited funding of family-planning projects offering abortion counseling, referral, or services, but no longer require that they offer a "broad range of acceptable and effective … family-planning methods" (the old requirement). Instead, they define family planning as "natural family-planning methods, adoption, infertility services and general reproductive health care, abstinence and contraception" – in that order. "Clinics" that offered only abstinence as a form of "natural" birth control could be funded under these regulations.[25] These regulations were reversed by President Clinton and reinstated by Bush II.

VII.

In the 1980s, a new reproductive issue moved to the center of political argument in the US: teenage pregnancy and out-of-wedlock childbearing. Through these issues, economic and social conservatives attempted to craft a unified perspective, possibly even bringing liberals into a coalition that argued concern for both public and individual welfare as well as sin. The coalition remains unstable, however.

Despite a great deal of research and publicity about teenage pregnancy, much of the popular discussion in the 1980s relied on the mistaken assumption that teenage fertility rates were rising. The fact is that these rates have been declining since 1960, nearing a record low in 1998 at 51 births per thousand girls aged 15–19. As of 1995, about 1/4 of the decline was due to increased abstinence and 3/4 to fewer pregnancies among those who were sexually active (Alan Guttmacher Institute 1999, 4). Also contrary to widespread misimpression, the decline was steeper among blacks than among whites, although blacks started from a higher teenage fertility rate.

So what prompted the 1980s panic that teenage pregnancies and childbearing were increasing? One reason is that adult births were falling even more than teenage births (Jencks 1989). More significant, however, is that the same cluster of conservative political attitudes expressed in anti-abortion campaigns, now applied to the issue of teenage pregnancy, led to an unnoticed misunderstanding. Accepting the rhetoric of Christian social conservatism, commentators fell into the mistake of not noticing teenage childbearing when the teenagers were *married*. In the 1950s, the birth rate to teenagers was higher than that of today, but those teenagers were much more often married. More recently, while teen births overall were decreasing, the proportion of teen births to the *unmarried* was increasing. The proportion of all teenage births that were out of wedlock increased about fivefold, from 17 percent in 1970 to 79 percent in 1998, while the proportion of all births that were out of wedlock rose eightfold, from 4 percent in 1940 to 33 percent in 1999.)[26]

In other words, the discourse about teenage childbearing typically rested on the hidden assumption that pregnancy among married teenagers is not objectionable – as if marriage somehow instantly makes teenagers into grownups. In fact, most of the negative consequences of teenage pregnancy pertain equally to the married and unmarried: teenagers have more difficult childbirths and less healthy babies, are worse parents, create more unstable marriages, and achieve less education and lower earning power and status. Ironically, during the 1960s, both scholarly and popular writing identified teenage marriage as the problem; by the 1980s the focus was on teenage pregnancy, with early marriage no longer considered problematic. In fact, some conservative commentators today recommend early marriage as a remedy, failing to recognize that for many poor young women marriage is unlikely to increase stability or standard of living (for example, Besharov and Quinn 1987;

Vinovskis 1988). It is worth considering that, while the rise of nonmarital pregnancies creates problems, the decline in early marriage is not a bad thing.

The racial subtext in the concern with unwed teenagers' pregnancies also fosters misunderstandings. While out-of-wedlock births among all black women are much more frequent than among white women, they are only slightly higher than those among whites of equal poverty. Furthermore, white rates of out-of-wedlock (not necessarily teenage) pregnancy are rising and black rates falling, among both adults and teenagers (Family Planning Perspectives 1987, 83–84; Ladner 1986, 70). African-American attitudes about teenage and out-of-wedlock pregnancies have gone through significant changes in recent decades. Following publication of the notorious "Moynihan Report" of 1965, which blamed black poverty on "pathological" family patterns, many black leaders responded critically, emphasizing the strengths of black extended-family networks and intergenerational child-raising, and criticizing the report's diversion of focus away from basic, structural racial discrimination. As Joyce Ladner put it, there was a "closing of the ranks" behind black families, making open discussion of teen pregnancy or lone-mother families appear as disloyal, as exposing one's weaknesses to the enemy. Indeed, the anxiety created by the Moynihan report and its spirit probably impeded open discussion of these problems (Ladner 1986, 69).[27] Since then, however, more black organizations have campaigned against teenage pregnancy, although they are as divided about solutions as white ones.

We can understand more by examining teenage pregnancy in a global context. The United States has substantially higher levels of teenage pregnancy, childbearing, and abortion than any other western industrialized country. U.S. teenagers are less likely to use contraception than those in other comparable countries. Furthermore, teenage birthrates have declined less steeply in the US – from 68.3 in 1970 to 48.7 in 2000 – than in other developed countries over the last three decades. These high rates in the U.S. correlate most exactly with the high rates of poverty and inequality in the U.S., which on the individual level mean less hope for upward mobility among the poorest teenagers who have most of the babies.

Teenage pregnancy often became a rhetorical surrogate for a larger 1980s discourse about single (or lone) mothers, welfare, and the "underclass." While public aid to lone mothers has long been more stigmatized than most other forms of public provision, conservatives stimulated even more hostility since about 1980. Conservative propaganda associated welfare recipients with a vaguely defined "underclass," said to be characterized by criminal activity, rejection of the work ethic, use of illegal drugs, reproductive irresponsibility and, if female, sexual immorality; with the unsaid but widely understood assumption that this underclass was largely non-white. The anti-welfare campaign argued that mainstream, hard-working, law-abiding Americans were supporting parasites with their tax money and that heavy taxes were responsible for the worsening economic conditions of the majority of Americans.

Single motherhood, poverty, and welfare receipt all create difficulties for both mothers and children, but the three factors need to be distinguished. Some lone mothers are prosperous, some have chosen this kind of family, and many suffer neg-

ligibly if at all from lack of husbands. Single motherhood in general is highly correlated with poverty – especially those single mothers who are heads of household,
and it is overwhelmingly because of poverty that female-headed households are correlated with lasting disadvantages for children.[28] Moreover, while early pregnancy
certainly adds to the mothers' problems, they are poor mainly because they started
off poor. Few would do much better even if they avoided early pregnancy; besides,
pregnancies do not occur randomly among teenagers, but affect those with the least
resources and hopes for the future. Moreover, poor girls of all races are more likely
to carry out-of-wedlock pregnancies to term than are more prosperous girls, who
have more abortions.[29] This should not be construed as minimizing the damages of
teenage pregnancy and parenthood. Many girls may be "choosing" to bear children,
either passively, in their lack of attention to birth control, or actively, as a means of
gaining status, but their "choices" emerge from a very limited range. For example,
a far higher proportion of teenage girls than of adults describe their pregnancies as
unwanted, and this is the case three times as often among blacks as among whites.[30]

Teenage pregnancy is unusual among reproduction-control issues in that nearly
everyone thinks it is a bad idea. But this consensus does little to promote agreement on policy. Liberals have argued for promoting contraception and increasing
access to it, but social conservatives fear that contraception will encourage teenage sexual activity which they consider immoral and harmful in itself. Since the
1960s, teenagers' sexual behavior became a symbol both of sexual immorality and
of parents' feelings of powerlessness. Perhaps because parents feel more helpless
to control the sexualization of the mass media and advertising, many are driven
to protest policies closer to home. The two Bush administrations have promoted,
and sometimes required, abstinence education to the exclusion of contraceptive
as well as abortion information. Although every evaluation has shown that abstinence education does not reduce sexual activity, it remains the dominant theme in
sex education for teenagers. Among the 70 percent of public school districts that
teach sexuality education, the vast majority (86 percent) require that abstinence be
promoted, either as the preferred option for teenagers (51 percent) or as the only
option outside of marriage (35 percent). Only 14 percent address abstinence within
a broader education program to prepare adolescents to become sexually responsible adults. In one-third of school districts, information about contraception is
either prohibited entirely or limited to emphasizing its ineffectiveness in protecting
against unplanned pregnancy and sexually transmitted diseases.[31]

By contrast, providing contraception in high schools does seem to work (Ladner 1986, 80; Fine 1983, 44; Tucker 1986). A St. Paul, Minnesota, school clinic cut
pregnancies by 30 per cent, for example. An evaluation of five different pregnancy
prevention programs found that the two that showed results were the two that were
most active in providing access to contraceptive services (Kirby et al. 1994, 339–
360; Moore et al. 1995). Moreover, there is wide public support for such programs,
and 23 states have legislated to give minors authority to consent to contraceptive
services for themselves.

But there is vociferous opposition to giving minors contraceptive access. In
1983, the Reagan administration promulgated a regulation (the "squeal rule") that

required clinics receiving Title X funds to notify both parents or the legal guardian of patients under the age of 18 within 10 days of prescribing a contraceptive. Advocates of this regulation maintained that family planning clinics had built a "Berlin Wall between the kid and the family," and that the squeal rule was a legitimate way to encourage family participation. It also argued that mandatory parental notification would protect minors from harmful side effects of contraceptives, deter some teenagers from having sex and improve the "consistency" of contraceptive use by teenagers who are sexually active. The regulations never took effect, enjoined by court injunctions, and the Reagan administration chose not to appeal.[32] But fear of opposition continues to limit teenagers' access to birth control. Of the 1135 school-based health clinics that existed in 1999, more than three-quarters were prohibited from dispensing contraceptives. The AIDS danger seems to be encouraging some of these three-quarters to make an exception for condoms, but this of course leaves girls dependent on boys for their protection.[33] Yet even conservative parents are ambivalent. For example, of the one-third of parents who believe that teenagers should be told to have sex only when they are married, 86 percent also want them to be taught HIV prevention and 71 percent, how to use condoms.[34]

VIII.

During these decades of controversy about reproduction control, another conservative social policy campaign gained ground with much less opposition: the campaign to "reform" what Americans call "welfare." Since the 1960s, "reform" had meant reduction of funding and/or more stringent eligibility requirements. By the mid-1990s, it came to mean repeal, and that is what happened in December 1996. By that time welfare had only a few not-very-influential defenders. Notably, none of the three major organizations representing constituencies with a direct interest in the welfare system – the key feminist lobbying organization, NOW; the labor unions; and the key civil rights organizations – made it a priority to defend the program.

This offensive is not only directed against the poor or otherwise weak – it is part of an attempt to create a much larger shift in our national political ideals. It is producing one of the most massive transfers of resources from the poor and the middle-class to the rich in American history. Repealing welfare, privatizing Social Security, reducing spending on medical care – all these rest on a similar ideological premise, sometimes explicit, sometimes implicit. The premise is that government neither can nor should try to solve social and economic problems or counteract increasing inequality. (Consider the principle upon which relief for the 9/11 victims is being paid out – on the basis of calculating the expected future income of the deceased or injured. So the survivors of partners in brokerages, who usually already have private insurance and who are usually people who will be high earners themselves, are receiving 40-50 times as much as the survivors of janitors.) This program takes us back to the "robber-baron" ideology of the late 19th century, which holds that markets are natural and supreme, their consequences irresistible. This agenda aims to strip government of the capacity to keep a floor under wages, provide jobs when the private sector doesn't, regulate economic instabilities, and curb business excesses. The attack on affirmative action is cut from the same cloth; it rests on the notion that only the market should determine who gets jobs and education, that discrimination cannot be challenged by regulating the market. The gendered and racial meanings of all this are central. Using the democratic state to move us closer to social, political and economic justice has been a central part of the historic labor, civil-rights and feminist programs. Today's government repudiates these traditions.

Reproductive rights issues played a central role in the development of the new Republican constituency on which the Bush administration rests. Starting in the late 1960s, a group of conservative thinkers who came to call themselves the "New Right" developed a new strategy for breaking apart the Democratic electoral majority that had been constructed by Franklin Roosevelt in 1932. The strategy called for appealing to white blue-collar and lower-middle-class voters on the basis of "social" issues rather than the two themes that had previously characterized the 20th-century Republican Party, conservative economic policy and virulent anti-Communism. The "social" issues were in fact mainly gender-and-sexuality issues: gay rights, abortion rights, sex education, the Equal Rights Amendment, pornography, racial integration of schools, illegal drugs. Opposition to "permissiveness" and feminism, support for "family values" and parental authority did in fact prove attractive to many voters, who became labeled the "Reagan Democrats." Republicans through the 1970s, 1980s, and 1990s hammered these issues continuously.

The teenage pregnancy/nonmarital childbearing panic contributed particularly to welfare repeal by dramatizing the old conservative argument that public support for poor children and their parents encouraged out-of-wedlock childbearing, combining appeals to sexism, sexual moralism, racism, and tax-cutting. With the selection of Bush II, a much broader agenda was disclosed. The conservative Republicans in power have as a goal nothing less than repealing virtually the entire welfare and regulatory functions of the US state.

Of course, the US welfare system rests on fissures that have been growing for a century. Through a two-level system, benefits aimed at the upper working class and middle class became installed as entitlements while benefits for the poorest groups – disproportionately women, children, and people of color – became constructed as charity, discretionary, and stigmatized. This structure discouraged political solidarity between the poor and those of other class positions, which made it easier to convince many voting Americans that the poor had themselves to blame for their poverty, and that cutting welfare provision would reduce taxes and increase the well-being of the non-poor. Promoted by a heavily funded propaganda campaign, the agenda first reached major success in 1996 with the repeal of the program (AFDC) for poor parents and children and the substitution of temporary assistance which typically requires that lone mothers take full-time or near full-time employment.

With Bush II's ascent to the presidency in 2001, it became clear that this repeal was only a beginning. Since then the administration and the Congress have been systematically repealing or relaxing government regulation in areas of environmental protection, occupational health and safety, food and drug oversight, transportation, fair employment practices, protection for labor unions, protection against sex and race discrimination, control of guns, etc.; and cutting back on social provision to education, health care, the elderly, the handicapped, children, and many other areas and groups. It constitutes a campaign to radically shrink the public sphere in every area except the military and those regulations designed to enforce "traditional" sex and gender values.

The attack on the public sphere is also an attack on political as well as social democracy. It can only further reduce the already low electoral participation in the US. Why should people vote if government makes so little difference in their lives? If most of our ills are defined as beyond political control?

The attack on the public sphere is also an attack on women, although not in the same way. For some women it is a direct attack, not only because they are struggling to raise children against formidable obstacles, but also because welfare has been a lifeline for women in bad relationships with men: high proportions of AFDC recipients have been victims of abuse. For prosperous women it is only an indirect attack, a disrespect for the social labor required to raise children. Welfare is, of course, a reproductive rights issue. It recognizes that not all mothers have husbands who can and will provide income enough to support the unpaid labor of mothering. Few American women have that privilege – in fact, it has *always* been only a minority of husbands who earned enough to support their dependents single-handedly. Yet the new welfare policy is essentially asking poor lone parents to be both mothers and fathers. Parents are supposed to work full-time *and* raise their children well, despite being unable to earn enough to pay for child care, medical benefits, and adequate housing – for that is the situation of the great majority of current and former welfare recipients.

A gender analysis of this conservative program should not assume that its sexism is parallel to its racism. AFDC's inferiority to old age pensions was not caused by misogyny but by a vision of the proper gender order. The authors of welfare repeal do not necessarily dislike and disrespect women. What is at issue is feminism, family, and sexual morality. The repeal of welfare was part of a worldwide backlash against feminism. The first sentence of the welfare repeal law, entitled the "Personal Responsibility and Work Opportunity Reconciliation Act of 1996," informs us that "The Congress makes the following findings: Marriage is the foundation of a successful society." Even leaving aside for the moment the relationships that this Congressional matrimony excludes, this credo rests on the assumption that poor women can find husbands who can keep them off welfare by single-handedly supporting a family – a demonstrably false assumption. The welfare repeal attempts to use support for children as a means of changing their mothers' sexual and marital behavior – something which has been attempted for centuries and which is always a failure.

We can misunderstand the passionate politics of reproduction control in the US, and miss what is at stake, if we remove it from its larger context. Reproductive rights have multivalent symbolic as well as practical implications. To supporters, they represent a necessary condition for women's equality and for democracy, a fundamental aspect of human rights and the right to privacy and freedom, and a further step in creating respect for a diversity of family and community bonds. To opponents, reproductive rights represent a weapon in an assault on the legally established family and the God-given gender system on which it rests; a capitulation to immoral, sinful sexuality and a rejection of God and Christianity as the foundation of American society; and a dangerous defiance of the proper relations of authority, power and property. The disagreements are fundamental and are unlikely to be resolved soon.

Notes

1   Full citations for the material in this paper can be found in my *The Moral Property of Women: A History of Birth Control Politics in America* (2002).
2   For the history of anti-abortion argumentation, see Brief of 281 American Historians as Amici Curiae Supporting Appellees, *Webster v. Reproductive Health Services*, 492 U.S. 490 (1989), No. 88–605.
3   Boardman; National Women's Health Network. 1988. National News, March–April: 1. On how these clinics worked see also Newsweek, September 1, 1986: 20; New York Times, December 17, 1986.
4   http://www.aclu-or.org/ppcase.htm and http://www.lektrik.com/PPvsACLA/home.htm
5   http://www.xs4all.nl/~oracle/nuremberg/aborts.html
6   Neal Horsley, quoted in *New York Times*, October 26, 1998, 10B. The website was taken off the web during a court trial, but could be visited under http://www.christiangallery.com/atrocity/aborts/ html at least until the end of February 2002.
7   In 2001, the following rules were effective in 50 US-states and D. C.: In 17 states a minor needed parental consent to obtain an abortion; 14 states required parental notification; 22 states required state-prescribed counseling; 14 states required a waiting period between counseling and abortion; 20 states banned abortions after the fetus was officially declared viable, except when the health of a women is in serious danger; 29 states refused Medicaid funds for abortions unless the woman's life was at risk or if the pregnancy had been caused by rape or incest; 28 states have prohibited so called partial-birth abortions: see http://www.agi-usa.org/pubs/abort_law_status.htm for updated information.
8   Maher vs. Roe, 432 U.S. 464 (1977); Beal vs. Doe, 432 U.S. 438 (1977); Poelker vs. Doe, 432 U.S. 519 (1977); Harris vs. McRae, 448 U.S. 297 (1980).
9   Davis 1988, 44. Studies conducted on the results of the cuts in public funding of abortions in California estimated that from 25 to 35 percent of women who wanted an abortion now carry their pregnancies to term; see Haddock 1989.
10 In *Roe v.* Wade, the Supreme Court required that any restrictions on a woman's decision would be subject to strict judicial scrutiny; in *Planned Parenthood of Southeast Pennsylvania v.* Casey, 505 U.S. 833 (1992), the Court upheld any restrictions that did not create an undue burden for the pregnant woman.
11 192 F.3d 1142 (8th Cir. 1999) und 120 S.Ct. 2597 (U.S. Supreme Court). Abstracts from the Supreme Court decisions are online at http://www.crlp.org/pub_fac_svcsum.html.
12 France, Austria, Belgium, Denmark, Finland, Germany, the UK, Greece, Israel, Luxembourg, Switzerland, and Ukraine.
13 Garb 1989; `Koop Challenged on Abortion Data,' New York Times Jan. 15, 1989.
14 ABC News/ Beliefnet survey, June 20–24, 2001.
15 ABC News/Washington Post survey, January 2001.
16 CNN/Time survey, January 2001.
17 Susan L. Norman for the Christian Broadcasting Network, quoted in Leatherman 1989.
18 ABC News/ Beliefnet survey, July 20–24, 2001.
19 Combs and Welsh 1982. See also Granberg and Granberg 1980; Cates 1977. It is important that – against the common assumption that African-Americans do not use contraception – recent stud-

ies argue that the decline in the black fertility rate since the late 19th century is mostly due to the use of contraceptives. See McFalls and Masnick 1981.

20 National Abortion Federation, Economics of Abortion Fact Sheet, January 1996, http://www.naral.org/medicaresources/publications/2002/funding.pdf. The study on North Carolina covers the period from 1981 to 1994.

21 Abortion Access Project, *Fact Sheet* at http://www.repro-activist.org.

22 Hospital Mergers: The Hidden Crisis. *Religious Pro-Choice Americans Speak Out*, Flugblatt; Washington, D. C.: Religious Coalition for Reproductive Choice, 2000, as well as http://www.rcrc.org/pubs/speakout/merge.html; National Abortion Federation, Fact Sheet, September 1997; Bucar 1998.

23 http://www.home.nycap.rr.com/deisley/quotes.html

24 Pater Paul Marx, Pro-Life/ Family Catalog, 1991, http://www.cs.unc.edu/allen/food.html.

25 Rosoff 1987; The U.S. International Family Planning Program under Siege, PPFA leaflet 1987; Klitsch 1988.

26 Ventura, Curtin, and Mathews 1999; Alan Guttmacher Institute, Welfare Law and the Drive to Reduce Illegitimacy. *Issues in Brief*, March 13, 2001, online http://www.agi-usa.org/pubs/ib_welfare00.html. Also, see two very different estimates in *Children's Defense Fund, Health of American's Children*, 27–29, and in *Family Planning Perspectives* 1987, 83–84.

27 The official name of the so called Moynihan Report was The Negro Family: The Case for National Health. Its author, Daniel P. Moynihan, was at that time deputy secretary of the Office of Policy Planning and Research im U.S. Department for Labor.

28 Among the numerous publications on the issue of single mothers and their children, see Luker 1984; Garfinkel and McLanahan 1986; on single mothers and the new poor, see Jencks 1989; McLanahan and Garfinkel 1989.

29 According to a survey published in 1994, 83 percent of teenage mothers were from poor families, as compared to 63 percent of those who decided to have an abortion and 38 percent of all teenagers. See Alan Guttmacher Institute 1994, 58. See also Pollack Petchesky 1984, 148–155. The allegation that there is a market for adoptions is wrong as respects babies of color.

30 Pratt and Horn undated; Advance Data from Vital and Health Statistics 108, 1985, summed up in: *Planning Perspectives* 17/6, November–December 1985, 274–275.

31 http://www.agi-usa.org/pubs/archives/newsrelease697.html; Alan Guttmacher Institue, School-based Health Centers and Birth Control Debate; http://www.agi-usa.org/pubs//ib_1200html.

32 Alan Guttmacher Institute, School-based Health Centers.

33 http://www.agi-usa.org/pubs/archives/newsrelease697.html; Alan Guttmacher Institute, School-based Health Centers.

34 Kaiser Family Foundation Briefing, Sex Education in America: A View from Inside the Classroom, September 25, 2000, http://www.kaisernetwork.org/health_cast/hcast_index.cfm?display=detail&hc=38.

References

Alan Guttmacher Institute. 1994. *Sex and America's Teenager*. New York.

Alan Guttmacher Institute. 1999. *Why Is Teenager Pregnancy Declining?: The Roles of Abstinence, Sexual Activity, and Contraceptive Use*. New York.

Antiabortion Violence. 1985. *Family Planning Perspektives*, 17/1, January–February: 4 (editorial).

Besharov, Douglas J., and Alison J. Quinn. 1987. Not All Female-Headed Families are Created Equal. *The Public Interest* 89, Fall: 48–56.

Blacks Agonize over Abortion. 1989. *Newsweek*, December 4: 63.

Boardman, Kathy. *BOGUS, the Consumer Scandal of the 1980s: Bogus Pregnancy Counseling Centers*. Unpublished manuscript.

Bucar, Liz. 1998. *When Catholic and Non-Catholic Hospitals Merge: Reproductive Health Compromised.* Washington, D. C.: Catholics for a Free Choice.

Cates, William Jr. 1977. Abortion Attitudes of Black Women. *Women and Health* 2/3, November–December: 3–9.

Cavanaugh, Michael A. 1986. Secularization and the Politics of Traditionalism: The Case of the Right-to-Life Movement. *Sociological Forum* 1/2, spring: 251–283.

Combs, Michael W., and Susan Welsh. 1982. Blacks, Whites, and Attitudes Toward Abortion. *Public Opinion Quaterly* 46: 510–520.

Davis, Susan E. (ed.). 1988. *Women Under Attack: Victories, Backlash, and the Fight for Reproductive Freedom.* Committee for Abortion Rights and Against Sterilization pamphlet No. 7. Boston: South End Press.

Dionne, E. J. Jr. 1989. Tepid Black Support Worries Advocates of Abortion Rights. *New York Times*, April 16.

Donovan, Patricia. 1985. The Holy War. *Family Planning Perspektives*, 17/1, January–February: 5–9.

Family Planning Perspectives 19/2, March–April 1987.

Fine, Michelle. 1983. Sexuality, Schooling, and Adolescent Females: The Missing Discourse of Desire. *Harvard Education Review* 58/1, February.

Garb, Maggie. 1989. Abortion Foes Give Birth to a `Syndrome'. *In These Times* Feb. 22-March 1: 3, 22.

Garfinkel, Irwin, and Sara S. McLanahan. 1986. *Single Mothers and Their Children: A New American Dilemma.* Washington, D. C.: Urban Institute Press.

Gordon, Linda. 2002. *The Moral Property of Women: A History of Birth Control Politics in America.* Urbana and Chicago: University of Illinois Press.

Granberg, Donald, and Beth Wellman Granberg. 1980. Abortion Attitudes, 1965–1980: Trends and Determinants. *Family Planning Perspektives* 12 5/September–October: 250–264.

Gross, Jane. 1989. Anti-Abortion Revival: Homes for Unwed Mothers. *New York Times*, July 23.

Haddock, Vicki. 1989. Hidden Costs of Denying Abortions for Teens. *San Francisco Examiner*, August 2.

Harding, Susan Friend. 2000. *The Book of Jerry Falwell: Fundamentalist Language and Politics.* Princeton, N.J.: Princeton University Press.

Harrison, Polly F., and Allan Rosenfield (eds.). 1996. *Contraceptive Research and Development: Looking to the Future.* Washington, D. C.: National Academy Press.

Henshaw, Stanley K. 1998. Abortion Incidence in the United States, 1995–1996. *Family Planning Perspectives* 30/6, November–December: 263–270.

Henshaw, Stanley K., and Kathryn Kost. 1996. Abortion Patients in 1994-95: Characteristics and Contraceptive Use. *Family Planning Perspectives* 28/4, July–August: 140–147, 158.

Jencks, Christopher. 1989.What Is the Underclass – and Is It Growing? *Focus* (University of Wisconsin Institute for Research on Poverty) 12/1, Spring–Summer: 14–26.

Kirby, D., et al. 1994. School-based Programs to Reduce Sexual Risk Behaviour: A Review of Effectiveness. *Public Health Reports* 109.

Klitsch, Michael. 1988. Courts Sink New Title X Regulations. *Family Planning Perspectives* 20/2, November–December: 96–98.

Ladner, Joyce. 1986. Teenage Pregnancy: The Implications for Black Americans. *The State of Black America 1986*. New York: National Urban League.

Leatherman, Courtney. 1989. Nearly 1 in 10 Female College Students Has Had Abortion. *Chronicle of Higher Education*, May 31, A23.

Luker, Kristen. 1984. *Abortion and the Politics of Motherhood*. Berkeley: University of California Press.

McFalls, Joseph A. Jr., and George S. Masnick. 1981. Birth Control and the Fertility of the U.S. Black Population. *Journal of Family History* 6/1, Spring: 89–106.

McLanahan, Sara S., and Irwin Garfinkel. 1989. Single Mothers, the Underclass, and Social Policy. *Annals of the American Academy* 501, January: 92–104.

Moore, K. A., et al. 1995. Adolescent Pregnancy Prevention Program: Interventions and Evaluations. *Child Trends*, June. Washington, D. C.

Neustadter, Roger. 1990. Killing Babies: The Use of Image and Metaphor in the Right-to-Life Movement. *Michigan Sociological Review* 4, 76–83.

Perkins, Spencer. 1989. The Pro-Life Credibility Gap. *Christianity Today*, April 21.

Pollack Petchesky, Rosalind. 1984. *Abortion and Woman's Choice: The State, Sexuality, and Reproductive Freedom*. New York: Longmann.

Pollack Petchesky, Rosalind. 1987. Fetal Images: The Power of Visual Culture in the Politics of Reproduction. *Feminist Studies* 13/2, Summer: 263–292.

Pratt, W. C., and M. C. Horn. Undated. *Wanted and Unwanted Childbearing: United States*, 1973–1982. Hyattsville.

Rosoff, Jeannie I. 1987. Taking Family Planning Out of Title X: The Impact of the Proposed New Regulations. *Family Planning Perspectives* 19/5, September–October: 222–226.

Ross, Loretta J. 1998. African-American Women and Abortion. In Rickie Solinger (ed.) *Abortion Wars: A Half Century of Struggle, 1950–2000*. Berkeley: University of California Press.

Tucker, Neely. 1986. Factions Spur Hodgepodge of Separately Funded Clinics. *Florida Today*, October 26.

Ventura, Stephanie J., Sally C. Curtin and T. J. Mathews. 1999. Declines in Teenage Birth Rates, 1991–98. *National Statistics Reports*, October 25. Atlanta: Center for Disease Control and Prevention.

Vinovskis, Maris A. 1988. Teenage Pregnancy and the Underclass. *The Public Interest* 93, Fall: 87–96.

Ann Shola Orloff

Explaining US Welfare Reform: Power, Gender, Race, and the US Policy Legacy

Introduction

US welfare reform, ushered in with the 1996 Personal Responsibility and Work Opportunity Reconciliation Act (PRWORA), has attracted notice across the developed world as a model – good or bad depending on the politics of the viewer – of social assistance when employment for all is fully embraced as a policy goal. Indeed, employment is the core of Temporary Assistance to Needy Families (TANF), the program that replaced Aid to Families with Dependent Children (AFDC), the old "welfare" (Weaver 1998, 2000; U. S. Committee on Ways and Means 1998; Ellwood 1999). TANF beneficiaries, whatever the age of their children, must participate in community service, better known as "workfare," after two months of receiving benefits, and must be employed within two years. Work requirements have been accompanied by increased funding for child care, yet caregiving has lost governmental backing when not accompanied by employment. The individual entitlement to social assistance, only firmly established in the 1960s and 1970s, was explicitly eliminated. Most strikingly, there is a lifetime limit of five years of benefits. Yet "welfare reform" should be considered along with other policy changes, such as the expansion of the Earned Income Tax Credit (EITC). Both changes may be credited with raising the employment rates of single mothers, but where TANF imposes new regulations and deterrent measures, the EITC works through the tax system and has helped to raise the incomes of poor employed parents, especially single mothers. Unlike AFDC, the EITC has been expanded several times over the course of the 1980s and 1990s. Claims for support are made in the course of filing tax returns, and are conditional on low income from employment and supporting children rather than on poverty, lack of employment and family status, as under AFDC. One might understand these changes as ending the "maternalist" strand of US social provision while expanding an employment-based strand, in the context of disentitlement and the expansion of the significance of the labor market for Americans' life chances and material conditions.

Welfare reformers' goals of reducing caseloads and increasing employment among single mothers seem to have been met: by 2000, the number of people on welfare had declined by over 50% since the legislation was signed into law in 1996 (U. S. Department of Health and Human Services 2000); studies of those who have left the welfare rolls show that most former recipients have found employment, albeit usually at low wages (Corcoran et al. 2000). Poverty decreased over this period, although the relative contributions of policy changes, including the expansion of EITC, and the buoyant economy of the 1990s are hard to separate. But while many conservative and liberal commentators both in and out of the academy proclaim that "welfare reform is working," there remain troubling problems. Poverty rates for children and for single-mother families – employed or not – remain high by international standards. Among lone mothers not in paid work, 93 percent are poor, while this rate drops to 43 percent for employed single mothers (again a poverty line of below 50 percent of median income) (Kilkey and Bradshaw 1999, 161). In the absence of other policy elements designed to "make work pay" which the Clinton administration supported, such as universal health insurance, the lives of poor single mothers combining employment and caregiving remain difficult. The racial and residential make-up of the caseload has changed: it is now overwhelmingly African-American and Latina, and located in urban centers; this indicates that the reforms have left behind those with more difficult problems in entering employment (DeParle 1998). EITC can only help those who are employed, unemployment insurance only those recently employed (and for sufficiently long to acquire coverage). When the business cycle next brings recession there will also be challenges for the states, for, unlike the old AFDC program under which the federal government funding to the states automatically expanded as demand grew during downturns, TANF's block grants are fixed and can only be expanded with explicit Congressional approval, in a context of politically-imposed budgetary constraints.

How can we explain this set of changes? Electoral and legislative politics were obviously significant (Weir 1998; Weaver 1998; Myles and Pierson 1997). But my interest here is slightly different. I am interested in the policy impact of changing balances of power and structural conditions, particularly long-term shifts in expectations about mothers' employment, including its racialized dimensions. Yet I also contend that these factors must be situated in the context of existing policy to make sense of how political actors, mainly in the Democratic Party, formerly committed to protecting welfare, began to embrace "welfare reform." Relations of race, class and gender shaped welfare reform, to be sure – but as mediated by the policy legacy and the larger political-institutional context. My approach fits within the rubric of historical institutionalism and policy regime analysis, which focus on the characteristics of policy regimes, and the politics engendered by these patterns (see e.g., Weir, Orloff, and Skocpol 1988; Weir 1992; Pierson 1994; Skocpol 1995; Orloff 1993a; Esping-Andersen 1990; Esping-Andersen 1999).

The Gender Effects of Welfare Reform

This set of social policy changes has had at least three notable effects on gender relations. First, the Personal Responsibility Act eliminated an entitlement – a conditional social right for poor single mothers to care for their children full time. This withdrawal of social rights affects all citizens, but is especially significant for groups which historically have depended disproportionately on public assistance: single mothers with poor earnings capacities and heavy caregiving burdens, and racial and ethnic minority people, who suffer from relatively high rates of poverty and unemployment. AFDC gave poor women the capacity to form and maintain autonomous households (Orloff 1993b) – an "exit option" from marriage or partnerships, and a safety net against unemployment that paralleled the exit option based on employment enjoyed by women with better labor market prospects. If social rights offer disadvantaged groups greater leverage vis-à-vis advantaged groups, this withdrawal diminishes their power. The EITC does offer public support to families in a non-discretionary manner, but only to those who are in the labor market and earning wages.

Second, PRWORA accomplished a shift in institutional relationships. By replacing an entitlement, or social right, to assistance, however encumbered with restrictions, with benefits granted on a discretionary basis, the state forces citizens and residents toward reliance on "private" sources of support, the labor market, families and charities. In terms of how care is organized, the new policy arrangements eliminate support for caregiving and reproduction when they are not linked to participation in the labor market – again emphasizing the importance of the market. While funding for child care services has been expanded, it remains insufficient to meet demand, and support for high-quality services has not yet been forthcoming. For those who do not gain access to the limited public support for care services, the availability and quality of care depend on market resources – thus disadvantaging those with jobs paying poorly or subject to high unemployment rates.

Third, this round of welfare reform accomplished a shift in the institutionalized expectations about the gender division of labor, in that women – or, more to the point, mothers – as well as men are now to be subject to the requirement of employment or work activities in claiming social assistance. Caregiving has been shifted to an even more marginal status within the US policy regime, as claims based on the status of family caregiver have been eliminated. The identity of "worker" has been strengthened, and the overall pattern of gender stratification reflects a greater emphasis on gender "sameness" – men and women both work for pay. But it must be noted that this is "sameness" on the male model of the unencumbered worker. Remaining gender differences in responsibilities for (unpaid) caregiving are occluded, partly because they continue to be relegated to the "private" sphere.

Explanations for Welfare Reform

Why has the US eliminated certain social rights of poor mothers? Why is employment to be expected of women – mothers – as well as men? Why has the state withdrawn support to caregiving and reproduction, except when it is accompanied by paid labor? I will briefly discuss alternative factors commonly invoked to explain welfare policy outcomes: first, power resources, and particularly the weakness of constituencies relying on welfare, here including the force of racism in US welfare politics; second, changes in gender relations, specifically women's increased labor force participation and increasing proportions of single-mother households; including racialized models of motherhood and employment. These were all implicated in the recent policy shifts around welfare. But I will argue that to understand fully the ensemble of policy changes, these factors must be understood in the context of the existing policies and processes of policy feedback. I will emphasize three aspects of that policy legacy, or "policy regime": (1) the residualism of US social provision, reflecting the weakness of the public safety net for the working-aged population; (2) the institutionalization in AFDC of a model of motherhood based on full-time caregiving when most women have had to enter employment to sustain households with or without partners, with little support from government programs; and (3) the racialization of welfare. The policy legacy gave rise to a politics in which work requirements were increasingly accepted, but also in which social rights to be supported while caregiving full time became increasingly tenuous.

Power Resources, Social Rights and the Policy Regime

Many analysts of the welfare state look to the strength, or power resources, of working-class forces as the central factor in the development of social rights (Korpi 2000). More recently, as race and gender have come to be understood as significant for policy outcomes, the strength of racism and gender discrimination as part of the overall constellation of power resources have figured in explanations for the character of US social policy (e.g., Quadagno 1994; Mink 1998; Boris 1995).

The relative weakness of social rights, the lack of generosity of American social programs for non-elderly people and the tight linkage of benefits to employment are often understood as reflecting the weakness of working-class forces and the strength of employers. Unions in the US have been relatively weaker than in Europe or the Antipodes, while the lack of a major labor, social-democratic or socialist party has been a notable feature of US political development. The US has had a relatively less-developed public system of supports for the working-aged population than has existed in other Western countries since at least 1950. Moreover, the position of employers has been strengthened over the last two decades by increased capital mobility and the opening of new low-wage labor markets in the developing economies (Esping-Andersen 1999). Also significant is the rise of neo-liberalism as an ideological force – and with it, a preference for private provision and for minimizing state interventions, reflected in pressures to keep taxes and social spending low. These factors have led to the retrenchment and restructuring of social programs everywhere, in order to make income support more closely conform to the "demands" of the new global economy – which is to say, of the employers in that economy (Rhodes 1996).

But while some might expect such a system to engender continuing but unfulfilled political support for the expansion of rights, this has not been the pattern of US social politics. Rather, limited social assistance has gone along with popular antipathy to welfare. Historical institutionalists and policy regime analysts have examined the political effects of the relatively strong private provision that characterizes the US and other "liberal" welfare states (Esping-Andersen 1990; Weir et al. 1988). Because US labor organization has been uneven, some sectors of the working class were able to wrest protections from their employers, creating a "private welfare state" for the better-organized segments of workers and their families (Stevens 1988), while leaving those who cannot get private coverage to a residual public system. This has produced weak political support for welfare provision aside from Social Security, the one US social program that covers almost the whole population. Poor single mothers on AFDC, disproportionately women of color, were a weak group, because the programmatic structure of the US welfare state politically isolated them and they commanded few political resources. While Medicaid involved the interests of medical providers or Food Stamps the concerns of agricultural interests, AFDC drew on no well-organized interests. This was particularly the case after mobilizations of poor people, especially women welfare recipients, died down after the early 1970s (Piven and Cloward 1977). However, poor single mothers have been a weak constituency for a long time, so one still needs to ask why in 1996 AFDC was vulnerable not just to cutbacks and the addition of deterrent provisions, but to elimination. In part, this means asking why more powerful political actors associated with the Democratic Party ceased to see the protection of welfare as an important goal.

Welfare reform reflects an androcentric bias in social politics. Caregiving, while socially necessary, is culturally and institutionally denigrated (Knijn and Kremer 1997). Political forces hostile to AFDC ignore the significance of unpaid, caring labor (especially but not only when performed by women of color), vilify welfare programs and construe any sort of dependency, or even interdependence, as pathological (Fraser and Gordon 1994; Roberts 1995; Naples 1997; Fineman 1995). The unequal valuation of caregiving as compared to employment embedded in welfare reform reflects a gendered imbalance of power. This complex of cultural valuations and power resources helps to explain the undermining of support to caregiving reflected in PRWORA.

A particularly influential view on how gender inequality is reflected in state social provision is that which sees welfare as bifurcated into two gendered "streams," "tiers" or "channels." The feminine tier is made up of inadequate social assistance programs, AFDC paradigmatically, serving a predominantly female clientele who make claims based on their family status, while the masculine tier is made up of relatively more generous contributory social insurance targeting a male clientele who make claims based on their status in the labor market (see, e.g., Pearce 1986; Nelson 1990; Fraser 1989). Because women are disproportionately responsible for care and domestic work, analysts once believed that all women should have had an interest in preserving and improving the treatment of such claims. Thus, the elimination of welfare rights could be seen as reflecting the political weakness of women. However, this view is hard to sustain when politicians recognize a gender gap in voting and when competition for women's votes has been intense. Moreover, the Clinton administration was quite supportive of the agenda of women's groups in many ways (e.g., personnel appointments, parental leave legislation, abortion rights). Programs of social protection aimed at covering the risks faced disproportionately by women, such as paid maternity or parental leave, are not well developed in the US (Gornick et al. 1997). But by many other indicators – declines in occupational sex segregation and gendered wage inequality, the strength of regulations prohibiting sexual harassment, or the broadness of the understanding of bodily, reproductive and sexual autonomy for women – many US women are relatively advantaged compared to their counterparts in other western countries (O'Connor et al. 1999). Perhaps it is not that women are politically weak, but that it is incorrect to characterize women's interests as united around welfare, or to assume that AFDC captured the pro-caregiving sentiments that many women express. And in fact, few women or women's equality organizations mobilized to protest against welfare reform.

Why did the proposed or actual elimination of AFDC not call forth popular protests similar to those that followed the 1989 Supreme Court Webster decision, when hundreds of thousands of women turned out to defend abortion rights? The Women's Committee of One Hundred, one of the few pro-welfare, feminist lobbying groups to appear when welfare was being debated, tried to mobilize under the slogan "a war against poor women is a war against all women" (Mink 1998). But it drew only hundreds in several demonstrations. In the case of defending abortion rights, women across the social spectrum saw this as an issue that engaged their interests; in the case of welfare reform, this did not happen.

We need to consider institutional factors to explain these events. Feminist descriptions of the "dual channel" US welfare state have tended to neglect the overall shape of the US welfare *regime*, with its large share of private provision for working-aged people. It is true that almost all adult recipients of AFDC and TANF were and are women, and in fact, women make the majority of family-based claims, while men's claims are almost all as workers (O'Connor et al. 1999, chap. 4). But most of these family-related claims are made by women in the upper-tier social insurance programs, principally old-age insurance. Before they reach retirement age, the majority of women, like most men, must rely on employer-provided or privately-financed services and benefits, or do without them. This includes the vast majority of single mothers, 84 percent of whom were in the labor force in 1997 (Meyer and Rosenbaum 1998). Women, particularly mothers of young children, do sometimes depend at least partially on male partners' income, but labor force participation has become the norm for women as well as men – in 1997, among married women with children under 18, 71 percent were in the labor force – not much below the rates for married men or single mothers, though rates are somewhat lower – around 63% – for married women with younger children; even among women with children less than a year old, half were in the work force (U. S. Bureau of Labor Statistics 1998). Women who identified their political interests and identities as those of "working (i.e., employed) moms" or taxpayers did not see themselves as potential welfare recipients. And while women exhibit more generous attitudes than do men vis-à-vis social spending, they did not defend "welfare as we knew it." Rather, there is sentiment for helping those who try to work for pay (Gilens 1999). Others would argue that most white women did not identify with welfare recipients because of racism. President Reagan and other Republicans mobilized these sentiments in the campaign against AFDC and "welfare queens" in the 1980s; this was the context for the Democrats move to the right on "wedge issues" (Dawson 1994; Williams 1998).

Today, there is little doubt that welfare politics has served as a mechanism for some whites' expression of racial antagonism toward African-Americans. African-Americans' political leverage has been blunted by the lack of competition for their votes, as Republicans could assemble winning coalitions based primarily on suburban and rural whites (Weir 1995; Dawson 1994). The media emphasized – to the point of distortion – African-American images in discussions of both poverty and welfare (Gilens 1999). Policy analysts have uncovered racial differences in patterns of welfare use that reflect the deeper and more chronic poverty of people of color, and their disproportionate share of unemployment and underemployment (Spalter-Roth et al. 1995; Pavetti 1997). As compared to white women, African-American and Latina women were more likely to depend on welfare for longer periods of time, either alone or cycling between welfare and employment. Whites tended to use welfare more intensively, for shorter periods of time. Welfare reform was designed to chase "short-term" would-be recipients to private sources of support, while subjecting potentially longer-term recipients to stringent new requirements, and it has – whites have been leaving the system faster than have minorities, with the consequence that the large majority of welfare recipients are now African-American and Latino (DeParle 1998).

Politicians did not have to discuss race explicitly for all to understand the racial impact of the new welfare legislation (Williams 1998). Yet social politics cannot be understood as a simple reflection of an underlying racial balance of power; rather, institutional factors conditioned how racial conflicts occurred (Quadagno 1994; Lieberman 1998). African-Americans were incorporated into national-level social insurance programs ("Social Security") with little conflict at the same time that their inclusion in welfare was being contested (Lieberman 1998). In state-administered welfare, the most conservative and racist forces had more influence than in federally-administered social insurance. Democrats worked hard to maintain their support among African-Americans (who vote for the party in Presidential elections at rates of over 90 percent), sponsoring a number of initiatives to this end. Clinton calculated that welfare reform would help him with white voters even if black voters would have preferred a different approach. Yet this was not simply a matter of blacks' lack of power but of a political context conditioned by the ambivalent policy legacy of welfare for liberals as much as by the racial make-up of the electorate. Indeed, even the Congressional Black Caucus did not make preventing welfare reform a high priority (Williams 1998).

The timing of welfare reform in the mid-nineties is especially interesting given that elimination of AFDC was politically not possible under President Reagan, who was certainly hostile to welfare. Democratic control of the House was a bulwark against the most radical retrenchment under Reagan; a Democratic President in 1995-96 was not a bulwark against the attempts of a Republican Congress to eliminate AFDC. It is not simply a matter of divided government, but a question of what deprived AFDC of political protection even among Democrats in 1996. Increases in women's employment made AFDC politically indefensible at worst, unattractive at best, even among many of those committed to women's equality (or racial justice). Having lost the commitment of those forces traditionally favorable to social provision, welfare became vulnerable to the right's campaign for repeal.

A comparison to Britain is instructive (Pierson 1994). Both the UK Income Support system, which supports poor lone mothers among other groups, and US AFDC were subjected to similar tinkering in the 1980s, but the programs' fates have diverged more considerably under Clinton and Blair. Clinton's election promise to put welfare mothers to work was very popular, and even the elimination of AFDC in 1996 did not bring popular or political outrage. In contrast, Blair's less radical proposals to cut lone mothers' benefits and to expand work incentives were greeted with resistance – in the former case, sufficient to force the administration to back down (Millar 1996; O'Connor, Orloff, and Shaver 1999, chap. 3-4). Mothers' full-time caregiving, at least until children are in school, remains legitimate and politically defensible in Britain, in a context where mothers generally are more likely to stay at home full-time or work part-time than in the US. In the US, the clamor for reform remained high through the 1980s and 1990s, despite the fact that US single mothers exhibit relatively high rates of labor force participation and low rates of welfare receipt and many US mothers cycled between paid work and welfare, in effect using AFDC as an unemployment benefit (Spalter-Roth et al. 1995). Yet in the US, a program assisting poor full-time caregivers could not call upon such popular and elite support. Why? To understand, we need to examine changing patterns of gender relations in work and family.

Changing Gender Relations: Motherhood, Employment and Race

The gender division of labor today is quite different than when AFDC was established in 1935, with higher rates of single parenthood, far fewer women staying home full-time to care for children, and large increases in women's, especially mothers', employment. Rhetoric championing the "traditional" family and attacking "illegitimacy" featured heavily in the welfare debates, drawing on reservoirs of hostility toward single mothers, particularly women of color. These sentiments were most notable on the political right, although liberals, too, claimed that single-parent families were harmful for children (e.g. McLanahan and Sandefur 1994). And these changes help to explain why work requirements for single mothers came to be seen as reasonable by policymakers, academics and the public. Benefits for single parents were established with the aim of allowing white single mothers to pursue the distinctive, non-commodified life pattern deemed appropriate for other white mothers in order to care for their children. Public provision construed single mothers as unemployable, as full-time caregivers rather than as potential workers, even as women's labor force participation, particularly among married mothers of children under age six, was accelerating (Reskin and Padavic 1994) and as the clientele of AFDC expanded to include more women of color. Work incentives were introduced into AFDC in 1967, so that women could combine employment earnings and welfare benefits, while retaining health coverage. While this was probably the outcome most favorable for beneficiaries in the short run, this line of policy development continued to leave the employed poor and most two-parent families outside the umbrella of social protection, which in turn left AFDC politically vulnerable (Weir et al. 1988). Then the Reagan administration enacted new restrictions against combining paid work and welfare, leaving in place a formal model of motherhood based on full-time caregiving, which over the course of the decade was increasingly out of sync with the behavior of most mothers, married or not (Reskin and Padavic 1994, 143-145). Furthermore, the "welfare poor" and the "working poor" were more clearly distinguished. The Family Support Act of 1988 at first glance might appear to have changed this formally institutionalized model of motherhood, as single parents were required to be at work or in training after their youngest child reached three years of age (Naples 1997). But because it was visibly ineffective in promoting employment among welfare recipients, it helped to bring the elimination of AFDC.

The emerging model of motherhood – as encompassing paid work – which we see expressed in US policies may also relate to the fact that US women of color have been held to requirements about combining motherhood and paid work that have differed historically from those applying to whites (Collins 1990; Glenn 1992). In the early years of AFDC, many women, particularly in the South, were excluded from the right to care for children full-time, as they were classified as "employable mothers" – and this had an unmistakable moral and racial cast, for it was unwed mothers and women of color who fell into these categories (Bell 1965; Lieberman 1998). But as these women came to be included in AFDC and its clientele was perceived as less white, the standards applicable to women of color were made requirements of all welfare programs, a trend reinforced by the increasing proportions of women of all races and ethnic groups entering the labor force. Perhaps the expectation that women of color should work for pay also reflects a lack of cultural valuation of their caregiving work, and of the reproduction of people of color (Roberts 1995; Mink 1998).

Mink (1998) has argued that single mothers are being singled out for harsh treatment in the new work requirements of TANF and that this reflects not a commitment to employment for all women, but special punishment for women who flout conventional household and sexual mores, with clear racial implications, given that women of color are far more likely to be unmarried mothers than are white women. She notes that in earlier welfare regulations forcing certain women – those who were "immoral," because unmarried (and therefore more likely to have been African-American) – to work for pay, "wage work became penance for illegitimacy" (Mink 1998, 37). And she argues that this is the impetus behind current welfare reform; women of color are being punished – by being forced to work – for their household and reproductive decisions, and because their caregiving work is not valued. This, she says is reflected in the fact that the PRWORA created a mandate for single parents to be in work activities, while requiring only one parent in two-parent families to be working, thus allowing housewifery in two-parent families receiving assistance (Mink 1998, 105-107). Indeed, unless a two-parent household claims child care benefits, one or both parents together must work the equivalent of 35 hours per week, while single parent households are required to be in work activities for 30 hours by 2000 (although states may limit this to 20 hours).

Should requiring employment be understood simply as racism? This is a hard argument to sustain in the context of the residualism of US social provision, and the fact that employment is the basis for most households' support. It does appear that two-parent families are to be allowed somewhat greater flexibility in making work and caregiving arrangements than are single-parent families – echoing the greater flexibility such families have outside the welfare system. Given the very small proportion of two-parent families that are even eligible for and receiving welfare assistance – never more than about five percent of the caseload (US CWM 1998, 410, 413, 451), the vast majority of two-parent families are forced to conform to economic exigencies in determining caregiving arrangements. The residualism of the system is significant. US families – in contrast to some of their European counterparts – do not receive any direct subsidy for full-time caregiving (Wennemo 1994). If a household's income permits, one parent can opt out of the labor market or cut back her/his hours. However, many fewer people are in this category than used to be the case, given the decline in jobs with family-supporting wages (in 1940, one-earner households comprised over 70 percent of US families; by 1980, they comprised 28 percent [Reskin and Padavic 1994, 49]).

The particular patterns of American women's labor force participation, the policy context within which these occur, and the disjunction between formal models of motherhood in AFDC and labor force participation patterns among women not on welfare made AFDC more problematic politically than sole-parent provision in other countries. American women are likely to work full-time – about 3/4 of all employed women are working full-time – and full-year (O'Connor, Orloff, and Shaver 1999, table 3.3). Perhaps most critically for the lack of political support for AFDC was that American women work with less *public* support, such as child allowances, child care or paid leaves, than do their counterparts in other parts of the West where women's employment is institutionalized in the policy regime (e.g., Scandinavia) (Gornick et al. 1997; Michel 1999). The US has not had programs of universal support for mothering while in much of Continental Europe, Britain and Australia, nationalism and pro-natalism helped to bolster social provision, creating a safety net in which motherhood was supported through near-universal programs – a set of provisions that in some places has been used by employed mothers in recent decades to ease caregiving-work conflicts, or, at the least, has eased the financial burden of childrearing. In the US, racial models of motherhood likely hastened shifts in the character of work requirements. In other English-speaking countries, there have been similar shifts toward encouraging employment, but the outcomes have been less severe given competing concerns about caregiving among policymakers and the public. However in the US, racism probably weakened the force of such competing concerns.

In the US, the logic of the market holds sway. There is widespread sentiment that mothers as well as fathers "must" work to maintain households, or, among the affluent, to maintain a proper standard of living, including education for children and the like. Staying at home full-time to care for children has come to be understood as something to be earned through one's efforts in the labor market – as a reward from an employer who gives paid leave – a benefit usually reserved for the best-off women, or supported through savings, help from parents or at the price of a normal consumption pattern (e.g., Christian conservatives argue that upholding "family values," including housewifery, requires resistance to middle-class consumerism). AFDC rules seemed to make possible staying at home to care for children at public expense for poor women – exactly what isn't guaranteed to any other mother or father. Against the backdrop of poorly-developed welfare state provision for non-poor working-aged people, politicians could paint welfare as a "privilege" and construe welfare reform as simply extending the compulsion of the market to welfare recipients.

Situating welfare reform in this context of wider policy developments relevant to gender relations – such as the regulation of labor markets and policy on re-production – makes clear that it reflects broader patterns characterizing the US policy regime and gender politics (Hobson 1994; O'Connor, Orloff, and Shaver 1999). Gender equality forces have defined employment and educational oppor-tunity as central to women's emancipation. Employment-equity legislation has, in combination with strong employer demand for women workers, helped to cre-ate much-enhanced possibilities for women's economic independence (Bergmann 1986); the gender pay gap has declined (McCall 2001). Reproductive rights are also understood as central to the equality project, at least partly because control of one's reproductive capacities is necessary to competing more equally in the labor mar-ket. The dominant understanding is that if all must work to support households, and in addition this furthers women's prospects, women on welfare, too, should be employed. I would argue that this is why women's organizations and organizations of African-Americans, including the Congressional Black Caucus, did not, in the end, make preventing welfare reform a high priority (Williams 1998). And once women, including mothers, are understood as workers, the logic of supporting their "choice" between employment and unpaid full-time caregiving collapses.

Welfare Reform and the Ending of Entitlement

Since the Reagan administration, the "reform" of welfare has meant increasing restrictions and work requirements, occasionally with enhanced child care serv-ices or training, or even elimination of the program. The political possibilities for more generous and more universalistic provision had collapsed some time earlier, with the defeat of Nixon's Family Assistance Plan in the 1970s. Welfare was a key "wedge issue" used by Republicans against Democrats throughout the 1980s, a key part of their strategy to separate white voters from African-Americans and Lati-nos. Democrats were put in the unenviable position of defending a deeply-flawed welfare program in order to defend poor people and a safety net, and lost support among traditional white working-class constituencies, among others, because of it (Williams 1998).

By the 1990s, Democrats had joined Republicans in taking advantage of the electoral popularity of welfare "reform." Clinton turned around his party's vulnerability among white voters with his famous 1992 campaign pledge to "end welfare as we know it," while promising to "make work pay." His approach could more easily accommodate EITC expansion than the defense of the existing welfare system. Poverty would be fought not with higher benefits or expanded coverage, but by getting everyone – including mothers – into employment, then improving pay and conditions. Clinton Democrats wanted to make AFDC more like unemployment insurance – a short-term benefit to help claimants "get on their feet" but premised on employment; in fact, this is how many women were using the program, although the formal rules obscured this (Edin and Lein 1997).

The elimination of AFDC became almost inevitable once Clinton made his famous promise. Although Democrats sought to retain control of the welfare issue, the call to end welfare was seized on mainly by Republicans, who moved the debate far to the right – to outright elimination of a right to assistance. After the Republicans captured the House of Representatives in 1994, President Clinton was challenged by Republicans to sign welfare bills much more restrictive and less generous that his own plan. After vetoing two bills, he ultimately signed the third. Did he have to do it? Critics point out that he could have continued his opposition; the Republicans probably could not have overcome a veto. Yet Clinton apparently worried about losing his healthy margin in the polls in the 1996 race with Bob Dole if he were to come before the electorate having failed in his promise to "end welfare as we know it" (Reich 1999).

Conclusion

The end of the entitlement to social assistance in 1996 coincided with a shift in formal expectations about women's employment and a withdrawal of (residual) support to full-time caregiving. Both the generally market-supporting and market-enhancing character of the US policy regime, and the articulation of feminist projects with women's employment helped to create a context within which welfare reform was likely to take a form which would support employment. And the neoliberal thinking in favor among political elites helped to ensure that welfare reform would encompass some shift of responsibilities from state to labor market, and tie assistance to work activities or to employment – so as to support, rather than undercut, the low-wage labor market. But this did not necessitate an end of entitlement – social rights could have been made conditional on employment.

Why were work requirements and the loss of social rights connected in the shifts in the US welfare regime? Requirements for recipients to seek employment were accepted by almost all who would reform welfare by the 1990s; the only questions left concerned the conditions under which they would do so. Even for political actors generally committed to women's equality, it was at best difficult or, more often, not politically compelling to defend AFDC strongly. But there was more contingency in the linkage of work requirements and the end of entitlement. American political and policy dynamics in the 1990s featured electoral pressures to move to the right on social spending and a "policy crisis" around AFDC. Quite simply, AFDC was utterly discredited among both policy and political elites and the public: public opinion polls after the 1994 election "showed that the public preferred *any* possible package of reforms over the status quo" (Weaver 1998, 375). There was mounting receptivity among the electorate for radical solutions to the "welfare mess." After all, this was not a system from which most voters gained any benefits – rather, they understood themselves to be supporting families with their own efforts. However much help middle-class Americans received through the tax system – and they do receive a fair amount (Howard 1997), this was not understood as "welfare," but in opposition to it, as a way of helping hard-working, "independent" taxpayers. The electoral victories of Republicans, along with a Democratic President determined to pass some version of welfare reform, created the conditions for the repeal of AFDC. Does the analysis of the origins of welfare reform suggest a way forward?

The centrality of employment for women as well as men in the US welfare regime has been reinforced through both welfare reform and the expansion of the EITC, but has been associated with a continuing lack of public support for caregiving. As many feminist analyses have pointed out, the lack of support to care – or to accommodating employment and care – has especially deleterious consequences for women, who still take up the bulk of this work, and for whom caregiving constrains employment opportunities and resources. But how should feminists encourage policies that make better accommodation for caregiving responsibilities and better support to care work? There are two different proposals (cf. Fraser 1994). The Women's Committee of 100 offers a "new maternalist" proposal: (income-tested) caregivers' allowances – in essence, an improved AFDC (without employment mandates) – which would allow poor women to have a measure of choice in making arrangements around caregiving and employment. This strategy, they hope, would speak to the needs of the most vulnerable, work to overcome racial inequalities in opportunities and resources for caregiving and reproduction, and valorize caregiving work (Women's Committee of 100 2000).

Although the aims are worthy, the new maternalist strategy is – in the contemporary US – a political dead end. While aimed at eliminating the caregiving-based dependency that characterizes many women's lives, it ignores the political vulnerability of targeted programs. Why should those who undertake caregiving in connection with employment, or who have partners, be ineligible? Those who are employed would essentially pay for their own caregiving supports such as child care, and pay taxes to support other women who care full time, while enjoying less leisure than those who stay at home. And as a matter of practical politics, note that this is exactly how welfare was interpreted, a fact that helped to undermine its political viability. Perhaps more generous family allowances (or family tax credits) could do some of the work of supporting the needs of those with caregiving responsibilities, but of course, they do not support full-time caregiving.

The dependence of so many women (and men) on employment, in the absence of reliable safety nets or supports for caregiving, points to a possible avenue for the development of more successful feminist policy alternatives. An "economic citizenship" approach would offer supports for combining employment and caregiving, on the assumption that both activities are critical for social and political participation, and that citizenship claims must be linked to employment to succeed politically (see, e.g., Bergmann and Hartmann 1995). Such an approach encompasses measures enabling poor single mothers to combine employment and caregiving, to be backed up by child care services, paid parental leaves, and an improved safety net. However, if strategies based on employment are the only politically viable option, one still must confront the fact that the workplace and the labor market remain deeply structured by gender, race and residence, and caregiving responsibilities create a number of problems for many mothers and other caregivers who are or would like to be employed, particularly when they are poor and un-partnered. Thus, any future policy reforms that would further gender equality must incorporate greater support for caregiving – through supporting care services and workers' rights to time to care, such as paid parental leaves – within the context of continuing efforts to create equal opportunities and rewards at work across gender, "race," ethnicity, sexuality and class.

References

Bell, Winifred. 1965. *Aid to Dependent Children*. New York: Columbia University Press.

Bergmann, Barbara R. 1986. *The Economic Emergence of Women*. New York: Basic Books.

Bergmann, Barbara, and Heidi Hartmann. 1995. A Welfare Reform Based on Help for Working Parents. *Feminist Economics* 1: 85-89.

Blank, Rebecca. 1997. *It Takes a Nation*. Princeton: Princeton University Press.

Boris, Eileen. 1995. The Racialized Gendered State: Constructions of Citizenship in the United States. *Social Politics* 2: 160-180.

Collins, Patricia Hill. 1990. *Black Feminist Thought: Knowledge, Consciousness, and the Politics of Empowerment*. New York: Routledge.

Corcoran, Mary, Sandra Danziger, Ariel Kalil, and Kristin Seefeldt. 2000. How Welfare Reform is Affecting Women's Work. *Annual Review of Sociology* 26: 241-269.

Dawson, Michael. 1994. *Behind the Mule: Race and Class in African-American Politics*. Princeton: Princeton University Press.

DeParle, Jason. 1998. Shrinking Welfare Rolls Leave Record High Share of Minorities. *New York Times* electronic edition, July 27.

Dionne, E. J. 1998. Up From the Bottom. *Washington Post* electronic edition, July 21.

Eardley, Tony, et al. 1996, *Social Assistance in OECD Countries: Country Reports*, U.K. Department of Social Security Research Report No. 46 and 47. London: HMSO.

Edin, Kathryn, and Laura Lein. 1997. *Making Ends Meet: How Single Mothers Survive Welfare and Low-Wage Work*. New York: Russell Sage Foundation.

Ellwood, David. 1988. *Poor Support.* New York: Basic Books.

Ellwood, David. 1996. Welfare Reform as I Knew It: When Bad Things Happen to Good Policies. *The American Prospect* no.26 (May-June): 22-29. http://epn.org/prospect/26/26ellw.html.

Ellwood, David. 1999. The Impact of the Earned Income Tax Credit and Social Policy Reforms on Work, Marriage and Living Arrangements. *Joint Center for Poverty Research Working Paper* 124. http://www.jcpr.org/wp/WPprofile.cfm?ID=129.

Esping-Andersen, Gosta. 1990. *The Three Worlds of Welfare Capitalism.* Cambridge: Polity Press.

Esping-Andersen, Gosta. 1999. *Social Foundations of Postindustrial Economies.* New York: Oxford University Press.

Fineman, Martha. 1995. *The Neutered Mother, the Sexual Family, and Other Twentieth Century Tragedies.* New York: Routledge.

Focus (newsletter of the University of Wisconsin Institute for Research on Poverty). 1998. The IRP Evaluation of the Wisconsin Works Child Support Waiver Demonstration. 19(2): 61-62.

Fraser, Nancy. 1989. Women, Welfare and the Politics of Need. *Unruly Practices:* 144-160. Minneapolis: University of Minnesota Press.

Fraser, Nancy. 1994. After the Family Wage: Gender Equality and the Welfare State. *Political Theory* 22: 591-618.

Fraser, Nancy, and Linda Gordon. 1994. A Geneology of 'Dependency': Tracing a Keyword of the US Welfare State. *Signs* 19: 309-336.

Gilens, Martin. 1999. *Why Americans Hate Welfare.* Chicago: University of Chicago Press.

Glenn, Evelyn Nakano. 1992. From Servitude to Service Work: Historical Continuities in the Racial Division of Paid Reproductive Labor. *Signs* 18: 1-43.

Gornick, Janet, Marcia Meyers, and Katherin Ross. 1997. Supporting the Employment of Mothers: Policy Variation Across Fourteen Welfare States. *Journal of European Social Policy* 7: 45-70.

Greenstein, Robert, and Isaac Shapiro. 1998. *New Research Findings on the Effects of the Earned Income Tax Credit.* Washington, D.C.: Center on Budget and Policy Priorities.

Howard, Christopher. 1997. *The Hidden Welfare State: Tax Expenditures and Social Policy in the United States.* Princeton: Princeton University Press.

Kilkey, Majella, and Jonathan Bradshaw. 1999. Lone Mothers, Economic Well-Being and Policies. In Diane Sainsbury (ed.) *Gender and Welfare State Regimes:* 147-184. New York: Oxford.

Knijn, Trudie, and Monique Kremer. 1997. Gender and the Caring Dimension of Welfare States: Toward Inclusive Citizenship. *Social Politics* 4: 328-361.

Korpi, Walter. 2000. Faces of Inequality: Gender, Class, and Patterns of Inequalities in Different Types of Welfare States. *Social Politics* 7: 127-191.

Leira, Arnlaug. 1992. *Welfare States and Working Mothers.* Cambridge: Cambridge University Press.

Lieberman, Robert. 1998. *Shifting the Color Line: Race and the American Welfare State.* Cambridge, MA: Harvard University Press.

McLanahan, Sara, and Gary Sandefur. 1994. *Growing up with a Single Parent: What Hurts, What Helps.* Cambridge, MA: Harvard U. Press.

Meyer, Bruce D., and Dan T. Rosenbaum. 1997. Welfare, The Earned Income Tax Credit, and the Employment of Single Mothers. *Joint Center for Poverty Research Working Paper,* May 1998 #2. Downloaded http://www.jcpr.org/labormothers. html.

Michel, Sonya. 1999. *Children's Interests/Mothers' Rights: The Shaping of America's Child Care Policy.* New Haven: Yale University Press.

Millar, Jane. 1996. Poor Mothers and Absent Fathers: Support for Lone Parents in Comparative Perspective. In Helen Jones and Jane Millar (eds.) *The Politics of the Family*: 45-63. Aldershot, UK: Avebury.

Mink, Gwendolyn. 1998. *Welfare's End.* Ithaca, NY: Cornell University Press.

Myles, John, and Paul Pierson. 1997. Friedman's Revenge: The Reform of 'Liberal' Welfare States in Canada and the United States. *Politics and Society* 25: 443-472.

Naples, Nancy. 1997. The "New Consensus" on the Gendered "Social Contract": The 1987-88 U.S. Congressional Hearings on Welfare Reform. *Signs* 22: 907-945.

Nelson, Barbara. 1990. The Origins of the Two-Channel Welfare State: Workmen's Compensation and Mothers' Aid. In Linda Gordon (ed.) *Women, the State and Welfare*: 123-151. Madison, WI: University of Wisconsin Press.

O'Connor, Julia, Ann Shola Orloff, and Sheila Shaver. 1999. *States, Markets, Families: Gender, Liberalism and Social Policy in Australia, Canada, Great Britain and the United States.* New York: Cambridge University Press.

Orloff, Ann Shola. 1993a. *The Politics of Pensions: A Comparative Analysis of Britain, Canada, and the United States, 1880-1940.* Madison: University of Wisconsin Press.

Orloff, Ann Shola. 1993b. Gender and the Social Rights of Citizenship: The Comparative Analysis of Gender Relations and Welfare States. *American Sociological Review* 58: 303-328.

Pavetti, LaDonna. 1997. How Much More Can They Work? Setting Realistic Expectations for Welfare Mothers. The Urban Institute. Downloaded from http://www.urban.org/welfare/howmuch.htm.

Pearce, Diana. 1986. Toil and Trouble: Women Workers and Unemployment Compensation. In B. Gelpi, N. Hartsock, C. Novak, and M. Strober (eds.) *Women and Poverty*: 141-162. Chicago: University of Chicago Press.

Pierson, Paul. 1994. *Dismantling the Welfare State? Reagan, Thatcher and the Politics of Retrenchment.* Cambridge: Cambridge University Press.

Piven, Frances Fox, and Richard Cloward. 1977. *Poor People's Movements.* New York: Vintage.

Quadagno, Jill. 1994. *The Color of Welfare: How Racism Undermined the War on Poverty.* New York: Oxford University Press.

Reich, Robert. 1999. Clinton's Leap in the Dark. *Times Literary Supplement* January 22, no. 4999: 3-4.

Reskin, Barbara, and Irene Padavic. 1994. *Women and Men at Work.* Thousand Oaks, California: Pine Forge Press.

Rhodes, Martin. 1996. Globalization and West European Welfare States: A Critical Review of Recent Debates. *Journal of European Social Policy* 6: 305-327.

Roberts, Dorothy. 1995. Race, Gender and the Value of Mothers' Work. *Social Politics* 2: 195-207.

Skocpol, Theda. 1995. *Social Policy in the United States.* Princeton: Princeton University Press.

Spalter-Roth, Roberta, Beverly Burr, Heidi Hartmann, and Lois Shaw. 1995. *Welfare That Works: The Working Lives of AFDC Recipients.* Institute for Women's Policy Research Report. Washington, DC: IWPR.

Stevens, Beth. Blurring the Boundaries: How the Federal Government Has Influenced Welfare Benefits in the Private Sector. In Margaret Weir, Ann Orloff, and Theda Skocpol (eds.) *The Politics of Social Policy in the United States:* 123-148. Princeton: Princeton University Press.

U. S. Committee on Ways and Means, House of Representatives. 1998. *1998 Green Book. Background Material and Data on Programs Within the Jurisdiction of the Committee on Ways and Means.* Washington, D.C.: U.S. Government Printing Office.

U. S. Department of Health and Human Services, Administration for Children and Families. 2000. Change in TANF Caseloads Since Enactment of New Welfare Law. http://www.acf.dhhs.gov/news/stats/aug_dec.htm.

Weaver, Kent. 1998. Ending Welfare as We Know It: Policymaking for Low-Income Families in the Clinton/Gingrich Era. In Margaret Weir (ed.) *The Social Divide: Political Parties and the Future of Activist Government:* 361-416. Washington, DC: Brookings.

Weaver, Kent. 2000. *Ending Welfare as We Know It.* Washington, DC: Brookings.

Weir, Margaret. 1992. *The Politics of Jobs.* Princeton: Princeton University Press.

Weir, Margaret. 1995. Poverty, Social Rights, and the Politics of Place in the United States. In Stephan Liebfried and Paul Pierson (ed.) *European Social Policy: Between Fragmentation and Integration:* 329-354. Washington, DC: Brookings.

Weir, Margaret (ed.). 1998. *The Social Divide: Political Parties and the Future of Activist Government.* Washington, DC: Brookings.

Weir, Margaret, Ann Shola Orloff, and Theda Skocpol (eds.). 1988. *The Politics of Social Policy in the United States.* Princeton: Princeton University Press.

Wennemo, Irene. 1994. *Sharing the Costs of Children: Studies on the Development of Family Support in the OECD Countries.* Stockholm: Swedish Institute for Social Research Dissertation Series No. 25.

Williams, Linda Faye. 1998. Race and the Politics of Social Politics. In Margaret Weir (ed.) *The Social Divide: Political Parties and the Future of Activist Government:* 417-463. Washington, DC: Brookings.

Women's Committee of 100. 2000. *An Immodest Proposal: Rewarding Women's Work to End Poverty.* http://hermes.circ.gwu.edu/cgi_bin/wa?A2=ind0007A&L=welfarem_l&P=R62.

Livia Popescu

Child Care, Family and State in Post-Socialist Romania

Introduction

During the 1990s, the welfare system inherited from the communist regime in Romania was transformed. Following the continental pattern, the present welfare arrangements preserve "the current status hierarchies via insurance-based systems and intervenes in the provision of welfare only as a last resort' (Makkai 1994, 203). The changes impacted the pattern of gender relations within the social protection system and the society in general. In addition, some of today's gender inequalities are rooted in the state socialist regime and possibly enhanced by recent developments. To an important extent, family benefits reflect the current trend of the welfare policy. The analysis of its present characteristics is framed by several theoretical approaches.

Sainsbury (1996) calls attention to the distinction between "male breadwinner" and "individual" models of social policy. At the empirical level, she compares the variations among welfare states by using several gender-relevant dimensions such as familial ideology, basis of entitlement, recipient and unit of benefit, taxation, unit of contribution, employment and wage policies, and sphere of care and caring work (p. 42). Korpi (2000) analyzes specific policy institutional characteristics in terms of dual-earner, general family support and market-oriented models. Generosity of paid maternity and paternity leaves, along with a high level of public day care provision for young children (and elderly) contribute to the dual-earner type. The preference for cash transfers and family tax credits together with public day care services for older children indicate a general family support, which favors the single-earner family. Finally, a low level of both publicly provided care services and state transfers leaves the women's welfare entirely dependent upon market forces.

For Singh (1998, 91), the duration of job-protected leave, the level of compensation during the period of child-bearing, publicly provided child care services, parental leave benefits and "gender role-sharing initiatives" are key aspects to the reconciliation of the public and private spheres and thus to the securing of women's autonomy.

Orloff (1993; 2002) suggests that people's capacity to form and maintain an autonomous household is essential for their relation to social rights. From this perspective, she looks at the extent to which paid employment and /or state support for full-time care work guarantee to both men and women their "personal independence vis-à-vis household formation." In this respect, the conditions faced by single parents and particularly single mothers are particularly relevant (Orloff 2002, 30).

The paper examines both the configuration and the outcomes of the current welfare policy in relation to the demographic and economic features of Romania. Subsequently, it attempts to draw the profile of the emergent family policy in the context of current discussion on gender(ed) welfare regimes.

Child Care, Family and Gender in State Socialist Times

Under the state socialism regime, Romania experienced a rapid pace of industrialization and urbanization. The process was accompanied by important changes in women's participation in the labour market. Between 1966 and 1977, the proportion of females among the urban active population increased from 37.5 percent to 43.0 percent. As the process continued, by 1992, the degree of urban concentration among active women exceeded that of active men: 57.9 percent and 54.2 percent respectively (Comisia Nationala de Statistica-CNS 1994, viii–ix). With the pursuit of a fast and mass-scale industrialization process as part of the state socialist engineering project, the employment opportunities for females increased steadily in all non-agricultural sectors. Between 1966 and 1992, women's activity rates in urban areas rose from 35.8 percent (1966) to 42.7 percent (1992), while the male population showed the opposite trend, namely a decrease from 60.1 percent in 1966 to 51.8 1992) (CNS 1994, xxxvi). Nevertheless, the modernization of the Romanian economy was never completed and a large part of the labour force was occupied in agriculture.

Despite Ceausescu's draconian pro-natalist policies, the birth rates followed the declining pattern which was specific to modern societies. State support for maternity and child rearing was modest compared to other communist countries. Maternity leave was paid for 126 days in proportion to the monthly wage, which varied between 55 and 85 percent, according to the duration of the woman's previous employment. Mothers were entitled to a paid leave in the case of a sick child under three years old. At the end of the maternity leave, many women managed to obtain sick leave by motivating the medical personnel with "gifts". They could also take an unpaid leave to care for a child up to the age of three.

Public services for children under three years old were crowded and notorious for their low quality care. Children enrolled in these "last resort' facilities made up 4.2 percent of the respective age group (Pop 2002). For the majority of working parents, the practical alternative to public nurseries was sharing child rearing with their extended family. This solution was adopted even if the child had to spend most of his/her pre-school years with the grandparents, oftentimes in the countryside. In urban areas, the majority of children aged three to six years of age were enrolled in kindergartens that provided predominantly part time service or what was the official "normal schedule." However, childcare facilities were less available in villages.

Families with dependent children under 16 (18, if attending school) received state allowances. These were included in company payrolls, and commonly paid to fathers, unless the dependent child lived with a single mother. The communist government encouraged women to have more than two children. A birthing allowance was paid to mothers after the second live birth and females with at least three children were entitled to a permanent benefit. Accordingly, the state allowance paid for the third and following children was higher than for the first two. From age 25 on, adults were additionally taxed if they had no children.

Under state socialism, families followed a specific pattern of reconciling child care and paid work, which emerged from a combination of formal, informal and at times illicit practices (e.g. unjustified medical leave). During the 1980s, an acute food shortage, and particularly the lack of formula products, dramatically worsened the children's quality of life. So did the under-funded health care system. In 1989, infant mortality and maternal mortality rates were the highest in Europe: 26.9 per 1,000 newborns and 168.1 per 100,000 newborns respectively (Unicef 2001, 63–64). Low-income families increasingly abandoned their children or put them in residential care. In 1989, the number of children in "institutions" exceeded 90,500 (3.9 per 1,000 inhabitants). About a tenth of them were less-than-a-year to three years old and represented 0.7 percent of the total children in the corresponding age group. (Zamfir et al. 1994, 54; Zamfir 1997, 88). In the aftermath of the 1989 Revolution, the high numbers of abandoned children and their terrible fate in the "orphanages" became emblematic for Romania.

Gender roles started to change in the 60's when an increasing number of women entered the labor market, thus becoming family breadwinners as well. They continued nevertheless to perform their traditional activities of caretaking and housekeeping along with paid work. State socialism encouraged women's participation in the formal economy, but the gender division of labour prevailed within the domestic sphere (Fodor et al. 2002).

Changes in Demographic Trends: Marriage and Childbearing in the 1990s

Marriage is monogamous and it is based on free consent of the spouses. Romanian law permits marriages exclusively between males and females. The minimum age of consent is 18 for a male and 16 or 15 (in case of "special reasons") for a female. In 2001, five percent of the women 15 to 19 years old were married, most of them living in rural areas or ethnic Roma. The average age for a first marriage increased constantly in the last decade. In 2000, it was 26.9 years for men and 23.6 years for women while the total marriage rate was 6.1 (per 1,000 inhabitants). Although relatively high compared to other European countries, this rate is the lowest recorded in post-war Romania (INS 2001a, 60). Marriages tend to be highly stable, as indicated by the average duration of 22 years and low divorce rates (NCS, UNDP 2000; INS 2001a).

Table 1: Changes in demographic indicators on marriage and child bearing (selected years within the 1989–2000 period)

	1989	1990	1996	2000
marriage rate (per 1,000 inhabitants)	7.7	8.3	6.7	6.1
age at first marriage	22.1(F); 25.3 (M)	23.7 (F); 26.9 (M)	25.8 (F); 26.2 (M)	25.4 (F); 28.5 (M)
women's average age at first birth	22.5	22.4	22.9	23.7
total newborn during first 2 years of marriage (%)	–	61.1	54.0	49.6
divorce rate (per 1,000 inhabitants)	1.56	1.42	1.57	1.37
divorces in families with children (% of total divorces)	–	54.9	52.8	48.6
fertility rate (per 1,000 women)	–	56.2	39.9	40.3
birth rate (per 1,000 inhabitants)	16.0	13.6	10.2	10.4

Source: INS 2001a; Unicef 2001, 62–65

Within the 1990–2000 period, the birth rate dropped from 13.6 newborns per 1,000 (1990) to 10.5 per 1,000 (2000). Also, a trend to postpone the birth of the first child is indicated by the decreasing proportion of newborns during the first two years of marriage: 49.6 percent in 2000 compared to 61.1 percent in 1990. According to a 1999 survey on reproductive health, women plan to have one child or two, at most. This preference has influenced the fertility dynamic, especially for the generation born after 1970 (INS 2001a, 27). Since 1993, more than half of newborns have mothers with a low education level (who have completed secondary school or vocational school at most). Within the same period, the proportion of housewives among females who delivered a child increased from 45.7 percent (1993) to 56.7 percent in 2000. A quarter of the total children are born out of wedlock, but most parents tend to legalize their union afterwards (INS 2001a, annexes 5, 9 and 10).

Half of Romanian households include children and the majority of them (56.2 percent) live in towns. Among households with children, 52.2 percent have just one child. This type of household constitutes the majority in urban localities and 46.6 percent in rural settings. Households with two children make up a third of total households in both milieus, while those with three or more children have a larger share in rural communities than in urban ones. Moreover, rural households with three or more children represent about two-thirds in the respective category (www.recensamant.ro/46.pdf).

Economic Environment and Women's Employment

The Romanian economy performed poorly in the last twelve years. In 2000, the GDP per inhabitant was estimated at 5,533 USD (PPP) for the general population and at 4,706 USD (PPP) for women. (UNDP 2002). Between 1990 and 2000, the dynamic of the GDP was negative while inflation reached peaks as high as 256 percent (1993). The economy started to recover only after 2000.

The employed population in different sectors is typical for underdeveloped economies: the largest share (38.1 percent) of the labor force is employed in the primary sector (agriculture). The remaining part of the population is almost equally distributed between services and industry (UNDP 2002).

In 2000, the employment rate (as a percent of the population 15 years old and over) was lower for women than for men: 52.8 percent compared to 65.1 percent (INS 2001b, 24). Among employed females, employees (53.7 percent) and the self-employed (16.1 percent) comprise less than three quarters of the total. "Non-paid family members" form the remaining 29.4 percent. If only employees and the self-employed are considered, the actual share of women in paid employment barely exceeds one third (about 34 percent) of the active female population. About 44.1 percent of the total of employed females work in agriculture and the overwhelming majority of these have a family helper status ("non-paid family member"). The men working in agriculture represent 35.9 percent of the total employed male population and they are either employed or independent farmers. In non-agricultural activities, women are employed as technical staff / clerical workers (21.6 percent), manual workers (10.4 percent), administrative staff (6.1 percent) and "specialists with intellectual occupations" (6.8 percent). Most of the males in non-agricultural occupations fall in the group of skilled and unskilled workers (33.4 percent), "equipment operators" (11.7 percent) and "specialists with intellectual occupations" (6.0 percent). The proportion of women who are in high managerial or administrative positions is less than half that of men's (INS 2001b, 27).

The gender composition of the employed labor force varies to a great extent by branch of economic activity. Women represent more than 70 percent of the employed population in health care, social services and pre-university education. Their share exceeds half of the employed labor force in banks and insurance companies, hotels, restaurants and retail trade. In recent years, women represented a slight majority among the people working in agriculture, but the 2000 Survey on Labor Force in Households (AMIGO) indicates for the first time a decrease of females below 50 percent (INS 2001b, 87). Farmers and non-paid family members in agriculture perform the typical part time work. About 53 percent of all part-time workers are women (INS 2001b, 28).

The women's unemployment rate was higher than that of men in the period 1991–1998. Since then, the opposite trend is in place, but women tend to remain unemployed longer than men, particularly those in the age group 35 to 49. (CNS, PNUD 2000; INS 2001b; Popescu 2003).

The 2000 Survey on Labor Force in Households (AMIGO) shows that women make up the majority (61.2 percent) of the inactive population (age 15 and above) and about a quarter of them are "housewives." Females are also prevalent among those who declare themselves available to take a job, but don't look for one because of anticipated failure (INS 2001b).

According to the 1992 Census data, the women's activity rate is not negatively influenced by marriage. The variation according to the number of children is nevertheless important, ranging between 58 percent for women with 1 or 2 children and 39 percent for those with 4 and more children. The lowest activity rates are recorded for young mothers aged 15 to 19 years old, followed by those in the 20-to-24 age-group (CNS 1994, XLIII).

Women's average pay is lower than that of their male co-workers in every salary-generating occupation (non-agricultural occupations, in general). In 2000, their gross salary represented 83.5 percent of men's. While the number of women in high-income categories is half of the men's, they constitute the largest proportion of the low- income groups (CNS, PNUD 2000, 36).

Gender Roles

At the beginning of the twenty-first century, 46.2 percent of the Romanian population lives in rural settings. In spite of the modernizing process that took place in post-war times, the patriarchal pattern of family life still prevails, particularly in the countryside (Zamfir 1995). Women are expected to be primarily committed to their husband's and children's well-being. They are expected to almost exclusively perform the domestic and caring activities. The idea of men's superiority is typical for the peasant family and it is embedded in the Orthodox religion. In the traditional pattern, as explained by Kligman (1998), men are the formal heads of families while women are assigned to household management. Men tend to be more active in community/public life and women spend more time in the domestic sphere. This traditional gender division of work was not essentially modified by the important participation of married women in paid work. Moreover, the general reduction of available jobs during the transition to the market economy discouraged women's employment rather than men's, thus increasing the number of "housewives". Extended parental leave combined with the absence of appropriate public daycare presumably enhanced the role of women as prime caretakers and housekeepers.

Romanian women have a very low presence in politics and the feminist movement is weak, if not totally absent (NHDR 2002; Popescu 2003, 538). Under these conditions, chances are that traditional gender roles will not be challenged, at least not in the near future. A 2000 public opinion survey showed that 63 percent of the representative sample believes that domestic activities are "mostly woman's rather than man's duty". Moreover, both the majority of female (82 percent) and male (86 percent) respondents agreed that "the man is the head of the family." Similarly strong support was declared for other defining elements of the traditional gender representations, such as the belief that the breadwinner role is mostly the man's; that the woman should "follow" her man; and that men cannot perform a child-rearing role as well as women do (Baromentrul de gen 2000; Popescu 2003).

Pregnancy, Maternity and Parental Rights

The communist Labor Code entitled pregnant female employees to claim the right to be transferred from dangerous work places or to be exempted from night work.

While the legal provisions were maintained during the 1990s, their enforcement was rather permissive. A very recent government ordinance on the protection of maternity at work places stipulates the employers' obligations towards the employees in case of pregnancy, and confinement of breast-feeding. Employers are required to give paid hours for pre-natal medical examinations and to protect pregnant women from exposure to harmful work conditions. If amelioration or change in the work conditions is not feasible, employees are entitled to a maximum of 120 days leave for maternal risk. The provision is insurance-based and amounts to 75 percent of the average previous income. A 25 percent reduction in working time with full pay is also granted if the health condition of the pregnant woman requires it. The governmental act forbids the dismissal of a person while on formal leave for maternal risk, maternity or child rearing (MOR 2003b).

Paid maternal and parental leave are insurance-based. Consequently, the benefits are provided to employed mothers/caretakers who actually contribute to the public insurance scheme. Its funding is based on shared payments of the employer and the employee. The minimum contribution period for maternity leave is six months out of the twelve months prior to delivery and ten months for the parental leave. Non-employed or self-employed persons can contribute to the insurance fund as well if their annual earnings equal at least three gross monthly wages (MOR 2000; MOR 2003a).

The entitlement continues after the contribution period if the delivery occurs within nine months after a woman loses her insured status. Women receiving unemployment benefits are covered for maternal leave as well. The maternal leave consists of 63 pre-natal and 63 post-natal days. The mother can combine the two periods and take only the post-natal leave. The leave counts as the employee's contribution towards all insurance schemes (pensions, health insurance and unemployment insurance.) The maternity benefit amounts to 85 percent of the mother's income base.

The leave for child care was enacted for the first time in 1991, allowing mothers to stay at home only until the child reached the age of one, and to be paid 65 percent of their previous income. In 1997, the government extended the leave up to age two of the child and raised the pay to 85 percent of the previous income. The basis of entitlement is contribution to the insurance fund (MOR 2000). For the first time, fathers (and any legal care-takers) became eligible for the parental leave as well, but those who actually take it are very few. Moreover, a 2003 ordinance for the protection of maternity, assumes that it is exclusively mothers who take parental leave (MOR 2003b). Recently, the government restricted the eligibility for parental leave, by increasing the minimum contribution period to ten months. At the same time, an upper limit for reference income was established. Hence, the amount to be paid for parental leave cannot exceed 85 percent of the net average wage that is calculated for the insurance system (MOR 2003a). The enactment of this limitation on pay was challenged by some amount of public opinion and the political opposition.

Table 2: Maternity and child care paid leaves

Characteristics	Maternal risk leave*	Maternity leave	Parental leave	Medical leave for sick child under 7
Basis of entitlement	contribution to the public insurance fund	contribution to the public insurance fund	contribution to the public insurance fund	contribution to the public insurance fund
Eligibility	employed pregnant women and mothers after compulsory post-confinement leave, if parental leave was not claimed	income-earning mothers	income-earning parent	income-earning parent
Minimum qualifying conditions	· health risks at work place · income equal to 3 national average wages · 10 months contribution	minimum 6 months contribution within 12 previous months	minimum 10 months contribution within 12 months before confinement	minimum 6 months contribution within 12 previous months
Status in the social security system	credited period	credited period	credited period	credited period
Duration	maximum 120 days	126 days (63 pre-natal and 63 post-natal or a cumulated period after confinement)	up to age 2 of the child	14 days per year
Amount	75% of the average earnings in the minimum contribution period	85 % of the average salary in previous 6 months	85 % of the average salary in previous 6 months, but not more than the standard average wage	85 % of the average salary in previous 6 months

Applicable from 2004
Source: MOR 2000; MOR 2003a; MOR 2003b; MOR 2003c

A parent (natural, foster and adoptive) or legal guardian also qualifies for a medical leave to care for a sick child up to age seven if the minimum six months of contributions has been paid. The benefit is granted for a maximum 14 days per year, per child and amounts to 85% of the average salary in the minimum contribution period (MOR 2000).

Although the number is not officially documented, many women do not qualify for the public insurance system and therefore do not get any financial support during the pre-natal and post-natal period. Housewives, non-paid family helpers and long term unemployed women are not entitled to benefits. Others, such as agricultural workers and those who are self-employed, run a similar risk for they might not meet the qualifying minimum income for the insurance scheme. Moreover, many women have temporary work contracts or they belong to the "illegal" labor market with no work contract at all. In either case, they do not meet the eligibility criteria for maternity and child care-taking benefits.

State Support for Families with Children

The state allowance for children up to age 16 or 18 was strictly linked to parents' employment during the communist regime, and therefore, eligibility was denied to self-employed, independent farmers and the jobless. The provision of family benefits continued in 1990 to 1993 in accordance with eligibility criteria inherited from the state socialist system. In 1993, the state allowance became a universal provision based on a child's right. The life benefit for mothers with three and more children was not adjusted for inflation and was eventually suspended in 1995.

At present there are three types of cash family benefits: birthing allowances, state allowances for children, and supplementary family allowances. All of these are universal benefits financed by the state budget. Mothers are entitled to a birthing allowance, which is a one-time flat sum provided for each of a woman's first four live births. The amount of money equals the minimum wage. By limiting to four the number of births for which a woman gets the birthing allowance, the 2001 law incorporates a discriminative provision against groups with a high birth rate and low income, such as Roma (MOR 2001).

The state allowance is actually provided as a universal right of the child. Any child who is raised either in his/her natural family or in foster care is entitled to this benefit up to age of 16 (or 18 if the child is attending school or is disabled). From the age of seven, eligibility is tied to school attendance. A parent or caregiver cashes the state allowance until the child gets his/her identity card (age 14). Every child gets the same monthly amount, regardless of his/her status within the family or of the family income (MOR 1999).

As its coverage became universal, the benefit's real value has dropped considerably. In 1989, the state child allowance represented 9.8 percent of the average wage and decreased to 7.3 percent in 1990 mostly as an effect of a general raise in salaries. Since 1991, the adjustment of the benefit to the inflation index was minimal. This policy resulted in a steady devaluation of the state allowance compared to the average wage, the sharpest among all transfers. After reaching its lowest level in 1996 (3.2 percent of the average wage), an increase in the real value of the state allowance occured in 1997 (Zamfir 1994; Zamfir 2001, 24).

The supplementary allowance for families with many children was enacted in 1997. The legal recipient of the benefit is the family who has at least two dependent children under the age of 16 (or 18). The amount depends on the number of children, but the progressive increase ends after the fourth child. School attendance is a qualifying condition as well (MOR 1997).

The sums to be paid as family benefits are decided by the government. Both the state allowance and the supplementary allowance have a rather irrelevant purchasing power as a result of their irregular adjustment to the inflation.

Special support is provided for wives (legally married) of men who are fulfilling their compulsory military duties. This is an income-tested benefit (the wife's income must be below the minimum salary) to which women are entitled to if either pregnant (from the 4th month on) or caring for a child seven years old or younger (MOR 2001). The monthly sum is tied to the minimum salary.

Table 3: The dynamics of the benefit as a share of the state budget and as a percentage of average net salary

	1989	1990	1991	1992	1993	1994	1995	1996	1997	1998	1999	2000
share of the state budget	–	9.8	4.7	3.0	3.0	3.1	2.3	2.1	3.6	4.0	2.8	2.3
state allowance (1st child) as % of the average net salary	9.5	7.3	6.1	4.9	5.5	4.0	3.7	3.2	6.3	5.5	3.9	3.3
state allowance + supplement. allowance (2nd child) as % of the average net salary	–	–	–	–	–	–	–	–	11.3	9.0	6.3	6.2

Source: Zamfir 1994; Zamfir 2001, 24; CASPIS 2002, 92; UNDP 2002, 127

The erosion of the child's benefit adversely affected primarily large families. In 1997, the provision of a new ("supplementary") allowance for families with two or more children was aimed at reducing poverty risk among this group of population. At the time, the value of the allowances received by a family with three children reached a peak of 46 percent of its 1990 level, but declined again to 23.7 percent in 1999. The share of the cash child benefits of the average household income varied, according to the number of dependent children, from 2.0 percent (household with one child) to 12.1 percent (household with four or more children). The redistributive impact of child allowances is rather low. While the first child diminishes the per capita income of the family by less than 5 percent, every additional one brings an average reduction of 15-20 percent, thus increasing the income gap between families with dependent children and those without (INS 2002, 29). The poverty rate among large families (three or more children) escalated between 1991 and 2001, when it reached its highest level: 58.4 percent for families with three children and 68.3 percent for families with four and more children (see table 2). For a small proportion of these families, child allowances have been effective in moving them from poverty conditions. In 1997, child allowances allowed 8.4 percent of people in households with two children and 10.7 percent of those in households with three children to stay above the poverty threshold (Unicef and INS 2001, 22).

Table 4: Poverty rates by number of dependent children in family (2001)

	Poverty	Severe poverty	2001 as % of 2000
Total population	29.0	11.9	- 3.3
Families with 1 child	27.4	10.4	-12.3
Families with 2 children	31.5	12.4	- 6.6
Families with 3 children	58.4	30.6	+10.8
Families with 4 and more children	68.3	44.2	+7.1

Source: CASPIS 2002

While their effectiveness in either granting the child well-being or poverty reduction was modest, child allowances remained universal until 2003. The most recent legislation shows a shift in government policy, which is consistent with the changed welfare paradigm or "the individualization of the social" (Ferge 1997). Hence, family provisions will become increasingly selective with the introduction of two benefits: a "complementary" allowance for low income families, which will substitute for the universal supplementary allowance, and a new "support" for low income single parent families (MOR 2003c). The amount to be paid is relative to the number of children, but the increase ceases after the fourth child.

In the last two years, the government displayed a preference for in-kind provisions, such as distribution of free formula milk for infants 0–12 months who are not receiving breast-feeding and school breakfasts for pupils in kindergartens and primary school. The universal provision of particular food items ("milk and croissant") as well as the practicalities of the distribution process raised public controversy.

Tax Credits for Dependent Children

Tax credits for children were first introduced in 1991, allowing for a 20 percent deduction from the parents' individual income. The policy proved to be highly regressive, and specifically very disadvantageous for low-income families, and was suspended in 1993 (Zamfir 1994, 56). A new approach was taken when global income taxation was adopted. At present, the basic monthly deduction (lump sum) from one parent's individual earnings increases by 35 percent for each of the first two children. With the birth of each additional child, a further 20 percent is deducted. Generally speaking, incentives for child rearing that are provided through the taxation policy are not significant. In principle, the system does not penalize the dual-earner family, since the taxation unit is the individual parent and not the family as a whole.

Child Care

The public child care system, which includes crèches or nurseries (for ages zero to three) and kindergartens (for ages three to six), preserved its structure from state socialist times. A 1991 government decision stated that public care facilities must provide instruction, education and medical assistance free of charge. For children enrolled in full-time facilities, parents pay up to 75 percent of the costs of food and service provision. The monthly fee depends on the family's earnings and the total number of children attending care facilities. Parents are charged for any supplementary activities such as foreign language teaching or swimming lessons that are organized by kindergartens. The cost of public child care was not entirely subsidized during state socialism either, but families paid a higher share of it in 1991 (82 percent) than in 1989 (69 percent). The fees as a proportion of the average wage doubled between 1989 (10.0 percent) and 1991 (21.4 percent). By 1992, family child care expenses dropped to 1989 levels, and then rose again in the following years. They remain among the highest in Eastern Europe (Zamfir et al. 1994, 21).

Under state socialism, nurseries for children aged two months to three years were notorious for overcrowding and for providing poor quality services. In the 1990s, the enrollment rate in public nurseries was as low as two percent, half of the 1989 figure (Fong and Lokshin 2000; Pop 2002). The enactment of paid parental leave to age one of the child, and then to age two, has certainly contributed to this reduction, along with an increase in the number of jobless mothers.

The decrease in public kindergarten enrollment was temporary and less dramatic. By 1999/2000, the net rate was 67.3 percent, slightly higher than in 1989 (INS 2001c, 68). About one third of pre-school children are kept at home, most of them being taken care of by grandmothers. Enrollment in private child-care facilities is rather exceptional, and amounts to 0.6 percent of all children in formal care (INS 2001c, 72). As shown by Fong and Lokshin (2000), placing children aged three to six in formal care is a common practice, whether the mother is working or not, because kindergartens provide pre-school education. Child care services are instrumental to mothers' employment as well. However, their function in allowing mothers to reconcile care and employment is incomplete. Most children aged three to six years old attend part-time kindergartens, which do not offer lunches. Subsequently, the care-giving for the remaining time is to be performed within the family, essentially by grandparents. During the primary school years, the extended family continues to be care/supervision providers, because children are not offered lunches and after-school programs are rather uncommon. Moreover, transportation of the children to and from public care services or schools is entirely the family's responsibility.

Fees for child care continue to be partially subsidized, but for some families, particularly low-income or families with many children, these services may be unaffordable because of the costs associated with kindergarten attendance, such as clothing and educational materials (Fong and Lokshin 2000). The "free milk and croissant" program in kindergartens, which was implemented in 2003, aims at encouraging low-income families to enroll their children in formal care.

Main Actors in the Transformation of Family Policy

The relation between social policy measures and the proclaimed ideological "color" of the post-socialist governments is rather confusing. Hence it is difficult to understand changes that occurred in family policies by strictly referring to the now classical distinction between social democracy, liberalism and conservative-corporatism (Esping-Andersen 1990). During the transition from bureaucratic state collectivism to democratic capitalism, conditions were rather inauspicious for the social democratic model, particularly in less economically developed countries, such as Romania. In his 1993 analysis, B. Deacon (1993) reflects that the social-democratic policy strategy is likely to be adopted in the Czech Republic, but even there, "only after an initial flirtation with liberal welfare capitalism" (p.193). In addition, the temporary form of (post-communist) conservative corporatism, which served as a model for Romania's welfare arrangements, will slowly evolve into liberalism as well (Deacon 1993).

In Romania, governing parties and trade unions shaped the emerging welfare regime. The role played by transnational organizations (such as the IMF and the World Bank) and foreign experts was important, but not decisive. As mentioned by Deacon (1993), it is debatable whether the post-communist parties – recently social-democratic – are genuine agencies of the "left". In the immediate post-socialist years, state protectionism was manifested primarily in salary policy and job preservation. The respective government decisions concurred with the trade unions' understanding of social policy. Social payments, particularly universal family benefits, were viewed as marginal by the main political actors. The most powerful trade unions, which were male-dominated, did not include the family payments issue on their agenda. A former minister of Labor and Social Protection recalls that during the discussion on reforming child allowances, trade unions did not actively support either an increase or extended coverage of the benefit (Zamfir 1995, 432). Otherwise, their strategy was successful in salary claims and compensation for collective redundancies, particularly in mining and heavy industry. The resulting inequalities together with new injustices induced by marketization worsened the situation of the powerless groups, one of them being children (Popescu 1998). During the centrist government (in fact a coalition between Christian-Democrats, liberals and reformist social-democrats), family support became a political issue. The government aimed at stimulating the birth rate by increasing child benefits and improving conditions for parental leave.

Since 2001, the government has adopted a more targeted approach to social policy in general, possibly based upon recommendations of the IMF and the World Bank. Selectivity with respect to child benefits combines with cuts or more restrictive eligibility for insurance-based parental leave. In addition, new regulations were adopted in line with EU standards for social inclusion of vulnerable groups and more specifically children's welfare in residential care.

Table 5: Summary of changes in family transfers and political orientation of the governments

Benefit	State socialism/ communism (until 1989)	Post-communist left (1990–1996)	Centrist (Liberal + Christian-democrat parties) (1996–2000)	Social-democrat party, formerly post-communist left (2000–2004)
birthing allowance	universal benefit from the second child	universal benefit from after the second child; increased value in 1995	universal benefit from the second child.	universal benefit; 2001: provided from the 1st child up to the 4th
life benefit for mothers with 3 or more children	universal benefit	· suspended in 1995	–	–
state child allowance	· related to parents employment status; · differentiated amount by child's rank/ birth order	· universal lump-sum benefit (since 1993); · significant devaluation;	· universal lump-sum benefit; · significant increase in 1997 and 2000	· universal lump-sum benefit; · increase in 2001
supplementary allowance for families with 2 and/or more children	–	–	· universal benefit, amount varies with number of children up to the 4th · increase in 2000	· universal benefit (same conditions as in 1997); · devaluation; · to be canceled in 2004
complementary allowance *	–	–	–	means-tested;
support allowance for single parent family *	–	–	–	means-tested
taxation credits	–	20 percent of the wage	2000: 1 st child: 35 % increase of the standard deducted sum	–
maternity leave	employment based; 126 days; paid at 55–85 percent	employment based; (same conditions as previously)	employment based; 126 days paid at 85 percent of previous wage	insurance-based; 126 days, paid at 85 percent of previous wage

Benefit	State socialism/ communism (until 1989)	Post-communist left (1990–1996)	Centrist (Liberal + Christian-democrat parties) (1996–2000)	Social-democrat party, formerly post-communist left (2000–2004)
parental leave	–	· up to 1 year · paid at 65 percent of previous wage	· extended up to 2 years; · paid at 85 percent of previous wage	· upper ceiling set at 85% of the standard average wage (2003); · increase of min. contribution period
maternal risk leave*	–	–	–	insurance-based up to 120 days

* to be provided from 2004
Source: MOR 1997; MOR 2000; MOR 2003a; MOR 2003b; MOR 2003c

The Orthodox Church took no explicit stand in the decision-making process, but its view on family matters (support for the traditional family model, anti-abortion statements) might influence the family policies in subtle, implicit ways.

With 9.7 percent women representatives in parliament and 6 percent in local councils, female political participation is among the lowest in Europe (HDRR 2001). Although female politicians tend to work through their own parties, occasionally they make a concerted effort to achieve gender-sensitive policies. In general, local women's agencies are lacking and feminist organizations very rarely tackle family policies (Popescu 2003). Actually, the present cabinet legislated the changes concerning child benefits and parental leave by ordinances, thus avoiding any parliamentary or public debate on the matters.

Some literature documents the fact that transnational agencies played a key role in the transformation of Eastern European welfare systems. In several transitional countries, the IMF and the World Bank recommended the reduction of child allowances, universal coverage and more targeting in benefit provision through income testing (Deacon et al. 1997; Ferge 1997). At the same time, the EU emphasized the need for candidate countries to improve their social protection schemes in the pre-accession phase (Deacon, 1997). The case of Romania is rather disconcerting. While the universality of child benefits was extended, its real value become irrelevant. During 1996–2000, the centrist Cabinets had liberal discourses and adopted economic policies inspired by the Bretton Woods institutions. They nevertheless allocated a record budget to family payments. Ironically, the policy changes envisaged by the present social-democratic government incorporated much of the IMF and World Bank thinking. EU pressures, which expressed almost the opposite approach to social protection, prompted substantial changes in the area of child welfare reform, equal opportunities and social inclusion of ethnic Roma.

Concluding Remarks on Child Care and the Emergent Gender Welfare Regime

Does the interplay of family, state and market in family policy indicate a specific gender welfare regime in Romania? Based on the examination on the current policy configuration and some of its outcomes, I tentatively hypothesize a mixed ("in-between") pattern or a dual-track policy model, especially if the urban-rural division is taken into consideration (see also Fodor et al. 2002).

Women's participation in the labor force is relatively high and the tax system does not discourage the dual-earner family pattern. Moreover the economic hardships encountered by most families make the second wage necessary. However, a significant portion of the female population works in the rural subsistence economy for low pay or no individual pay at all.

Paid maternal and parental leaves are based on insurance, and women qualify for them only if they have an employment history of at least six to ten months. In order to receive protection and be paid for their child-rearing work, women are encouraged to participate in the labour market before pregnancy. They also receive minimum job protection in the period following the maternity and parental leaves. Mothers without an employment record are not eligible for any financial support other than the one-time lump-sum paid at delivery. Their economic dependency upon their husbands/families is therefore unavoidable and this is especially the case among women with a low level of education. Taxation is based on the individual while giving credits for dependent family members, children and spouses. Universal benefits are too meager to provide for the basic needs of children. Moreover, supplementary allowances do not increase after the fourth child, thus discriminating against larger families. The income-based benefits, which will be enacted in 2004, bear the same "racist undertones" and will potentially enhance the social exclusion of ethnic Roma (Fodor et al. 2002).

The introduction of an upper limit for parental leave benefit will probably compel women with above-average incomes to resume their careers before the end of the two years. Moreover, care-giving work is also symbolically devalued, thus further de-motivating fathers to take the leave. Since services for young children are rare, most mothers share child-rearing responsibilities with the extended family. It is commonly accepted that this is a grandmother's job and women's lower retirement age has somehow legitimized these expectations. The state's responses to gaps or failures in family and/or market provisions are rather inadequate. They sometimes create worthiness distinctions among categories of women and among families as well.

For females with employment records, insurance-based leave benefits maintain a proportion of their income while the day services for older children (above age three) support, to some extent, the return to their employment commitment. Even in these circumstances, the extended family is expected to provide child care on a regular basis. It will soon be the turn of today's mothers to care for their aged parents, since day services for elderly people are underdeveloped. With respect to services in particular, the welfare arrangements bear salient "familialistic" features (Esping-Andersen 1999).

Romanian family policies do not entirely correspond to either Korpi's (2000) dual-earner type or Sainsbury's individual models, especially because of the low level of public day care provision for young children (and the elderly). The traditional gender division of care-giving is an additional factor of divergence. In the near future, high-income women will increasingly purchase day care services on the market. On the other side, the deviation from the "general family support" is also important; the family allowances and tax credits are economically irrelevant and fail to encourage the single-earner type (Korpi 2000). However, the single-earner type tends to prevail among poorly educated and/or Roma families as a result of those women's respectively low employability. The marginal occupational status of the females in the subsistence rural economy is reproduced in the welfare system with similar negative consequences.

Until now, a specific policy for single parents has been lacking. The envisaged benefits for this category are both income-tested and restrictive for large families. In addition, free of charge, full-time day care services have reduced coverage. For women, entering marriage is hardly a choice freed from economic constraints, and single parents face a serious poverty risk. In conclusion, the capacity to form and maintain an autonomous household, as defined by Orloff (1993), is minimal and will continue to be so, at least in the near future.

References

Barometru de gen (Gender Barometer). 2000. Bucuresti: Fundatia pentru o Societate Deschisa.

CASPIS. 2002. *Planul National Anti-Saracie si Promovare a Incluziunii Sociale* (National Plan Against Poverty and for the Promotion of Social Inclusion). Bucharest: Romanian Government.

Deacon, Bob. 1993. Developments in East European social policy. In Catherine Jones (ed.) *New Perspectives on the Welfare State in Europe*: 177–198. London: Routledge.

Deacon, Bob, et al.1997. *Global Social Policy*. London: Sage Publications.

Esping-Andersen, Gøsta. 1999. *Social Foundations of Postindustrial Economies*. New York: Oxford University Press.

Ferge, Zsuzsa. 1997. The Changed Welfare Paradigm: The Individualization of The Social. *Social Policy and Administration*, vol. 31, No.1, March 1997: 20–44.

Fodor, Eva, et al. 2002. Family policies and gender in Hungary, Poland and Romania. *Communist and Post-Communist Studies*, 35: 475–490.

Fong, M., and M. Lokshin. 2000. *Child Care and Women's Labor Force Participation in Romania*. http://wbln0018.worldbank.org/research/workpapers/nsf.

Human Development Report-Romania. 2002. www.undp.org.ro/pdf.

Institutul National de Statistica (National Institute for Statistics) – INS. 2001a. *Analize demografice. Situatia demografica a Romaniei in anul 2000* (Demographic Analyzes. Romania' s Demographic Situation in Year 2000). Bucuresti: INS.

Institutul National de Statistica (National Institute for Statistics) – INS. 2001b. *Ancheta asupra fortei de munca in gospodarii in anul 2000 (AMIGO)* (Household Survey on the Labour Force in Year 2000). Bucuresti: INS.

Institutul National de Statistica (National Institute for Statistics) – INS. 2001c. *Starea sociala si economia Romaniei in perioada 1997–1999* (Social Situation and Economy in Romania within 1997/1999). Bucuresti: INS.

Institutul National de Statistica (National Institute for Statistics) – INS. 2002. *Coordonate ale nivelului de trai in Romania. Veniturile si consumul populatiei* (Coordinates of the living standard in Romania. Income and expenditure of the population). Bucuresti: INS.

Kligman, Gail. 1998. *Nunta mortului: Ritual, poetica si cultura populara in Transilvania* (The wedding of the dead: ritual, poetics and popular culture in Transylvania). Iasi: Polirom.

Korpi, Walter. 2000. Faces of Inequality: Gender, class and patterns of inequalities in different types of welfare states. In *Social Politics*, No.7: 127–191.

Lewis, Jane. 1992. Gender and Welfare Regimes: Further Thoughts. *Journal of European Social Policy*, 2/3: 159–73.

Makkai, Tony. 1994. Social Policy and Gender in Eastern Europe. In Diane Sainsbury (ed.) *Gendering Welfare States*: 188–205. London: Sage Publication.

Monitorul Oficial al Romaniei – MOR (Official Gazette). 1997. Nr. 149/11.06.1997.

Monitorul Oficial al Romaniei – MOR (Official Gazette). 1999. Nr. 56/08.02.1999.

Monitorul Oficial al Romaniei – MOR (Official Gazette). 2000. Nr. 140/01.04.2000.

Monitorul Oficial al Romaniei – MOR (Official Gazette). 2001. Nr. 401/20.07.2001.

Monitorul Oficial al Romaniei – MOR (Official Gazette). 2003a. Nr. 167/17.03.2003.

Monitorul Oficial al Romaniei – MOR (Official Gazette). 2003b, Nr. 750/27.10.2003.

Monitorul Oficial al Romaniei – MOR (Official Gazette). 2003c. Nr.747/26.10.2003.

Orloff, Ann Shola. 1993. Gender and the Social Rights of Citizenship: State Policies and Gender Relations in Comparative Perspective. *American Sociological Review* 58(3): 303–28.

Orloff, Ann Shola. 2002. *Women's Employment and Welfare Regimes. Globalization, Export Orientation and Social Policy in Europe and North America*. UNRISD.

Pop, Luana (ed.). 2002. *Dictionary of Social Policy*. Bucuresti: Editura Expert.

Popescu, Livia. 1998. State and Market in Romanian Social Policy. In Demetrius S. Iatridis and June Gary Hopps (eds.) *Privatization in Central and Eastern Europe: Perspectives and Approaches*: 155–168. Westport, Conn.: Praeger.

Popescu, Livia, and M. Roth. 2002. Variabila gen in analiza dezvoltarii umane din Romania (Gender variable in the human development analysis in Romania). In G. Cosma et al. (eds.) *Prezente feminine. Studii despre femei in Romania* (Female Occurrences. Women's Studies in Romania): 453–477. Cluj: Editura Fundatiei Desire.

Popescu, Livia. 2003. Romania. In Lynn Walter *The Greenwood Encyclopedia of Women's Issues Worldwide: Europe*: 529–545. Westport: Greenwood Press.

PNUD/Programul Natiunilor Unite pentru Dezvoltare in Romania, Comisia Nationala de Statistica-CNS. 2000. *Femeile si barbatii in Romania* (Women and Men in Romania). Bucuresti: PNUD.

Sainsbury, Diane. 1996. *Gender, Equality and Welfare and Welfare States*. Cambridge: Cambridge University Press.

Singh, Rina. 1998. *Gender autonomy in Western Europe: an imprecise revolution*. Houndmills: MacMillan Press Ltd.

Unicef, INS. 2001. *Familia si copilul in Romania* (The Family and the Child in Romania). Bucuresti: Edit. Extreme Grup.

Recensamantul populatiei si locuintelor din Romania (Census of population and dwellings). 2002. www.recensamant.ro/46.pdf.

Zamfir, Catalin, et al. (eds.). 1994. *Romania '89–'93. Dinamica bunastarii si protectia sociala* (Romania '89–'93. The dynamics of well-being and the social protection). Bucuresti: Editura Expert.

Zamfir, Catalin (ed.). 1997. *Pentru o societate centrata pe copil* (Toward a child-centered society). Bucuresti: Edit. Alternative.

Zamfir, Catalin. 2001. Politica sociala in Romania (Social Policy in Romania). In Elena Zamfir, Ilie Badescu, and Catalin Zamfir (eds.) *Starea societatii romanesti dupa 10 de ani de tranzitie*: 13–33. Bucuresti: Ed. Expert.

Adriana Baban

Women's Health and the Politics of Reproduction: The Case of Romania

Introduction

The recognition of health as a function of the interactions among biological, psychological, social, cultural, familial, environmental, occupational, and spiritual factors is the key to diminishing or eliminating health problems (Hoffman and Massion 2000). Women's health problems cannot be accurately detected and effectively resolved separately from the complex context in which they occur. It is important to recognize that political, economic and social systems have the power to diminish or eliminate some specific women's health problems or to create, exacerbate or ignore them.

Good health is one of the most vital conditions for women's full participation in social, political, economic and family life, as well as for the subjective feeling of fulfillment and well-being. During the last decade, two landmark events for women's health occurred: the 1994 International Conference on Population and Development in Cairo, Egypt and the 1995 World Conference on Women in Beijing, China. Both conferences reaffirmed reproductive rights as fundamental human rights, and established a link between such rights and women's physical and psychological health. Reproductive health is an essential element to women's empowerment and dignity, as it was defined by the International Conference on Population and Development: "[…] reproductive health is a state of complete physical, mental and social well being and not merely the absence of disease or infirmity, in all matters relating to the reproductive system and its functions and processes. Reproductive health therefore implies that people are able to have a satisfying and safe sex life and that they have the capability to reproduce and the freedom to decide if, when and how often to do so." (ICPD 1994)

In line with the above definition, reproductive health cannot be viewed strictly in biological terms. Unfortunately, the women's health approach has inherited a model of health care that reflects both the Cartesian duality of mind and body and a philosophy of medical science based on biological reductionism. A comprehensive understanding and care for women's reproductive health requires the contribution of other elements of analysis, such as: subjectivity, culture, politics, economy, social and gender relations, ethics and values. The main argument of this chapter is that reproduction is complexly linked to political and social processes, state policies and economic changes; reproduction is an area where the state can exercise its power, and control can become visible.

According to Gordon (2002), birth control is women's "moral property", and this property, like all other property, has been and remains the object of political conflict. Having access to information, the means for controlling reproduction health, and the motivation to adopt particular behaviors, are all shaped by political negotiations. Most of the time these negotiations are so far out of individual control that most people are unaware how decisions are being made. Reproductive policies are among those areas of public policy that bridge the gap between the private and public spheres of life. The study of sexuality and reproduction is a study of the manner in which politics interacts with individual life. Addressing political attempts to restrict reproduction rights becomes a key element on the international health agenda for women (Denious and Russo 2000).

Romania has long been an extreme case in the field of public population policies and the responses they elicit in private sexual and reproductive behavior. Romania's history of liberalization, restriction, and re-liberalization of abortion laws provides a stark demonstration of the impact that legislation, political institutions and public discourse can have on women's health (see Baban 1999 for a more comprehensive analysis of reproductive politics in Romania).

The aim of this chapter is to provide a contextualized analysis of the relationship between the legal, political and social contexts and women's reproductive health. I will analyze the topic of reproduction, both as a problem of discourse of the political establishment, and as a question of everyday practices. I will examine the kinds of policies and programs that are proposed by political actors for women in the name of these discourses, and how they shape women's choices. I will highlight how the psychological experience of abortion and contraception are inevitably socially constructed. Using examples from qualitative research on women's reproductive health, I offer an illustration of how personal narrative can be heard and read as both individual and social accounts. The qualitative data are drawn from 112 individual interviews with women and men, and three focus groups, carried out from 1993 to 2001 (see Baban and David 1994, Baban 2000, Baban 2003). My analysis is also based on secondary materials, including published articles, documents, reports, and census data.

Reproduction and Policies under State-Socialism

Romania's demographic policy before 1990 was over-determined by ideological interests, with each trend strongly influencing women's behavior and attitudes towards sexuality, reproduction and their bodies (David and Baban 1996). In the socialist period, the ideological doctrine formally promoted women's equality, which was to be achieved by abolishing private property and providing productive employment for women (David and Skilogianis 1999). It was only after the 1960s that women's dual roles as workers and mothers become the subject of considerable debate in Romania. This debate was brought by concern over the continuing decline of birth rates (Kell and Andreescu 1999). The maximization of women reproductive capacities became the political objective of the legislation. In this way, women were caught between two identities assigned to them by the socialist-state, (mothers and workers), whereas they did not question their role as housewives.

This cast women in the triple roles (and triple burden) of devoted mother, full-time worker, and sacrificing wife.

The right of the nation to mobilize all of its resources, even its unborn members, was a key issue in the official discourse of state-socialist Romania, according to which giving birth was considered a patriotic duty and any attempt to avoid fulfilling this duty was perceived as a threat to national continuity (Kligman 1991). Ceausescu's dictum that "the fetus is the socialist property of the Romanian nation" is eloquent in this respect.

By defining women primarily in terms of their reproductive capacity, the exploitative socialist-state opened ways for "disciplining" women's bodies and set restrictions to women's right of self-determination (Kligman 1998). A strict anti-abortion law and repressive surveillance aimed at monitoring private behavior were adopted. Legal abortion was restricted to women who were over 45 years of age, or who already had at least five children, all under the age of 18. At the same time that the regime restricted access to abortion, couples were also denied the means to prevent unwanted pregnancies. Modern methods of contraception were banned, insertion of IUDs for medical reasons was prohibited, and surgical sterilization was forbidden. In order to gain legitimacy for these policies, the prevailing discourse was that of scientific proof of the medical risks of modern methods of family planning. Illegal abortion became a common method of fertility regulation.

During those 23 years of draconian pro-natalist policy, the state strengthened its mechanism aimed at taking reproductive decisions away from women. New measures to enforce the law were introduced: taxes for unmarried people over 25 and on childless couples, quarterly monitoring of women at reproductive age through compulsory gynecological examination, investigation of all spontaneous abortions by the Romanian State Security police. Abortion providers (medical and non-medical), as well as women who self-induced abortions or who obtained illegal abortion by other means, were subject to imprisonment. This situation of fear and suspicion forced women to stay away from hospitals if they had medical complications after an illegal abortion.

Many women persisted in their quest for terminations of unwanted pregnancies, regardless of potential consequences for their health. Interviews conducted after 1990 revealed a sizeable proportion of women who had had 20 to 30 abortions during Ceausescu's pro-natalist policy. Women's accounts reflect their strong will to terminate an unwanted pregnancy at whatever cost or risk to their well-being, as a way to protect and secure their existing family. They accepted illegal abortions as a form of sacrifice and devotion towards their already struggling families, holding the conviction that they were doing the right thing: "As a woman I had to learn not only to cook, to sew, and to raise my children, but also how to induce an abortion." (Baban and David 1994, 32) or: "I made a catheter using an electric cable from which I extracted the metal wires. I tried several times to insert it by myself and finally succeeded." (Baban and David 1994, 50). Another woman: "Nobody and nothing could stop me in my making the decision to get rid of my pregnancy. I assumed all risks involved; I did what I felt I should do for my family, in order to bring up my children." (Baban and David 1994, 55)

Women's bodies were treated as state property and perceived as machines that produced the state's future workers. In other words women's bodies were "nationalized", and put under the state control for its ideological goals (Tsagarousianou 1995). Despite the claim of the rhetorical slogan "women equal rights with men", citizenship rights for women were in fact undermined by this specific representation of women as reproductive resources. Such legislative regulation and discourses of political actors favored social antagonism not only between the state and the population, but also between men and women, and sometimes between women and their own bodies. The psychological cost of lack of reproductive rights, and the perceived trauma of coping with unwanted pregnancies was severe. Many women interviewed expressed frustration, regret or sadness: "After abortion I thought I could no longer make love again. I looked at my husband as an enemy." (Baban and David 1994, 53) And: "It was enough only to see my husband enter the bedroom, and I already felt that I was pregnant." (Baban and David 1994, 37) Or: "I hated my body, my uterus, my ovaries. I wished to reach 45 and be over with this monthly dreadful fear." (Baban and David 1994, 45)

Each time the regime intensified its drive to raise fertility, its success was more limited than in the previous attempts, as the population found more and more ways to escape the demands of the fertility bureaucracy. The health effects of reproduction policies that denied access to reproductive rights were dramatic for women, couples and families. Nearly 10,000 women died over the previous 23 years from complications related to illegal abortions, and many more were physically damaged as a result of unsafe, unhygienic procedures. Maternal mortality (170/100,000) was ten times higher during the communist regime than the average for the rest of Europe, with 86 percent of deaths due to illegal abortions. As for the percentage of maternal deaths from all causes, abortion-related deaths rose from 20 percent in 1965 to nearly 90 percent in 1989 (Stephenson et al. 1992). In addition to claiming lives, unofficial estimates suggest more than 20,000 children becoming orphans as a result of maternal mortality due to illegal abortions. More than 20 percent of Romania's women of reproductive age became infertile, more than twice the proportion expected for a population that size (Hord et al. 1991). As Kligman (1995) notes, banning abortions does not stop women from having them; it only makes abortion "invisible".

It was not only women who had paid a high price. The infant mortality rate was also affected by the abortion restrictions (28.9 infant deaths per 1,000 live births in 1987). In 1990, Romania recorded Europe's highest infant mortality rate (David 1990). Of those children who survived unintended conception and unwanted births, thousands were abandoned to state care in public orphanages. There were over 90,000 abandoned children living in state care institutions. Epidemiological studies of these children showed a considerable increase in the incidence of psychological and neurological disorders. After 1990, Romania was confronted with a boom in HIV-infected children, most of whom lived in institutions and were probably infected before 1990.

From No-Option to Pro-Choice Strategies

"The human rights of women include their rights to have control over their body and to decide freely and responsibly on matters related to their sexuality and reproduction, free of coercion, discrimination and violence." (Fourth World Conference on Women 1995). These words recognize that reproductive rights are fundamental for women's quality of life and well-being.

The fall of the communist regime in Romania, in 1989, brought to worldwide attention the dramatic consequences of one of the most repressive reproductive policies, which drastically denied women their right to have control over their body and to decide freely, with no coercion, on matters related to their sexuality and reproduction. Confronted with the epidemic maternal mortality and morbidity, the new government revoked all prohibitions against abortion and contraception in its first day in power. It authorized the production, sale and import of modern contraceptives and legalized first-trimester abortion on request, if performed by an obstetrician-gynecologist in a hospital, clinic, or private office. Terminations without charge were provided for women having four children, for medical reasons and for women having no income (Baban 2000).

The liberation of women's bodies from the control and coercion of the state was considered of paramount importance for the democratization of Romanian society and for women's health (Kligman 1992). This legislative change has had beneficial effects on women's health, reflected in the drop in maternal mortality in 1990 to 83 deaths per 100,000 live births, almost half the ratio of 1989. By 2000, maternal mortality rates had dropped further to 40 deaths per 100,000 live births, of which 50 percent were due to abortion (Serbanescu, Morris, and Marin 2001). While progress in reducing maternal mortality has been considerable, Romania continues to have the highest rate in Europe in this respect. It is widely believed that clandestine abortion continues to be the major cause of abortion-related maternal mortality.

Today, many women perceive the legalization of abortion as their "reward" for having endured the suffering and humiliation caused by Ceausescu's regime. The right to abortion has become emblematic for the new democracy: "We have suffered enough for several generations. Nobody can possibly realize what we really went through, unless one experiences the same humiliation and violence that we did." (Baban 2000, 233) And: "The right to abortion was gained at the expense of thousands of women's lives, who died during the Ceausescu regime, as well as of the blood of those who died during the December 1989 revolution." (Baban 2000, 233) Or: "I do not plead for abortion, but it is a human right that must be respected. Especially in Romania! The young generation today does not know what it was like, to be afraid every time you made love." (Baban 2000, 235)

After 1990, as abortions became legal, Romania rapidly became the country with the highest abortion rate in Europe. Almost one million abortions were reported in 1990, when it was estimated that a physician performed 30 abortions per day. The abortion rate climbed to the highest recorded rate in the world (almost 200 per 1000 women aged 15–44 in 1990). The abortion rate was 3.2 for every live birth.

In spite of a gradual decrease over the last three years, abortion rates remain very high (Johnson, Horga, and Andronache 1993). The proportion of repeated abortion is also very high in Romania; a report of the Ministry of Health estimates that the lifetime abortion rate per woman was almost 5 in 1990, declined to 3.4 in 1993, and further to 2.2 in 1999. The highest rate of abortion occurred among women aged 25–29, followed by women aged 30–34 years. The abortion rate per woman is inversely correlated with education and socio-economic status.

With access to legal abortion restored in 1990, and confronted with the economic difficulties of transition, Romanian couples decided to have smaller families. The total fertility rate dropped from 2.19 per woman in 1989 to 1.3 in 1999. Notably, fertility among Romanian adolescent women is 3 to 6 times higher than in Western European countries (Serbanescu, Morris, and Marin 2001).

In the economic context of transition, abortion is constructed as a response to the precarious conditions of daily life. The relationship between the social construction of abortion and women's experience of it can be highlighted by the reasons given by women for choosing abortion. The tension engendered by the decision to abort is normalized by some women interviewed in their consideration that: "It is better to choose abortion over abandoning a child you cannot afford to bring up." (Baban 2000, 235) "I never thought I did something wrong when aborting. I am confident that God understands what I was doing and I am not afraid of His curse." (Baban 2000, 235) And: "There is a big difference between wanting children and being able to provide them with a decent living." (Baban 2000, 236)

Since 1989, the conditions of everyday life have grown more uncertain, influencing decisions regarding marriage and family size. People must contend with poverty, unemployment and inadequate housing, among other things. In 1999, 90 percent of the families with three children and 60 percent of the families with two children lived below the poverty line. In the absence of socio-economic measures to protect families with children, and in the absence of a more efficient method of education on modern contraceptives, abortion is one answer to the circumstances of living in transition in Romania.

The legacy of the old regime's reproductive policies silenced critical discussion about abortion and population policy in the immediate post-Ceausescu years. Most researchers considered Romania an exception in the region, from this perspective. However, since the fertility rate in Romania has dropped below the replacement level, women have been often defined in public discourse as murderers of the nation, as their exercise of control of their reproduction function: "There mustn't be any war in Romania; Romanian women bring death to millions of lives." (Malanescu 1992) And: "To remain passive and not react against the millions of annual abortions is to consent to your people's extinction." (Valcu 1995)

The decline of the birth rate is seen by some political actors and religious leaders as a national disaster, and women are regarded as mainly responsible for it. The Romanian Orthodox Church understands this and has responded to this demographic situation by calling for the reintroduction of the abortion ban. In an open letter to the president, the cabinet and the parliament, Patriarch Teoctist argued that abortion equals national genocide, saying that: "the adoption of a law against abortion [...] will cease the national infant genocide" (cit. in Tsagarousianou 1995, 289). In this rhetoric, the figure of women emerges as ignorant and unconscious in the face of a "demographic catastrophe". Again, in a manner similar to that during the Ceausescu regime, women are not considered rational individuals capable of making important decisions about whether and when to have children. Einhorn (1993) has argued that the invocation of reproduction responsibility is being used in East Central Europe as a way to get women out of the labor market, as a way of dealing with unemployment.

The fear for the "death of the nation" is usually accompanied by xenophobia towards other groups, defined as different, that are reproducing faster. Anxiety about Romania's demographic future is aggravated by what is presumed to be a higher birthrate among the Gypsy communities. Through this kind of public discourse, abortion is now less linked to women's autonomy and power to decide about reproduction, but rather involves notions such as national identity and the nation's future vitality.

Barriers to Reproductive Health

Despite the major positive changes in reproductive policy, Romanian women confront different obstacles in achieving good reproductive health. In countries with well-established, comprehensive family planning programs, elective abortion is usually a last resort, employed when contraception fails to protect women from unintended pregnancies. In the early 1990s Romanian women relied more on abortion than on contraception to control fertility. This situation has been attributed to health care providers' unfamiliarity with contraceptive methods after more than 20 years of medical isolation, to lack of available contraceptives, concerns about the health risks associated with certain modern methods, and to the easy access and low cost of abortions. Reproductive health care personnel tend to perceive their role as one of treating women as patients instead of offering counseling. (Johnson, Horga, and Andronache 1996)

Even though abortion rates have gradually declined (from 182 abortions per 1,000 women in 1990, to 47 per 1,000 in 1998; the abortion-to live-birth ratio decreased from 3 abortions for each live birth in 1990 to 1.5:1 in 1998), Romania continued to report widespread use of induced abortion. Among other Eastern European countries and newly independent states, the rates are comparable with those of the Russian Federation and higher than most other former Soviet-block countries (Morris 2003). Even though induced abortion is widely available, both in public and private facilities, illegal induced abortions still exists (in 1998, 224 illegal abortions were reported).

The results of the Romanian Reproductive Health Survey (RRHS; Serbanescu, Morris, and Marin 2001) conducted on a sample of 6,888 women and 2,434 men, aged 15–44 shows that 51.8 percent of women living in legal union do not use any kind of contraception; 35 percent rely on traditional methods (withdrawal and calendar) and 29 percent use modern methods. Although the prevalence of unwanted pregnancies decreased by twelve percent from 1990, unintended conceptions continue to prevail (60 percent). The report also documents that almost 9 out of 10 unwanted pregnancies are aborted.

The answers given by the 2,434 men involved in the RRHS (Serbanescu, Morris, and Marin 2001) reflected a low level of knowledge on the use of modern contraceptives, and one that is lower than women's. Only 47 percent of men stated they knew how to use pills, 43 percent IUDs, 16 percent spermicides and 13 percent emergency contraception, while 88 percent said they know how to practice coitus interruptus. A significant minority of the young respondents under the age of 18 did not know there is such a thing as contraception. With regards to assessing the efficiency of contraceptive methods, more than half of the men (52 percent) believed coitus interruptus to be an effective method. However, the most serious aspect is the reduced prevalence of the use of modern contraception, although this is the natural consequence of the low level of knowledge of and of attitudes towards such methods. The RRHS (Serbanescu, Morris, and Marin 2001) revealed that 49 percent of men did not regularly use any method of contraception. Out of the 51 percent who declared that they usually resorted to contraception, 28 percent relied on traditional methods, and only 23 percent on modern ones. Under the circumstances, it is not surprising that coitus interruptus is by far the most widely used method by men, accounting for 42 percent of the total prevalence of contraception; eleven percent of men rely on the calendar, nine percent use condoms, eight percent birth control pills, and six percent IUDs.

Even though contraception is theoretically available through the state health system, Romania remains what has been called "abortion cultural" (David 1999). There are many reasons which could explain this situation. Romania remains the only country in Eastern Europe not manufacturing any kind of contraceptives. Contraceptive supplies, including condoms, must be imported and are too expensive for many women and men. Birth control pills cost up to two or three times as much as an abortion. The number of family planning clinics is inadequate, and the absence of clinics in rural areas and poor access to affordable contraceptives deprives women of family planning options. There is no comprehensive reproductive health policy that promotes women's health throughout their lives, and sexual education in schools is limited and sporadic.

Negative perceptions of modern means of contraception were often reported by women and men during in-depth interviews. Many of them explicitly expressed reluctance to use pills or resort to an IUD. These methods were constructed as "chemical, so unnatural substances", or as a "foreign body", therefore dangerous for the woman's health. Such a construction mobilizes a discourse in which fear of the side effects of contraceptives often turns out to be the main reason for not using them. It was widely believed that pills cause liver and heart disease, cancer, growth of body hair and sterility after long-term use. Also, it was thought that pills could negatively affect the health of children, by increasing the risk of giving birth to children with disabilities or various malformations: "These modern pills never interested me; they do good in one respect and they are harmful in 10 others." (Baban 2003, 193)

Condom use was perceived by men interviewed as incompatible with long-term relationships, and was associated with a certain type of sex, significantly with sporadic sexual encounters, and with casual sex. Condoms are constructed as having symbolic meanings: "the accidental", "the mistrust", "the illicit sex". Different constraints operating on men impede their ability to practice safe sex by using condoms. First, there is the existing "natural contraceptive culture" in the context of the Romanian legacy. Various forces and traditions have come together, along with what Holland (1994) called the value of "spontaneity" in making love, to obstruct the use of condoms. Another constraint experienced by men is the perception of the condom as a disruption of sexual satisfaction and a diminishment of pleasure: "Condoms diminish the pleasure. It is like going into the garden to smell the flowers while wearing a mask over your face." (Baban 2003, 194)

The strongest rejection reaction was engendered in men by the possibility of male sterilization after having had the number of children they wanted. Most men cannot mentally cope with sterilization, which is believed to cause loss of virility and manliness. Only three of the men interviewed (out of 50) said they would accept sterilization, and one man said he would accept it "only on one condition: that I can have my semen frozen". The words used by respondents regarding male sterilization, firmly placed respondents within a context of being incompatible with such a "drastic and radical" method of contraception: "Why take away a part of yourself? It makes you not feel like a whole man anymore. You would be taking away your manhood. It would make me feel handicapped." (Baban 2003, 192) Or: "I would never adopt such a method. You are not allowed to give up on the gift you have received from God. It is a pure violation of human nature." (Baban 2003, 192)

In order to reduce tensions between their current sexual practices and the potential negative consequences for their health, most men invoke different reasons (medical, social, economic, psychological) in order to rationally justify their behavior, whereas others adopt a life philosophy of "carpe diem" or "Russian roulette": "Everything is a risk in life. I run the risk of losing my job, of getting sick; I take a risk every time I step out of my home. Why shouldn't I take risks in a sexual relation as well? One risk more or less, it doesn't make any difference. Sometimes risking may be agreeable and exciting." (Baban 2003, 193) And: "You cannot be cautious all the time. If you think only about being cautious, you won't do anything anymore. If I had thought that I could have handicapped children, just as it happens to some people, I wouldn't have had any children at all. Sometimes you should forget about the rules, at least in the bedroom." (Baban 2003, 193)

The ways in which modern contraceptives are constructed by men call for consideration of the options left for women to oppose and challenge these constructions. Although the participants believed that men and women should carry equal responsibility regarding contraception, the pattern of women relying substantially upon men for using withdrawal as the main measure of contraception has emerged from the individual accounts, but also from Romanian Reproductive Health Survey (2001). The frequent failure of natural methods is one of the direct causes for the high incidence of unwanted pregnancies and abortions.

A major concern for public health authorities is the rise, among adults, of sexually transmitted diseases, especially syphilis and AIDS. The increasing incidence of syphilis recorded over the last few years is quite alarming; the reported syphilis rate (new cases) has increased almost 5 times between 1986 and 1996 (Romania/MOH 1997). In Romania, AIDS is mainly considered a disease of children, however, the number of young adults with AIDS has increased steeply during the past 10 years, and seems set to continue to rise, since it is estimated that only nine percent of sexually active women in Romania use condoms. The most significant increases in HIV/AIDS cases were reported in women: 391 cases in 2000 versus 37 cases in 1991 (Antoniu 2000). Currently, the total number of HIV/AIDS patients is approximately 11,000. Unfortunately, the lack of concern about AIDS is widespread.

Although knowledge of HIV/AIDS and other STDs, and awareness about transmission and prevention is high among Romanian young people, risk-taking behavior or denial of risk is manifest in this field as well. According to the Romanian Youth Narratives Survey (RYNS; 1999) the majority of young people (75 percent of females and 69 percent of males) think their own risk of contracting HIV/AIDS is below average. A breakdown by number of lifetime partners shows that self-perceived risk is not directly related to sexual behavior. For instance, only ten percent of males with four or more lifetime partners believe they have an above-average risk of infection. Under the circumstances, it is not surprising that Holscher noted: "The 1999 RYNS shows that young Romanians are gambling with their sexual health. Many of the young men are sexually active, they have multiple partners, they know about HIV/AIDS, but they are still not protecting themselves from this disease and against unwanted pregnancies." (Romanian Youth Narrative Survey 1999)

This situation is partly due to the lack of institutional sex education. The responsibility for disseminating sexual and reproductive knowledge, as well as providing necessary advice and counseling for young people, has been perceived in conflicting ways by different agencies, including educational institutions, public health providers, school teachers, as well as by parents. Some potential actors even believe that sex education may encourage sexual experimentation and lead to higher risk sexual behavior in the young, and thus should not be advocated. Although the non-governmental organizations have made efforts to send volunteers to high schools to deliver lectures on methods of birth control and sexually transmitted diseases, these lectures are sporadic and insufficient.

Addressing Gender Issues

Equal relationships between women and men in matters of sexual relations and reproduction, including full respect for the integrity of the person, require mutual respect, consent and shared responsibility for sexual behavior and its consequences. (Fourth World Conference on Women 1995)

In the post-Cairo and Beijing era, it is not sufficient to explore the links between women's health and reproductive rights. Rather, it is necessary to go beyond this, clarifying the connections of gender with sexual and reproductive health, and particularly with reproductive and sexual rights. This triangle (gender, sexuality, reproduction) is defined by the social discourses and norms, by the ideology and religious doctrine, and by the biomedical perspective on health and illness. The gender approach to sexuality and reproduction should take into consideration the role of complex interactions between women and men in promoting, protecting and impeding health. Gender norms shape the family planning experience by determining who has access to reproductive health information, who holds the power to negotiate contraceptive use or to withhold sex, who decides on family size, and who controls the economic resources to obtain health services.

According to Watson (1993), the transition of Eastern Europe societies to liberal capitalism has resulted in the rise of masculinism, which appears to be the primary characteristics of gender relations in Eastern Europe today. It has been argued that the emergence of masculinism does not affect only patterns of behavior among males, but at the same time it also shapes and reconstructs femininity. The masculine ideology is expressed in sexual and reproductive behavior and in gender relationships. A preventive sexual behavior is bound by gender power relations that define and limit negotiation between partners, whereas sexual and reproduction negotiation and communication assume an equality position across genders, a goal which has not yet been attained in Romania (Baban 2002).

The Romanian Reproductive Health Survey (RRHS; Serbanescu, Morris, and Marin 2001) of a nationally representative sample of young people aged 15 to 24 found that there is a major gender difference in the timing of the first intercourse. In boys, sexual activity begins much earlier than in girls. Approximately 25 percent are sexually active before the age of 16, a figure which increases to 57 percent before the age of 18. There is also a significant gender difference in the lifetime number of sexual partners: while only seven percent of the females reported having four or more partners, this is the case for 62 percent of males, and among the latter, 27 percent reported having had more than ten partners. Moreover, 34 percent of the males aged 20 to 24 reported having had two or more sexual partners over the past 3 months, as compared to 2 percent of the females aged 20 to 24.

The masculine ideology was also expressed in the ways men endorsed the view that male sexuality is different in many ways from female sexuality. "Sex as learning experience" within the process of male development was mentioned as an essential indicator of men's maturity, therefore as one of the priorities on their agenda. The same attitude was perceived as inappropriate for women, and those who accepted it, ran the risk of being devalued as women: "Nature created us to be different. The woman needs affection and stability, whereas the man needs experiences and adventures. A behavior that is natural and normal in men, is bad taste and not refined in a woman." (Baban 2003, 184)

Violence against women has been recognized as having serious consequences for women's health, including their reproductive health. Women subjected to partner violence may be unable to use contraception effectively and may lack control and negotiation skills that would enable them to avoid sexually transmitted disease or to plan pregnancies. Romania proved to be one of the Eastern European countries with the highest incidence of domestic violence abuse (Serbanescu and Goodwin 2003). The Romanian Reproductive Health Survey (Serbanescu, Morris, and Marin 2001) shows that almost one in two women reported verbal abuse by a partner at some time in their lives; 29 percent of women reported lifetime experience with spousal physical violence, while 10 percent reported physical abuse from a partner during the past twelve months. Sexual abuse by a current or former partner was reported by seven percent of women. An interesting result is that young women reported more physical abuse in the current relationship than did women aged 35 years and over. The level of physical abuse against their partners reported by males was as high as the abuse reported by women. Although these results are proof of the consistency and validity of research data, they are disturbing in the way they reveal that Romanian men consider domestic violence a socially acceptable behavior in order to express gender power and maintain gender inequity. Data from RRHS (Serbanescu, Morris, and Marin 2001) also illustrate the possible association between domestic physical abuse and induced abortion and the current unmet need for contraception. Women who reported physical abuse by the partner were significantly more likely to have had an induced abortion than women who did not report physical violence.

An important step to improving women's reproductive health is the involvement of men in reproductive health education. Health programs should educate men regarding responsible sexual and reproductive behavior and the role they can assume in family planning, whether by using contraception themselves, supporting their spouses' decision to begin contraception, or supporting their spouse while she is using contraception. Health programs should offer counseling to help men and women improve their communications and decision-making skills based on gender equity and respect.

Concluding comments

The discursive and practical effects of debates about reproduction provide one lens to understand how politics is being reshaped in East Central Europe. As Gal and Kligman (2000) note, such debates project women as political actors and as an integral part of social and political actions.

Romania's case is a real life demonstration of the impact of reproductive policy on women's health. My analysis has demonstrated how historical legacy, political, culture, demographic and socio-economic conditions as well as women's own agency can shape and reshape experiences of reproduction. The pro-natalist policy drastically advocated by the Romanian socialist-state did not enable women to make proper choices regarding their reproductive behavior and health. By denying women the right and means to control their fertility, the state produced the highest maternal and infant mortality rates in Europe.

Major changes relating to sexuality and reproductive rights have taken place in Romania in relation to access to contraception and abortion since December 1989. However, between political regulations and the process that put a policy into practice, there are important gaps, contradictions and compromises. In viewing the interaction between the legal rights and the difficulties encountered in translating those rights into everyday realities, a major barrier in Romania seems to be the traditional attitude of men and women regarding fertility planning behavior. Apparently, men are less willing to accept methods they cannot control, whereas women are more willing to approve male-controlled methods for preventing pregnancy. Men downplay the importance of their behavior by denying its risk and by creating distance.

Despite a Romanian government commitment to improving women's reproductive health, quality of care and well-being, outcomes may be compromised where the socially and culturally accepted legitimacy of sexuality and reproduction remains unchallenged and where issues of gender power are neglected. The analysis of the issues surrounding Romanian women's reproduction health raises challenges to redefine social norms about women and men, if there is a genuine desire to empower women to make proper decisions for themselves and their families.

There is evidence to support the claim that reproductive entitlements are under negotiation not only in official policy but also more broadly in society as a result of cultural, economic and social changes, through the networking and service provision activities of non-governmental organizations, and through women's everyday strategies. Although debates surrounding reproduction are multidimensional, involving political, social, economic, feminist and religious dimensions, all equally important, women's health issues must never be forgotten.

References

Antoniu, Sorin. 2000. Concern about rise in AIDS in Romanian adults. *Lancet* 356: 1090–1091.

Baban, Adriana. 1999. Country report: Romania. In Henry P. David (ed.) *From Abortion to Contraception. A Resource to Public Policies and Reproductive Behavior in Central and Eastern Europe from 1917 to the Present*: 191–221. Westport: Greenwood Press.

Baban, Adriana. 2000. Women's sexuality and reproductive behavior in post-Ceausescu Romania. In Susan Gal and Gail Kligman (eds.) *Reproducing Genders. Politics, Publics and Everyday Life after Socialism*: 225–255. Princeton: Princeton University Press.

Baban, Adriana. 2002. Social construction of femininity and masculinity: social and individual practices in Romania. In Gizela Cosma, Eniko Magyari-Vincze, and Ovidiu Pecican (eds.) *Women Study in Romania*: 43–76. Cluj-Napoca: Editura Desire.

Baban, Adriana. 2003. The social construction of men's sexuality. In Ionela Baluta and Ioana Carstocea (eds.) *New Trends and Topics in Women Studies in Romania*: 179–203. Bucharest: New Europe College.

Baban, Adriana, and Henry P. David. 1994. *Voices of Romanian Women: Perceptions of Sexuality, Reproductive Behavior and Partner Relations during the Ceausescu Era*. Bethesda, MD: Transnational Family Research Institute.

Boyle, Mary. 2000. The experience of abortion: a contextualist view. In Jane Ussher (ed.) *Women's Health: Contemporary International Perspective*: 339–355. Leicester: BPS.

David, Henry P. 1990. Romania ends compulsory childbearing. *Population Today*, 18: 4–10.

David, Henry P. 1999. Overview. In H. P. David (ed.) *From Abortion to Contraception. A Resource to Public Policies and Reproductive Behavior in Central and Eastern Europe from 1917 to the Present*: 3–21. Westport: Greenwood Press.

David, Henry P., and Adriana Baban. 1996. Women's health and reproductive rights: Romanian experience. *Patient Education and Counseling*, 28: 235–245.

David, Henry P., and Joanna Skilogianis. 1999. The woman question. In Henry P. David (ed.) *From Abortion to Contraception. A Resource to Public Policies and Reproductive Behavior in Central and Eastern Europe from 1917 to the Present*: 39–47. Westport: Greenwood Press.

Deniuos, Jane, and Nancy F. Russo. 2000. The socio-political context of abortion and its relationship to women's mental health. In Jane Ussher (ed.) *Women's Health: Contemporary International Perspective*: 431–441, Leicester: BPS.

Einhorn, Barbara. 1993. *Cinderella Goes to Market: Citizenship, Gender, and Women's Movement in East Central Europe*. London: Verso.

Fourth World Conference on Women: Platform for Action. 1995. Beijing, China, United Nations.

Gal, Susan, and Gail Kligman. 2000. *The Politics of Gender after Socialism*. Princeton: Princeton University Press.

Gordon, Linda. 2002. *The Moral Property of Women*. Chicago: University of Illinois Press.

Hoffman, Eileen, and Charlea Massion. 2000. Women's health as a medical specialty and a clinical science. In Lorraine Sherr and Janet St. Lawrence (eds.) *Women, Health and the Mind*: 3–16. Chichester: J. Wiley & Sons Ltd.

Holland Janet, Caroline Ramazanoglu, Sue Sharpe, and Rachel Thomson. 1994. Power and desire: the embodiment of female sexuality. *Feminist Review* 46: 21–38.

Hord, Charlotte, Henry P. David, France Donnay, and Merrill Wolf. 1991. Reproductive health in Romania: reversing the Ceausescu legacy. Studies in Family Planning 22: 231–240.

ICPD: Program of Action. 1994. Cairo, Egypt, United Nations.

Johnson, Brooke R., Mihai Horga, and Laurentia Andronache. 1993. Contraception and abortion in Romania. *The Lancet* 341: 875–878.

Johnson, Brooke R., Mihai Horga, and Laurentia Andronache. 1996. Women's perspective on abortion in Romania. *Social Science and Medicine* 42: 521–530.

Kell, Thomas, and Viviana Andreescu. 1999. Fertility policy in Ceausescu's Romania. *Journal of Family History* 24: 478–493.

Kligman, Gail. 1991. Women and reproductive legislation in Romania: implications for the transitions. In George Breslauer (ed.) *Dilemmas of transition in the Soviet Union and Eastern Europe*: 141–166. Berkeley: University of California Press.

Kligman, Gail. 1992. The politics of reproduction in Ceausescu's Romania: a case study in political culture. *East European Politics and Society and Societies* 6: 364–418.

Kligman, Gail. 1995. Political demography: the banning of abortion in Ceausescu's Romania. In Faye D. Ginsburg and Rayna Rapp (eds.) *Conceiving the New World Order: the Global Politics of Reproduction*: 234–255. Berkeley: University of California Press.

Kligman, Gail. 1998. *The Politics of Duplicity. Controlling Reproduction in Ceausescu's Romania.* Berkeley: University of California Press.

Malanescu, Rodíca. 1992. The Tree Without Fruits. *Doína* 7: 11.

Morris, Leo (ed.). 2003. *Reproductive, Maternal and Child Health in Eastern Europe and Eurasia: a Comparative Report.* Atlanta: Center for Disease Control.

Romania/Ministry of Health Bulletin. 1997. Bucuresti.

Romanian Youth Narratives Survey. 1999. Bucuresti.

Serbanescu, Florina, Leo Morris, and Mona Marin. 2001. *Reproductive Health Survey in Romania: Final Report.* Atlanta: Center for Disease Control.

Serbanescu, Florina, and Mary Goodwin. 2003. Physical and sexual abuse. In Leo Morris (ed.) *Reproductive, Maternal and Child Health in Eastern Europe and Eurasia: a Comparative Report*: 211–220. Atlanta: Center for Disease Control.

Stephenson, Patricia, Michael Wagner, Mihaela Badea, and Florina Serbanescu. 1992. The public health consequences of restricted induced abortion-lessons from Romania. *American Journal of Public Health* 82: 1328–1331.

Tsagarousianou, Rosa. 1995. "God, patria and home": reproductive politics and nationalist (re)definitions of women in east/central Europe. *Social Identities* 2: 283–296.

Valcu, Tudor. 1995. The Extinction of Romanian People. *Echinox* 4: 3.

Watson, Peggy. 1993. The rise of masculinism in Eastern Europe. *New Left Review* 198: 71-82.

Yelena Kulagina

Socio-Economic Problems of Families in Russia: Gender Aspects

Introduction

The gender situation in Russia is presently undergoing significant changes. The transition of the society to a market economy is accompanied with growing gender asymmetry. The country is carrying out democratic transformations – Russian legislation is being modified with due regard for the principles of international law. Amendments have been introduced that regulate equality of men and women in the sphere of labour legislation, family legislation, parenting, etc. However, the measures intended to ensure gender equality have turned out to be ineffective.

This chapter deals with gender aspects of socio-economic problems of urban Russian families with children under the new economic conditions, as well as the impact of gender-related issues on the reproductive sphere of the population. I will start with a short review of the gender policy of the Soviet state. Then I give a description of the current socio-economic situation in Russia and economic position of families. Special attention is paid to forms of state support for families with children and then a consideration of the gender aspects of families' adaptation to the changing economic conditions follows.

The paper is based on information from the Institute for Socio-Economic Studies of Population RAS, Moscow Center for Gender Studies, All-Russian Center for Public Opinion Research (VCIOM), Institute of State and Right RAS, RF Ministry of Labour and Social Development, Russian Statistics.

Retrospective Review of the Gender Policy in Russia: Traditions of the Soviet Lifestyle

Gender relations in Russia have been and remain asymmetrical. According to historically established traditions, women kept the house and raised children. Men were breadwinners. The present-day division of parents' responsibility for raising children and earning a living includes more sophisticated forms of gender inequality. They have been mainly formed under the influence of the communist ideology of the Soviet state. Radical changes in the sphere of childrearing, distribution of parental roles and functions and employment of women took place with the establishment of Soviet power. The following illustrates the most significant of these.

Initially, the Soviet state policy was aimed at discrediting the role of family. The main idea of a communist upbringing of all children at the expense of the state, the so-called "public upbringing," was put into practice. Absurd ideas, such as the nationalization of children, circulated among the Bolsheviks. They believed that neither family nor separate individuals nor groups could fulfil the colossal task of communist upbringing as rationally as the whole society and the whole state (Nechayeva 2000). The state was proclaimed the supreme tutor (guardian) of every child. Acting in this capacity, the state regarded parental power as a subordinate form of care for minors: "state but not family determines a minimum level of education, care and welfare necessary for children" (Nechayeva 2000).

Another important moment was the emancipation of women from family oppression and their mass involvement in public production. Only one month after the revolution of 1917, Russian women were freed from all restrictions concerning children and wealth by the dissolution of marriage. They were given the right to a free choice of professions, residences, and education, as well as the right to equal payment for equal work. In 1920, the right to abortion was legally recognized. (Ayvazova 1998) Soon, "free" women became a source of cheap labour at socialist construction sites in the country. Public labour for the welfare of the state became an obligatory facet of their existence, but in order to allow them to combine their maternal and labour responsibilities, it was necessary to solve the problem of children. The Bolsheviks treated this task quite formally: "if we do not release women from babies or older children, [...] we shall not be able to involve a required quantity of women in productive activity" (Nechayeva 2000).

One more important change of that time was belittling the role of the father. The state committed itself to providing care for mother and child, and Stalin became "Father of all nations" for all citizens. The notions of "father" and "fatherhood" gradually disappeared from official documents. Under the conditions of general poverty and fear, men lost their positions in the family (Ayvazova 1998).

It is evident that at that time it was very difficult to support and balance all the above changes by social policy measures for development of social infrastructure, personal services and child care. The weakening of family foundations resulted in growing numbers of homeless children. It negatively affected demographic development, bringing about a decline in fertility and threatening the normal reproduction of the population.

The Stalin Constitution of 1936 changed attitudes towards the family, strengthened the protection of mother and child through the introduction of state assistance to families with many children and single mothers, granted paid maternity leaves to women, and established a network of maternity centers, nurseries and kindergartens. That year a law prohibiting abortions was passed, and the procedure of divorce was complicated. Divorce came to be regarded as an indication of the "moral unsteadiness" of a citizen (Ayvazova 1998).

Since that time, a new stage of the state policy with regard to the family began to develop. The state took guardianship over the family as a "cell of society", the basis of stable social relations, morals and order. With the beginning of the Second World War, a need for firm support of the family and stable family relations emerged. The role of the woman as a true wife and keeper of the Soviet family rose even higher (Ayvazova 1998). In 1944, the title of Mother-Heroine, the Order of Mother Glory and the Medal for Maternity were established. At the same time, researchers note that families did not get any real help because their material support was insignificant (Nechayeva 2000).

These sorts of tough, family-related policies were loosened only after Stalin's death. In 1955, abortion was again legalised. Later, the procedure of divorce was simplified and alimony obligations were regulated. However, the responsibility for raising children was officially placed on women's shoulders and no family status was attributed to fathers willing to take on family duties in order to give women-mothers the opportunity to work. Therefore, the policy aimed not at strengthening the family, but rather at continuing the creation of a wider range of child care establishments for children (Nechayeva 2000).

Throughout the Soviet years, men were excluded from the sphere of family problem-solving. Women were the object of social policy concerning family, as their active participation in public production was advantageous for the state. Employment of women was advertised in the USSR at all levels of mass consciousness. In the 1970s and 1980s, 92 percent of Soviet women were working or studying. Beginning with the mid-60s, 59 percent of women were among the specialists with secondary and higher education. The idea of a woman not working disappeared completely from Soviet public consciousness. Modern sociologists define the character of gender relations at that time as the "contract of working mother" (Ayvazova 1998).

During the Soviet era, the state constantly implemented measures aimed at helping families and assisting women (not men) in every possible way with performing their dual socio-demographic functions – worker and mother. The purpose of these measures was to promote women's labour activity in the national economy, on the one hand, and to render them maximum support in keeping the house and bringing up children, on the other hand (Rimashevskaya 2001a, 278). This was ensured by a growing number of pre-school and out-of-school educational establishments, flexible forms of part-time employment, special measures of social protection (e.g. provision of maternity leave), guaranteeing jobs for pregnant women, reservation of jobs for three years after childbirth, paid sick leave to care for a child up to the age of 14, etc.

In fact, there was no equality. Women had to work and bear responsibility for their children and family. There was no equality in payment for work and employment in different branches of the economy, no equal access to political decision making, etc.

Research carried out in the late 1960s (Taganrog – I, 1967–1968) produced results contradicting the official propaganda. Analysis of the socio-demographic characteristics of married couples showed that, despite a certain tendency to equalize the position of spouses, there was clearly a factual social inequality of women. The whole complex of transformations aimed at securing equal opportunities did not guarantee their equal realization by men and women. Among the spouses in the same age group, only 40 percent had equal education levels, about one-third performed work with the same qualifications, and slightly over one-fifth of married couples received equal work payment. The contribution of working women to the family budget was significantly lower than that of men; therefore, women were partial "dependants" (Rimashevskaya 2001a, 282). Research of the late 1970s (Taganrog – 2, 1977–1979) showed that by the time of marriage, spouses have approximately equal "starting" social potentials. However, in the course of married life, after giving birth to children, women begin to "lag behind" and their rate of professional growth decreases. They are twice as unlikely to improve their professional skills, and they prefer to economize. The ratio of average earnings by men and women is 3:2 (Rimashevskaya 2001a). Research of the late 1980s (Taganrog – 3, 1988–1989) revealed gender asymmetry of decision-making in the family. While men played a decisive role at work, women had the final say in family mattters. In case of divorce, the child was left with the mother (99 percent), and the father's responsibilities were reduced to paying child support (Rimashevskaya 2001a, 290).

Beginning with the early 1990s, "maternal" leave for taking care of children was granted to fathers, grandmothers, grandfathers and other relatives. Gradually the RF Labour Code was amended so that the parental rights of both mothers and fathers were taken into consideration.

Summing up the Soviet historic experience, we should acknowledge some progressive results influencing women's self-esteem. During the period of Soviet rule, women accumulated invaluable experience in economic independence, high levels of education and active participation in productive activity. In addition, a powerful social infrastructure was created, making child care easier for many families.

Socio-Economic Situation in Russia: Distribution of Gender Indicators

It should be stressed once again that the current stage of development is extremely difficult for Russia. Not a single country across the world has experienced such a severe economic crisis. Total losses in GDP over a period of twelve years (from 1989–2000) amounted to approximately three and a half times the 1989 GDP (Afanasyev 2002). It is no coincidence that in recent scientific publications, there has been a tendency to compare Russian demographic and social indicators with USSR data from the period of the Second World War.

The present socio-economic situation in Russia can be illustrated by selected data on population incomes, unemployment, the social protection system and social infrastructure. The statistical data will be considered from the point of gender issues.

The present state of Russian society is characterised by the impoverishment of most of the population due to a sharp decline in incomes. The drop in earned incomes is one of the crucial factors. It has not only lowered the population's living standards, but has also restrained the economic development of the country on the whole. In 2001, the average per capita income of the Russian population was 96 USD[1] (Goskomstat 2002).

The numeric value of average per capita income is only twice the subsistence minimum that is regarded as poverty level in Russia[2]. According to the Goskomstat data, the subsistence minimum in 2001 was 50 USD a month (Goskomstat 2002). The amount for food constitutes only half of this sum. The subsistence minimum ensures merely physiological survival. Therefore people with incomes below this level do not meet the conditions for survival. The percentage of the population with incomes below the subsistence minimum, or poverty level, is variously estimated by official statistics and experts. The estimates range from 28 percent to one third of the total population. In a large country such as Russia, this share amounts to 40 to 50 million people. These circumstances foreground the task of poverty alleviation as one of the most important issues of socio-economic policy (Rimashevskaya 2002a).

Let us consider the main causes of low income levels: The first cause is a decline in wage levels. Real wages in 2000 amounted to only 32 percent of those in 1990 (Ovcharova 2002). In 2001, the average nominal wage was 100 USD and minimum wage was about 9 USD (Goskomstat 2002). Low levels of wages and social benefits result in a situation where unemployed and homeless people, and even employed workers, are among the poor. A considerable portion of the population experience great deprivation. They have to economise by even reducing their spending on food. As wages are distributed between men and women quite unevenly, women find themselves in the group of the discriminated. According to the data from VCI-OM, in 2002, women's wages totaled 56 percent of men's wages (Baskakova 2002).

The second cause is unemployment. During the years of socio-economic transformations in Russia, there was a general reduction of employment – the number of jobs for men decreased by ten percent, and those for women by 20 percent. The officially registered unemployment rate reached its peak in 1998: 13 percent. In recent years, this figure has declined to 8.4 percent (Khotkina 2002). During the entire period of crisis, female unemployment has been somewhat lower than male unemployment. Still, the point is not the quantitative but qualitative differences. Unemployed men find new jobs more quickly, and most women remain jobless for a long time. The loss of a job usually results in women leaving the sphere of economic activity or exiting the official labour market (Khotkina 2002).

The third cause of low income levels in Russia is a low level of pensions, benefits and stipends, and the degradation of the social sphere branches. In the course of market reforms, the state has sharply reduced financing for social protection and the social sphere. Funding has been reduced, while the number of recipients of social benefits and exemptions has increased owing to improvement of the legislation on the basis of the democratic principles of international law[3]. At present there are over 140 kinds of benefits and exemptions granted to almost all residents of the country (Rimashevskaya 2002a). However, the level of current funding remains so low that all the elements and the system as a whole have become inefficient, and attained a rather formal character. The system of social protection has actually been destroyed.

Here are some examples of monthly social payments and their relation to the subsistence minimum:
- The monthly child allowance (the main kind of support for families with children) now amounts to 4.5 percent of the subsistence minimum, which is equal to around 2 USD;
- The average old age pension amounts to 61 percent of the subsistence minimum, or 27 USD;

• The minimum stipend is about eight percent of the subsistence minimum, or 3.5 USD (Rimashevskaya 2001b, 13).

Another cause of the decline in living standards is the growing cost of social services (education, health care, etc.). For example, in Soviet times, health services were rendered free of charge and funded from the state budget, but now funding is divided between the state budget (45 percent), health insurance funds (16 percent) and households (39 percent) (Rimashevskaya 2002a).

Degradation of the social protection system and social infrastructure has the most negative effect on women for the following reasons:
• As the social sphere is a traditional "female" sphere of employment, its underfunding first affects women working there – doctors, teachers, social workers, etc.
• The reduction of the social support for the elderly, children and disabled persons usually places the responsibility for their welfare on women, who are willing to assume more responsibilities, take other jobs, or even quit working if need be.
• The decline in the level of pensions also has a greater impact on women, since their old age pensions are significantly lower that that of men.

Socio-Economic Position of Families with Children

Among the serious shortcomings of the official statistics is the lack of data relating to the position of Russian families. In Russia, there are actually no gender statistics, particularly in the field of "family" issues. Therefore, the presented materials are based on the data from long-term research carried out by the Institute for Socio-Economic Studies of Population RAS in the city of Taganrog.

Income levels of families

Family incomes are a function of family type. Data from the Taganrog surveys show negative trends in the dynamics of the economic welfare of separate household types over the period from the late 1980s to the present. Table I shows that, irrespective of changes in the methods of estimation of the minimum living standard, the share of households below the poverty line has continuously increased.

Table 1: Percentage of poor households by demographic types (the case of Taganrog)

Demographic type of household	1989	1993	1998	2000
Married couples without children	8.5	18.3	37.9	46.6
Two-parent families with children	16.9	49.4	71.6	61.4
One-parent families with children	32.0	61.9	76.3	68.5

Source: Zhenshchina 2001

In the late 80s, single-parent families with children were in the most difficult economic position. About one third of them were poor. The proportion of poor among two-parent families was lower – it amounted to one sixth of that group. Gradually, the proportion of poor two-parent families with children increased, and the gap between one-parent and two-parent families diminished. From 1989 to 2000, the number of poor single-parent families doubled and that of two-parent families increased 3.6 times. In 2000, the share of poor single-parent families was 68.5 percent and that of two-parent families reached 61.4 percent. So it is that we can speak about an "equality of the overwhelming majority of families at the lowest income level" (Prokofieva 2001).

State Benefits for Families with Children

The current legislation provides for many kinds of state support for families with children in monetary and non-monetary form: child allowances, maternity benefits, targeted social assistance to under-provisioned families, subsidies and privileges (for food, transportation, housing and communal services, medical services, pre-school educational establishments, etc.)

The most widespread form of state support of poor families is the state allowance for children up to 18 years of age. By the end of 2001, about 58 percent of children were recipients of this benefit. It is worth noting that its amount is 2 USD per month, but it is quite often impossible to receive even this small sum because of systematic payment arrears. By the beginning of 2002, the total amount of delayed payments in 33 regions exceeded the yearly sum of resources necessary for payment of the allowances (Ministry of Labour 2002).

Another widespread form of state support is presented by maternity benefits. The "largest" among them is a lump-sum benefit to pregnant women (about 9 USD) and a single payment on the birth of a child (about 140 USD). In the first quarter of 2002, the monthly benefit to mothers staying at home to look after their children up to 18 months of age amounted to one fourth of the subsistence minimum for adults. In 2001, 58 percent of the families receiving these monthly benefits were poor (Ministry of Labour 2002).

Poor families are entitled to targeted social assistance paid out from regional budgets. Benefits in cash and in kind are granted to families with per capita income at the level of 50 to 70 percent of subsistence minimum. The amount of benefits ranges between 1.5 and two USD a month. Social assistance in kind includes food, clothing and services which are subsidized or free of charge (Rimashevskaya 2002b, 89). In 2001, over 40 percent of families with children up to 18 years old received subsidies and privileges (Ministry of Labour 2002). The amount of state support is not sufficient to provide substantial assistance to families – the money value of in-kind subsidies and privileges accounts for only two percent of disposable resources in households with one child, and ten percent in families with four children or more (Ministry of Labour 2002). The average value of subsidies for housing and communal services amounts to only 24 percent of the total bills. Families raising children with disabilities and families with many children receive maximum benefits and privileges without arrears. However, despite state support, they traditionally are among the poor.

Thus, on the one hand, there is a legislative base providing for a wide range of state payments, and there is a certain mechanism for the allocation of resources. On the other hand, however, there is no funding for these payments. The reproductive sphere is left to its own resources.

Being left without state support, people in the reproductive sphere finds itself in a vicious circle: having many children, or a small child, or a child with disabilities reduces a mother's chances to earn money. But if the mother is not working, the economic position of family deteriorates. Since there is no reliance on state support, caring for children is a private problem for each separate family. In conditions of severe poverty, giving birth to a child becomes impossible for parents. As a result, we have a deterioration in children's quality of life as well as a reduction in fertility.

Socio-Economic Adaptation of Families to the Changing Economic Conditions

Research data show that the success of family and household adaptation to the new conditions is determined by a complex of factors (Zhenshchina 2001). We shall consider gender aspects of adaptation.

First, adaptation takes the form of an increase of the total workload for both men and women. Working time and incomes of households are directly related to each other – an increase in working time is connected with a growth of earnings. People are actively using secondary employment – holding a second job, rendering personal services, etc. A considerable amount of labour is now transferred to the household sphere. Households' economic functions have increased through development of various forms of private activities ensuring additional family incomes and saving resources, including private subsidiary activity, and replacement of communal consumer services with self-service – repair of housing, appliances, clothing and footwear. Increase of the total labour burden on the population has resulted in a considerable reduction of leisure time. This necessarily has an impact on the physical condition, cultural and spiritual development, and upbringing of children. Thus, now only 28 percent of parents devote some time to children every day or almost every day (2002 survey data) as opposed to 43 percent in 1990 (Poletayev 2002).

Second, one of the characteristic features of the vital activity of families with two working parents is a growing gender asymmetry in the distribution of time between gainful employment and housework. This is linked to a considerable extent with increasing employment of men (Alexeeva 2000). As the economic position of families is deteriorating, the burden of housework performed by women is increasing. Women spend much more time than men on housework, including private subsidiary production, keeping the house and looking after children. Thus, in 1997/98 the women: men ratio was 2:1 (Alexeeva 2000).

Third, discrimination processes in the labour market and in the sphere of reproductive policy are clearly demonstrated by the emergence of a social category of housewives in Russia. In 1999, their number amounted to 5 million. But only one third of them had left their jobs and returned to the family voluntarily. The remaining three and a half million wanted to work (Khotkina 2001). Most importantly, the ousting of women from the labour market is connected with the crisis in the economy – reductions of the employment sphere, unemployment, severe conditions of competition in the labour market, etc. Further, women are experiencing ideological pressure. The idea of equal participation in the national economy is being replaced by the idea of a biological predestination of women as housekeepers. The image of housekeeper is actively imposed on women, although as they have before, most of them measure their life success with a professional career (Arutyunyan 1998). They cannot leave their jobs, since with the present income levels, it is impossible to rely solely on a husband's wage. And finally, women's retreat from the labour market is a strategy for the adaptation of families with small or disabled children to the new economic conditions.

Here are some of the circumstances which persuade women to join the ranks of housewives: First, parents are not satisfied with the quality of care and upbringing of children in pre-school establishments, or with the costs involved for the children's stay there. Second, under the conditions of severe competition on the labour market, women have no opportunity to work part time or get flexible working days. Therefore, it is difficult to combine gainful employment and care of children. Almost half of preschool-age children – 45 percent – are raised at home. During the nineties, the number of children in pre-school educational establishments dropped by eleven percent (Breeva 2002). Third, another reason why women cannot work is a general deterioration of children's health. At present, healthy children make up ten to twelve percent of pupils in younger groups, eight percent in middle groups, and five percent in older groups at school (Breeva 2002). At the beginning of 2002, there were 658,000 disabled children in the Russian Federation (Ministry of Labour 2002). The poor condition of children's health is the result of the declining quality of life. Fourth, spouses in well-off families prefer to distribute labour functions in a traditional way: men earn money and women keep the house.

Conclusion

Gender asymmetry is a factor hampering the adaptation of families. First, total family incomes are decreasing due to the reduction of women's share in them. Against the general background of low levels of incomes and wages, the low earnings of women or their absence result in increasing poverty. Poverty of families has a negative effect primarily on children's health and on the whole reproductive process.

Second, the social status of women is declining. Such changes lead to a worsening position of women in the family, and this, in turn, results in instability of family relationships and marriage, and a deterioration of their quality. The current economic crisis has a negative effect on the reproductive sphere, where women traditionally play the main role. The lack of effective state support of families with children at various stages of the reproductive process should be regarded as a threat to the whole process of population reproduction.

Notes

1   The value of per capita income is overstated for most of the population in such a vast country as Russia. For our purposes, it has to be sufficient to consider the difference between incomes and savings. Thus, the difference in wages between the upper and the lower deciles of income distribution – the upper ones amounting to the 32-fold of the lower ones – is very large. Savings distribution is also very uneven: 40 percent of households have no savings at all, and five percent of households possess only three fourths of a saving fund (Rimashevskaya 2002a).
2   Subsistence minimum is a cost value of the food basket which guarantees a minimum number of calories, as well as the cost of non-food goods and services, taxes and obligatory payments for low-income people.
3   For example, rehabilitation of victims of the Stalin repressions expanded the list of medical indications for classifying persons as invalids, the age interval for children was raised to 18 years, etc.

References

Ayvazova, Svetlana G. 1998. *Russkiye zhenshchiny v labirinte ravnopraviya* (Russian Women in the Labyrinth of Equality): 75, 77, 78, 82–86. Moscow.

Afanasyev, Vladen. 2002. Velikiye depressii SShA i Rossii. Opyt sravnitel'nogo analiza (Great Depressions in the USA and Russia. Comparative analysis). *Economist*, No 3: 80.

Alexeeva, Olga A., and Katarina Katz. 2000. Deyatel'nost' domokhozyaystv: time characteristics (Household activities: time distribution). *Narodonaseleniye*, Moscow: ISESP RAS, No 4: 27–35.

Arutyunyan, Marina. 1998. Muzhchiny i Zhenshchiny: Modeli uspekha (Men and Women: Models of Success). *Narodonaseleniye*, Moscow: ISESP RAS, No 1: 81.

Baskakova, Marina E. 2002. Gendernye razlichiya v zarabotnoy plate. (Gender disparities in wages). *Sotsial'no-ekonomicheskiye pokazateli gendernogo neravenstva* (Socio-economic indicators of gender inequality): 52. Report prepared by ISESP RAS for the RF Ministry of Labour and Social Development.

Breeva, Yelena B. 2002. Deti i reformy (Children and Reforms). *Rossiya: 10 let reform. Sotsial'no-demographicheskaya situatsiya* (Russia: 10 Years of Reforms: Socio-Demographic Situation): 170. Moscow: ISESP RAS.

Goskomstat Rossii. 2002. *Rossiiskiy statisticheskiy yezhegodnik 2002* (Russian Statistical Yearbook 2002): 173, 189, 196, 175. Moscow.

Khotkina, Zoya A. 2001. Gendernyi podkhod k analizu truda i zaniatosti (Gender approach analise of labour and Employment). *Gendernyi kaleidockop* (Gender mosaic): 368. Course of lectures. Ed. M. Malysheva. Moscow: Academia.

Khotkina, Zoya A. 2002. Gendernye razlichiya v zarabotnoy plate (Gender Disparities in Wages). *Sotsial'no-ekonomicheskiye pokazateli gendernogo neravenstva* (Socio-economic indicators of gender inequality): 35. Report prepared by ISESP RAS for the RF Ministry of Labour and Social Development.

Nechayeva, Alexandra M. 2000. *Rossiya i eye deti* (Russia and her children (child, law, state)): 89, 108, 103, 126, 144. Institute of State and Law RAS. Moscow.

Ministry of Labour and Social Development. 2002. *O polozhenii detey v Rossiiskoy Federatsii* (On the Position of Children in the Russian Federation). National Report: 6–8. Moscow.

Ovcharova, Lilia N. 2002. Bednost' v gendernoy proektsii v stranakh s perekhodnoy ekonomikoy (Gender aspect of poverty in transition economies). *Narodonaseleniye*, Moscow: ISESP RAS, No 3: 27.

Poletayev, Yury A., Irina E. Palilova. *Dosyg – nedosug* (Leisure time). www.vciom.ru.

Prokofieva, Lidia M. 2001. Material'naya obespechennost' otdel'nykh tipov domokhozyaystv (Economic welfare of separate types of households). *Zhenshchina, muzhchina, sem'ya v Rossii: poslednyaya tret' XX veka* (Woman, Man, Family in Russia: the Last Third of the 20th Century. Project "Taganrog"). Moscow: ISESP RAS: 52–55.

Rimashevskaya, Natalia M. 2001a. Gendernaya asimmetriya rossiiskogo sotsiuma: dinamika poslednikh desyatiletiy (Gender asymmetry of the Rusian socium: dynamics of the last decades). *Zhenshchina, muzhchina, sem'ya v Rossii: poslednyaya tret' XX veka* (Woman, Man, Family in Russia: the Last Third of the 20th Century. Project "Taganrog"). Moscow: ISESP RAS.

Rimashevskaya, Natalia M. 2001b. Strategii sotsial'noy zashchity naseleniya Rossii (Strategies for social protection of the Russian population)". *Narodonaseleniye*, Moscow: ISESP RAS, No 1.

Rimashevskaya, Natalia M. 2002a. Gendernye aspekty sotsial'no-ekonomicheskogo razvitiya Rossii. (Gender aspects of the socio-economic development of Russia). *Ekonomika i sotsial'naya politika*: *Gendernoye izmereniye* (Economics and Social Policy: Gender Dimension): 11–12. Course of lectures. Ed. M. Malysheva. Moscow: Academia.

Rimashevskaya, Natalia M. (ed.). 2002b. *Sotsial'naya zashchita naseleniya* (Social Protection of Population). Moscow: ISESP RAS.

Zhenshchina, muzhchina, sem'ya v Rossii: poslednyaya tret' XX veka (Woman, Man, Family in Russia: the Last Third of the 20th Century. Project "Taganrog"). 2001. Moscow: ISESP RAS.

Michele Rivkin-Fish

The Politics of Reproduction and Nationalism in Russia

In the aftermath of the Soviet era, reproductive politics has become a key vehicle for nationalist revival in Russia. Public debate on reproduction focuses on two interconnected concerns: first, the "problem" of low fertility, described as contributing to the country's serious "demographic crisis"; and second, the perceived breakdown of morality in sexuality and family life. Portraying both of these situations as profound threats to the survival of the Russian nation, conservatives and nationalists persistently advocate interventions to increase childbearing, restrict access to family planning and abortion, and "raise the level of morality" among the population. After successfully inhibiting the work of sex educators and derailing federal funding for family planning services in the late 1990s, by August 2003, this coalition had succeeded in severely restricting the official criteria for accessing abortion in the second trimester.

The campaigns and achievements of Russian nationalists are neither surprising nor unique, but have reflections in both neighboring Eastern European contexts and the Soviet past. This chapter begins with an historical overview of Soviet demographic concerns over fertility, and the factors contributing to a moral panic over women's roles and sexuality in the late 1980s and 1990s. I then present the contemporary contours of reproductive politics, highlighting the close connections between governmental, Church and "patriotic" social movements' efforts to raise the birth rate, hinder family planning programs, and develop a nationalist revival after state socialism.

Demographic Politics Under the Soviet Regime

To understand the significant kinds of events that have occurred over the last decade in Russian reproductive politics, it is first necessary to examine state programs and policies during the socialist era. Two overarching strategies characterized state socialism's approach to reproductive politics: an unwavering pro-natalist stance, and the creation of what has been called an "abortion culture," involving the "adaptation of the society to the widespread provision of abortion as the primary and even only method of regulating" childbearing (Popov and David 1999). I discuss each of these and their interrelations below; it is important to note here, however, that the Soviet Ministry of Public Health's dual agenda of promoting childbearing while making abortion the main method of fertility control involved multiple contradictions and hypocrisies that have long taken a toll on women's health and lives.

A firm pro-natalist stance and a normative expectation that the population would consistently (if only moderately) increase characterized demographic policy under state socialism. Eastern European states rejected Malthusian theories concerning the need to limit population growth due to finite resources and stressed instead that human capital – meaning labor supplies – were among society's most valuable resources. In this way, policy makers followed Leninist thinking on population. They believed that socialism's guarantees of the basic human needs of food, shelter, and employment removed material obstacles to childbearing, and made the limitation of reproduction unnecessary. Yet to ensure that moderate increases in fertility did result, the state expended substantial efforts on the surveillance of reproductive practices and the engineering of family life in ways compatible with "society's" population needs. State efforts took different forms at various historical moments and in various contexts. In Bulgaria, for example, the hope of raising fertility rates led the state to restrict abortion for married women with fewer than two children (Daskalova 2000). As Adriana Baban discusses in this volume, coercive pro-natalist politics were most insistently and thoroughly established by the Ceausescu regime in Romania. Ceausescu's incessant need to control biological and social reproduction led him to criminalize abortion and to enforce an obligation for every woman to bear at least four children in what altogether entailed a twenty-three year campaign to achieve absolute population control in its most literal sense (Baban 1998).

Within Russia itself, the state exerted control over women's bodies in a variety of different ways. When the Soviet regime embarked on its industrializing frenzy in the 1920s, reproductive capacities were scrutinized scientifically and evaluated in terms of "productive outputs"; women's pelvic sizes and the quality of their menses were societal matters made analogous to the outcomes of factory work (Hyer 1996). In the later decades of Soviet rule, when concern over low fertility and high divorce rates led many to suggest that the public no longer valued family life, state surveillance focused on women's reproductive motives through surveys comparing their "ideal" number of children and their "expected" number, in addition to their reasons for limiting their fertility. This booming survey industry was accompanied by educational efforts to instill in youth the importance of stable marriages with two to three children in order to ensure both personal happiness and society's vitality.

Pro-natalism coincided with abortion policy in numerous ways. In 1920, the Soviet Union became the first country in the world to legalize abortion, a decision justified as necessary for realizing the emancipation of women from the domestic sphere and their full incorporation into the labor market. The legalization of abortion was part of broader Bolshevik experiments to radically transform the structure and role of the family in a socialist society. Yet physicians and other experts opposed contraception, on the grounds that its widespread use could lead to depopulation (Gross Solomon 1992). Moreover, the progressive possibilities inherent in legalizing abortion and transforming the family quickly fell victim to the state's obsessive concern with establishing control over individuals, raising the birth rate, and expanding its ideology about moral purity into the personal sphere (Goldman

1993). In 1936, Stalin criminalized abortion again with the explicit purpose of increasing the population. In a single legislative act, abortion was prohibited while maternity hospitals, day-care centers, and children's homes were increased (Gross Solomon 1992). As is well known, the strategy achieved its desired goals only temporarily: the birth rate increased from 33.6 per 100,000 population in 1936 to 39.6 in 1937, but declined again almost immediately as women resorted to illegal abortions in massive numbers (Lorimer 1946). The tragedies endured during the 18 years in which women were denied legal access to abortion left a searing impression in the collective memory of the Soviet public. On this basis, the majority of Russians have long expressed opposition to criminalizing the procedure.

When Khrushchev reversed the ban on abortion upon coming to power in 1954, he maintained a firm commitment to pro-natalism. Without legitimizing or promoting the practice, he legalized abortion due to the dangers it posed to women's health when left uncontrolled and provided underground, and thus to facilitate a rise in fertility. With legalization, then, the "fight against abortion" formed the basis of state ideology: official health promotion literature railed against the dangers of abortion, and "education for family life" and "sex education" courses conducted by obstetricians and gynecologists in medical institutions emphasized that abortion often leads to infertility (Field 1996). At the same time, the Ministry of Public Health made very few efforts to promote the use of contraceptives in place of abortion. Although the Soviet state strongly advocated the acquisition of proper habits of "personal hygiene" (such as physical cleanliness) as part of a sweeping disciplinary program to transform its citizens into "civilized" and "cultured" modern subjects, it neither advocated nor facilitated the active prevention of pregnancy as a routine part of daily life (Peterson 1996). Instead of promoting women's health in and of itself, pro-natalist ideology dominated "the fight against abortion," making it synonymous with the promotion of motherhood. At the same time, physicians reaped substantial financial benefits from providing abortions, through (often illicit) payments made to obtain improved care, confidentiality, or to obtain abortions that did not fit the legal criteria. This financial incentive entailed another reason for physicians' (and the Ministry of Public Health's) reluctance to replace the procedure with widespread contraceptive use.

By the late 1960s, demographers realized that in the two decades since the end of World War II, there had been no significant or sustained rise in fertility. Despite official hostility to abortion, data from the late 1980s revealed that approximately seventy percent of pregnancies in Russia were terminated (Remmenick 1991; Popov and David 1999, 244). Women resorted to abortions twice as often as they gave birth throughout the 1990s. And the official abortion rate of 52 per 1000 women (as of 2001) (Vishnevskii 2002, 55) is considered to be an underestimate of the actual numbers (due to large amounts of unregistered abortions and abortions provided "under the table" for extra fees, or as favors to friends). By contrast, the US rate in 2000 was 21.4 per 1000 women; in Belgium in 1997, it was 6 per 1000 (Finer and Henshaw 2003; Alan Guttmacher Institute 2000). Nonetheless, the Soviet state did not officially recognize that women and men perceived a need to control their fertility until the 1970s. Having rejected Malthusian thought as "bourgeois cannibalism," in Khrushchev's words, experts toed the Party line that under socialist conditions, where basic economic necessities were guaranteed, moderate fertility increases should "naturally" occur (Desfosses 1976). Soviet leaders construed low fertility as problematic, since, as mentioned above, they viewed labor supplies as one of the country's key economic resource. Moreover, they sought control over fertility as part of their perceived need to plan the socialist state, predict and organize labor supplies, pension resources, and military power. Planners viewed population growth as essential for maintaining the Soviet Union's stature as an international superpower. No less importantly, the fertility rate was also interpreted as a measure of social stability, and declines in childbearing were read in conjunction with rising divorce rates as a sign that marriages were unstable and individuals were not sufficiently committed to realizing "societal interests" in and through their family life (Warshofsky Lapidus 1978, 293–295; Perevedentsev 1968).

Yet demographers did not agree on either the causes of low fertility, or how best to increase childbearing. One explanation noted the difficulties women faced in managing daily domestic tasks under conditions of poor and cramped housing, few household amenities, and constant deficits. Proponents of this perspective recognized that women limited their births because poor material conditions made bearing and raising children immensely difficult (Piskunov and Steshenko 1974; Volkov 1986; Kuznetsova 1989). Without advocating that men assume equal responsibilities for childrearing and domestic life, they did suggest offering more services to working mothers, socializing childcare more completely, and reducing women's work responsibilities by offering part-time options and longer maternity leaves. Using survey data that showed many women had fewer children than they ideally wanted due to 'material constraints,' these scholars asserted that improving the conditions of everyday life would solve the problem of low fertility. This approach cannot be labeled "feminist" in any Western sense, focused as it was on achieving the state's pro-natalist goals. However, it did represent a progressive effort to introduce what proponents termed "the needs of the family" into discussions of reproductive policy. In the Soviet context, where ideological orthodoxy remained rather strictly enforced, I argue that such analyses of fertility patterns and policy recommendations offered oblique critiques of state dominance over personal life as experienced under the Soviet regime (Rivkin-Fish 2003).

Another group of fertility specialists opposed this approach virulently. These sociologists and demographers insisted that policy makers implement direct interventions to increase the fertility rate immediately, and establish the goal of increasing childbearing as the centerpiece of a national demographic politics. Their discourses portrayed women as consciously refusing to bear more than one or two children out of a selfish rejection of family life and their society's demographic needs. Some experts considered the possibility that women's "emancipation" into the labor force had resulted in the loss of their "maternal instinct" (Kvasha 1981). The policy recommendations they offered discounted the value of improving living standards as a means of raising fertility, because, as one prominent specialist emphasized, higher economic conditions are associated with lower, not higher fertility (Antonov 1980). Rather, pro-natalists sought to mobilize the state's arsenal of propaganda tools in order to promote the status of motherhood, to raise the popularity of having many children, and to celebrate the importance of home life (Antonov 1986). These experts portrayed women's concerns and perceived obstacles to childbearing as at best misguided, and at worst morally corrupt. During the Soviet era, state ideology held that all of society had shared interests, and experts were best suited to discern these interests and establish appropriate policies for furthering them. The official position on population therefore viewed each individual and family as having the same demographic interests as society (and the state) as a whole; professional demographers were assigned sole responsibility for interpreting these interests, while Party elites would develop a national demographic policy based on their assessment of this work. Clearly, this perspective denied the possibility that women and/or families could have legitimate interests that contradicted the needs of society as a whole. Scholars maintaining this perspective argued that demographic policy should center on establishing a norm of two to three children per couple in European regions of the USSR (Kvasha 1981, 116–117). Notably however, Central Asian republics of the USSR, where fertility rates were substantially higher, were targeted with programs to "modernize" and "emancipate" women from their traditional domestic roles (Massell 1974), partly in order to maintain ethnic balance among diverse sectors of the multiethnic Soviet state.

As debate over fertility continued throughout the 1970s and 1980s, the popular media increasingly depicted childbearing as women's "most important biological and social function," as well as the "family's obligation to society" (Antonov 1980). In the view of one prominent fertility specialist, Anatolii Antonov, small families (defined as those with one or two children) were a deviant and dangerous phenomenon which had arisen from the combination of two main factors: the loss of children's economic value to family survival, and the rise of a destructive, self-indulgent consumer mentality (Antonov 1980). Antonov persistently urged the government to combat what he identified as the one-child family mentality [odnodetnaia sem'ia] that was sweeping the educated and professional classes and threatening the moral and demographic base of the society (Antonov 1980; Antonov 1982; Antonov 1995; Antonov and Medkov 1987). To some extent, policy makers listened: it was certainly cheaper and easier to generate messages about family values than to resolve housing shortages and invest in childcare resources.[1] Educational policy makers adjusted the high school curriculum to include "sex-role socialization" courses, aiming to ensure that young women would cultivate their "maternal instinct" and that all young adults would embrace traditional stereotypes about women and men's characters and societal roles (Attwood 1990). Few part-time opportunities or other improved conditions for women's employment materialized, but Soviet leaders extended maternity leaves to facilitate women's exit from the work place and their deeper connection with the domestic sphere. Images of mothers and nurturers came to dominate media representations of women (Posadskaia 1992). Such representations were not coincidental: they often consciously remarked on the need to replace early socialist representations of women as the physically and mentally strong equals of men with a renewed feminine image of maternity and domesticity. As we will see below, the strategy these demographers and policymakers applied of using propaganda about traditional gender roles to raise the birth rate, did not achieve its desired effect. Fertility continued to fall throughout the 1990s and into the 2000s. Yet this strategy laid the groundwork for further interventions in the post-Soviet era, by helping legitimate nationalist attacks against women's reproductive rights.

From Family Planning to Family Values: The Campaign Against Reproductive Health

The right to abortion was legally guaranteed by the Russian Federation Law passed on 23 June 1993. Article 36 of the law states:

Each woman has the right to make the decision about motherhood independently. The artificial termination of pregnancy is provided on the woman's demand up to 12 weeks of pregnancy, for social reasons up to 22 weeks pregnancy, and in the case of medical indicators and with the woman's agreement, without regard to the time of gestation (Ballaeva 1998, 37).

"Social reasons" included circumstances established in 1987 by the then Soviet Ministry of Health, and included severe injury or death of one's husband, divorce, incarceration of the woman or her husband, loss of parental rights, having three or more children already, and pregnancy resulting from rape. In 1996, the Russian Ministry of Health tacitly acknowledged the exacerbation of economic hardship among the vast majority of Russians amidst post-Soviet reforms, and expanded the list of acceptable "social reasons" to include a woman's unmarried status, homelessness, refugee status, a disabled husband or disabled child to care for, loss of the woman's or her husband's job, and having a salary lower than the minimum living standard for one's region (Aleksandrovna Mishle 1998, 356). Yet, despite this recognition that economic constraints often lead women to seek abortions, actual availability of the procedure was increasingly limited due to the state's rapid withdrawal of funding for health care generally, and new, legal loopholes enabling local governments to exclude abortion services from the list of insured medical procedures (Ballaeva 1998, 41–47).

Given the long-standing reliance on abortion for fertility control, and the historical lack of contraceptive technologies during the Soviet era, there was virtually no family planning infrastructure in Russia at the time the Soviet Union collapsed. Nor was the government's hypocrisy towards birth control entirely reversed. The state did not undertake extensive measures to ensure that contraceptives would be available to all women and men; it largely left this task to the newly emerging market and Western humanitarian agencies. And these 'foreign' institutions – mainly Western pharmaceutical companies and development agencies – seized the new opportunities availed by Russia's opening to deliver contraceptive supplies. Some local physicians also realized the need to reduce abortions through promoting contraception, and gradually began establishing clinics or programs, mostly for women. Both international and local government support figured in their efforts, but these funding streams represented different ideological perspectives. Whereas international agencies cited the need to advance women's rights, or reduce abortions as a matter of preserving 'human life', the Russian government maintained its concern with demographic issues. Thus, in 1992, when The Russian Family Planning Association, an affiliate of the global International Planned Parenthood Federation, was founded as the country's first NGO devoted to promoting birth control, Yeltsin's administration included it in the Presidential Program "Children of Russia" and allocated one million rubles for its efforts.[2] Yet rather than supporting reproductive choices, it justified this funding as helping realize the organization's goals of resolving the country's demographic crisis through improved reproductive health and a higher birth rate.

Ten years later, Russia showed significant progress in reducing abortions: Whereas in 1990 official data revealed 206 abortions for every 100 live births, by 2001, that rate was reduced to 154. Viewed in other terms, the number of abortions per 1000 women of childbearing age steadily decreased for all age groups. In 1991, there were 100 abortions for every 1000 women aged 15–49, and in 2000, that number had decreased to 55. Viewed by age group, the decreasing abortion trends are as follows:

Ages	15–19	20–34	35 and older
1991	69	153	51
2000	37	100	24

Source: Naselenie Rossii 2001, 57

The Russian Ministry of Public Health further classifies the following "types" of abortion based on method of accessing the procedure: self-induced, legally induced (at the woman's request, up to 12 weeks gestation), medically indicated, criminal, socially indicated (those past twelve weeks), "mini-abortions" (performed before six weeks) and those with unknown sources. Data from 1992–2001 reveal interesting changes in the frequency of these various approaches to accessing the procedures. Criminal abortions, meaning those performed outside of a licensed institution, decreased from .3 percent to .1 percent of the total number of abortions; decreases were also seen in the proportion of legally induced abortions – which account for the vast majority of abortions performed – from 61.4 percent of all abortions in 1992 to 57.3 percent in 2001. On the other hand, the proportion of self-induced abortions increased from 6.3 percent of all abortions in 1992 to 9 percent in 2001, and abortions accessed on the basis of social indicators increased from .8 percent in 1992 to 2.2 percent in 2001 (Demoscope Weekly 2003). These trends are particularly interesting to examine in light of the Ministry's 2003 decision to severely restrict second trimester abortions. Most notably, the category of social indicators, which involved factors related to poverty and social marginalization (such as homelessness, unemployment, single motherhood, and divorce), increased by almost three times between 1992 and 2001. Nonetheless, these late abortions still account for fewer than 3 percent of the total number of abortions performed, which strongly suggests that women resort to second-trimester abortions only in the most difficult personal and financial circumstances. Why, then, did the Ministry of Health severely restrict the social reasons for accessing abortion in August 2003?

Reproductive Politics after Socialism: Following the Eastern European Trend

Any simple explanation of the 2003 decree is impossible, inasmuch as the decision was made in a top-down, hasty fashion, which allowed virtually no time for public debate and discussion. A handful of specialists in women's health expressed opposition to the new regulations soon after they were issued. The *Demoscope Weekly* electronic bulletin of the Institute for Demography and Human Ecology devoted an entire issue to the question of abortion use soon after the Ministry's decree, and quoted the reactions of several top specialists in reproductive health. The chief obstetrician-gynecologist of Moscow, Professor Iuri Bloshanskii, asserted, "I am categorically against the reconsideration of social indicators for terminating a pregnancy. And if we are going to reconsider them, then it must only be in order to expand them. I'll explain why. In a country where abortion is permitted, it must be done solely on the basis of a woman's request. That means there must not be any limitations. In a country where abortion is legal, there must not be the situation in which an abortion after twelve weeks is dangerous for women because doctors are not skilled in this procedure."

The Assistant Director of the Research Center of Obstetrics and Gynecology of the Russian Academy of Medical Sciences, Academic Vladimir Serov, expressed similar dismay with the decree, and then questioned why the social indicators for abortion should even be a question that medical experts should decide:

Social indicators for abortion exist in no country in the world. The operation is either permissible or prohibited. It cannot be any other way [inogo ne dano]. And these twelve weeks, by which we are limiting the period for performing an abortion, are nothing else but a prohibition. And if we believe it is allowed in our country, then there must not be these poorly received twelve week limits on it. And if we are discussing social indicators, then that is not at all a medical issue and is not the business of doctors – it's a matter for the social organs, the leaders of the government. It's simplest of all to throw the issue to doctors. But was it they who created women's misfortunes, made her homeless, deprived her of a normal salary, condemned her to poverty, and forced her to terminate a pregnancy? To reduce or increase the social indicators for abortion – it's not our doctors' matter (Krasnopol'skaia 2003).

Press reports on the new regulations linked it with the hope of increasing the birth rate, as the headline of one article announcing the changes stated, "Doctors limit late abortions in the hope of raising the birth rate." (Timashova 2003) The expense of abortions to the government was also raised in one report that noted that five percent of all public health expenditures was spent on abortions. On the other hand, representatives of the Ministry of Public Health cited neither the demographic nor financial issues, but spoke of their commitment to improving women's health and the "need" to increase women's sense of responsibility in their reproductive lives. The Chief of the Department of Obstetrical and Gynecological Care of the Ministry of Public Health, Dr. Liudmila Pospelova, asserted that there had been a decrease in the number of abortions over the last few years. Nonetheless, she explained that the decision to place restrictions on social indicators was made after observing the fact that 30 percent of maternal mortality cases are linked to complications stemming from this late stage abortion. She stated: "The Ministry had to take steps to reduce abortions at late stages of pregnancy, preventing its harmful outcomes and establishing women's responsibility for their health and the health of their children." (RIA Novosti 2003)

Yet if the Ministry's goal was truly to reduce maternal mortality resulting from later term abortions, one wonders why it did not implement re-training courses to improve physicians' skills, rather than prohibiting the procedure and risking the possibility that women would resort to illegal and unsafe abortions.

This author believes that understanding the new abortion regulations requires contextualizing them within Russia's broader political context, shaped by the Soviet history of pro-natalist politics and a decade of vibrant activism on the part of Russia's anti-abortion lobby. These activists have strongly linked opposition to abortion with the need for both moral renewal and nationalist revival. This tactic is far from unique to Russia. Throughout the 1990s, virtually all Eastern European states attacked abortion symbolically and legislatively, in ways that directly equated the de-legitimation of abortion with a progressive retreat away from the socialist legacy (see De Soto 1994; Eberts 1998; Fuszara 1993; Funk 1996; Gal 1994; Verdery 1994). Polish parliamentarians sympathetic to the Catholic Church drafted a bill banning abortion unconditionally as early as 1989; by 1992, restrictions on the procedure were put into place, and by 1993 they were legally codified. After continued debate and reversals, abortion was again re-criminalized in 1997. Efforts to restrict abortion have also been pursued in the Czech Republic and Slovakia, in Hungary, Serbia and Croatia, and in reunified Germany[3]. In all these contexts, opposition to abortion became a key discursive means of signaling difference from the socialist past, and establishing a new moral foundation for the nation. Even in Romania, where the end of socialism brought an immediate end to such repressive policies, nationalist anxieties over negative population growth have led some demographers to call for restricting abortion again (Baban 2000, 238–239).

Theorizing about these and related changes concerning gender amidst post-socialist transitions, Susan Gal and Gail Kligman demonstrated that addressing reproductive issues facilitates several political goals for elites (Gal and Kligman 2000, 15–36). It helps them reconfigure the relations between citizens and the state, establish new criteria for states to assert their political and moral legitimacy, and construct women as certain kinds of citizens whose roles and responsibilities may be defined through politically useful categories (such as biology/nature, social norms, or liberal ideologies of the rational subject). Additionally, reproductive politics enables those vying for power to pursue campaigns for nationalist supremacy against ethnic others defined as outsiders and threats (Gal and Kligman 2000, 15–36). Reproductive issues are thus important for post-socialist political contenders in part because, as elsewhere in the world, the nation is defined as a biological entity, with the national essence (blood, genes, etc.) transferred and preserved – or lost – through the physical process of procreation (Borneman 1992; Brubaker 1992; Herzfeld 1992; Ginsburg and Rapp 1995). In this paradigm, the nation's continuity cannot be achieved through cultural or social processes alone. Childbearing is deemed necessary, resulting in the constant monitoring of fertility – both of one's own nation and that of others. Slobodan Milosevic, for example, warned Serbs of the threat posed by Albanians' high birth rate in order to instigate a sense of national vulnerability and to justify pro-natalist measures (Gal 2000, 27). Similarly, nationalists in Bulgaria view Turks and Roma as ethnic others whose higher rates of reproduction must be combated to save "the Bulgarian nation" (Daskalova 2000, 351).

The commonalities found in reproductive politics in Eastern Europe are instructive. They suggest that as socialism increasingly becomes a part of the past, a resurgence of nationalism is occurring throughout the region. Indeed, overcoming the socialist past is often equated with the development of nationalist identities and politics (Verdery 1996). And the struggle for control of women's bodies, in Russia as elsewhere, is a central tactic of nationalist revivals.

A Moral Panic Over Women, Sexuality, and the Reproduction of the Nation

A vibrant campaign for nationalist revival after socialism, however, was not an inevitable occurrence (Verdery 1996). Again, it is necessary to consider how social and political-economic changes of the last decade worked in tandem to produce a disturbing sense among many Russians that Westernizing reforms were the cause of their country's moral and physical deterioration. Since glasnost in the mid-1980s, many Russians experienced shock and revulsion as the new openness in public discourse and an end to censorship became equated with sexually explicit films on prime time television, pornographic literature filling street corner newspaper stands, and the displacement of chaste Russian movies with Western-made graphic violence and sex in the cinemas. As many scholars have noted, Russians had a very different interpretation of the new "democratic freedoms" so celebrated in the Western media. Many lamented the unraveling of strict laws and state controls as leading to the degradation of moral order and propriety, the advent of lawlessness, chaos, and depravity (Kon 1995; Ries 1997). Older Russians and conservatives claimed opposition to these socio-cultural changes as antithetical to the nation's spiritual legacy and its moral foundations. And they linked the emerging (im)moral public atmosphere directly with Westernizing reforms.

Moreover, democratization and market economics did not have cultural effects alone. The harsh economic losses associated with the end of price controls, full employment, and a substantial welfare safety net resulted in a range of public health problems that register as statistically significant changes among the majority of the population. Morbidity rates in almost all categories of disease rose over the last decade, not infrequently reaching epidemic proportions (Feshbach 2001; Field 1995). Diagnosed cases of active tuberculosis, for example, increased 2.2 times between 1991 and 1998, reaching a rate of 76 cases per 100,000 population (in comparison with U.S. rates of approximately 10 per 100,000); children and adolescents experienced significant rises in morbidity as well: cancer in this demographic age group, for example, rose 2.9 times between 1991 and 1998, and diseases related to the endocrine system, digestive system, and immune system rose 3.9 times in the same period (Naselenie 2000, 90). Life expectancy for men fell from approximately 64 years in 1987 to 57 years in 1994, rising again to 61 years in 1998 (Naselenie 2002, 99). These devastating deteriorations in public health indicators seemed to confirm that Russia's perceived moral degradation had physical correlations. For conservatives and nationalists opposed to democratization, all of these changes could be blamed on the West.

Moreover, such nationalist sentiment became explicitly gendered. Demographic and public health experts, politicians, and the media linked girls' and women's health directly with the reproduction of the nation, and followed the indicators of these groups' health particularly closely. When the Soviet Union collapsed, the already low birth rate plunged further. The average number of children a woman would bear in her lifetime (the total fertility rate, or TFR) fell from 1.87 in 1979–80 to 1.34 in 1995 and then to 1.24 in 1998.[4] Sexually transmitted diseases (STDs) rose astronomically, with syphilis reaching a rate of 277.6 per 100,000 population in 1997 (an increase of 64.5 times since 1989) (Naselenie 1999, 85–86). The press most frequently reported the health crisis in sensationalist ways, omitting discussion of the methods and problems of a given study to highlight the alarming trends it represented. In a typical example, the newspaper Kommersant announced that, "Only 6.3% of teenage girls in Russia today can be considered healthy, while 10 years ago the figure was 29%…" (Alekseyeva 2002). Without precise definitions of "healthy," or details of the predominant illnesses, their causes, and methods of data analysis, such reports cannot be critically assessed. But they do achieve a different kind of cultural work. They contribute to a moral panic that links girls' and women's health with nationalist anxieties over Russia's decline. The Kommersant article, for example, concluded that a necessary solution to this crisis involved introducing education on the ethics of male-female relations in schools (Alekseyeva 2002). As I have shown elsewhere (Rivkin-Fish 1999), Russian courses on sex education and family life contain strong moral messages about women's need to maintain sexual purity, which is said to be necessary both to ensure proper maternal relationships with their children and to sustain life itself.

The panic over women, sexuality, and the nation increased in 1992, when high male mortality and sharp decreases in fertility resulted in a net population decline in Russia. The Russian popular press began announcing an impending national demographic catastrophe (Field 1995). Typical statements in newspapers and other media outlets announced, "The demographic situation…is called a crisis. That's not accurate. It's not a crisis, it's a national catastrophe…. The annihilation [ubyl'] of the population has acquired a stable pattern" (Semenov 1996). Headlines in mainstream newspapers announced that "Russia has 100 Years to Live," or offered ominous announcements such as "Distressing Diagnosis – Health Problems Plague More Than Half of Russia's Children" (Derzhavina 1998; Sukhaya 2002). Terms such as "dying out" [*vymiranie, ubyl'*] depopulation [*depopulatsiia*], and degeneration [*degredatsiia*] pervade newspapers. Such discourses resonate with a key cultural image of Russia and its people as long-suffering, enduring, and tragic, ironically reaffirming a central part of Russian identity (Ries 1997). At the same time, women's health is narrowly viewed as a matter of reproductive potential alone; extremely little attention is paid to the health of women past reproductive age, while health issues unrelated to reproduction for younger women tend to be discussed in terms of their effects on their future childbearing (Bassom 1999).

For nationalist and communist activists, rhetoric on "the death of the nation" serves several political purposes. It offers a means of impugning Western inspired market reforms and advocating a return to Soviet-style rule or nationalist alternatives. One prolific Communist demographer blamed market economics for "sentencing Russia to extinction" in part through "the feminization of poverty." He has called for the eradication of the market, a return to price controls, and the reinstitution of a socialist welfare system (Khorev 1995). In fact, the Communist Party introduced impeachment proceedings against Boris Yeltsin in part for perpetuating the "genocide of the Russian people" through his economic reforms. Poverty, induced by market economics, had brought sickness, disease, and death to the Russian nation, they argued.

Rhetoric on the impending "death of the nation" also justifies calls for state support that preserves "the nation," frequently defined as a biogenetic entity. The business newspaper *Delovoi Peterburg*, for example, invited a range of community leaders and concerned professionals to a roundtable discussion in the summer of 2000 to discuss the demographic crisis and necessary steps for resolving it. "Petersburg knows how to make babies, but can't," mourned the headline for an article about the roundtable discussion, which was described as a conversation about "the degree of the tragedy and measures for raising fertility" (Kak 2000). While the newspaper announced in its introduction that the survival of the nation was at stake, the specialists participating in the discussion emphasized the need for government programs to preserve the Russian "gene pool" (Kak 2000).

Anxiety over low fertility and demographic decline, framed in terms of a biogenetically-defined Russian nation, further serves to legitimize hostility towards non-Russians. These include both ethnic groups who have been long-time citizens of former Soviet republics, and recent immigrants to Russia from other parts of the world. Indeed, at the same time that Russian nationalists advocate the implementation of immediate pro-natalist measures to save the Russian people from extinction, the mass media reported and expanded upon the public's dismay over the presence of non-Russian migrants. People from the Caucasus and former republics of the Soviet Union with largely Islamic populations are seen as posing particular threats to the pre-eminence of the Russian people due to their higher fertility rates and supposed inclinations towards religious fundamentalism (Shumilin 2000). Street violence against persons with dark complexions, often carried out by organized skinhead gangs, has substantially increased; not infrequently, their actions find support among ordinary residents, police, and political leaders (Russian 2003; Russia 2002; Lepina 2002; Kostyukovsky 2002; Rotkevich 2002). The Krasnodar Territory Legislative Assembly and Governor, for example, instituted "measures to eliminate excessive migration in the region." The stated goal of the measures was to deny residence registration to "persons of Caucasian nationality." The blatant racism of this policy is evident in the fact that it was not solely targeted at immigrants. The number of years people were residences of the Territory was considered irrelevant. One report on this policy in the newspaper Noviye Izvestiia stated that the Governor had organized special training for officials "in lawful methods of restricting immigration."

> According to human rights advocates, [Governor] Tkachov has already indicated what the guidelines for the training will be. Specifically, he has offered tips on how to distinguish a desirable immigrant from an undesirable one. Look at the surname. If it's Armenian, Georgian, or Azerbaijani, deny entry. If the surname is Russian, the person may be allowed into the Kuban... (Tselms 2002).

To ensure that this policy is realized, the governor has enlisted police and local Cossack units to "step up their activity" and to check passport status on a daily and nightly basis. Those found without the proper registration will be immediately deported from Russia within 72 hours (Tselms 2002). Deportations of illegal migrants have also become a frequent policy in Moscow, targeting workers from countries such as China and Vietnam (Sukhov 2002).

Many observers advocate policies that will encourage the "return" of ethnic Russians from outside the Russian Federation to combat the demographic and social effects of non-Russian migration into Russia. Nationalists and others (referred to in local parlance as 'patriots' and 'Russophiles') also openly criticize intermarriage between Russians and non-Russians as threatening the continuation of the Russian "gene pool" (Stoliarenko 2000; Goble 2001; Santana 2003). For example, the Moscow-based Union Against Illegal Immigration lobbies for measures to restrict illegal immigration and for the deportation of illegal immigrants. The organization's head, Alexander Belov, invoked the fear of national extinction when he stated that immigrants were out-populating Russians by having more children. "Soon we'll be able to read about Russians only in history books," he said (Santana 2003). Even moderate observers who see a need for migration as a solution to Russia's labor force needs often show little tolerance for the needs of immigrants, and expect their full assimilation into Russian society as the price for residency. Aleksandr Khramchikhin, the head of the Analysis section of the Moscow-based Institute for Political and Military Analysis, has argued for the necessity of a civil society and civil notion of citizenship, rather than one based on biogenetic notions of inclusion. Still, he asserts that immigrants must show acceptance towards the native-born population rather than receiving rights to retain their own ethnic and cultural identity. "They must integrate fully into the general Russian identity and adopt Russian patterns of behavior." He endorses the American melting pot system, with the concept of a single, unified nation based on citizenship, not blood; the "melting pot will smelt [immigrants of non-Russian ethnicity] into Russian citizens," he asserted (Khramchikhin 2002).

The Politics of Reproduction and Nationalism

The panic over national decline and moral depravity fed directly into conservative campaigns to debilitate family planning, sex education, and abortion services. As mentioned above, 1992 marked both the founding of the Russian Family Planning Association and the beginning of a demographic trend in which high male mortality rates and declining fertility resulted in a net population loss for Russian society. Although negative population growth unquestionably resulted from factors other than family planning efforts, such as alcohol-related traumas, violence, suicide, and emigration (Zakharov 1999), nationalists and other opponents of western supported reforms decisively linked the two together in public discourse. Hostile political protest thus confronted family planning work nearly from its inception. Even when the RFPA's activities received official approval from the Yeltsin regime in the form of a Decree sanctioning its establishment, the legitimacy of family planning work was defined strictly in terms of improving the country's fertility rate. As the decade wore on and population decline continued, those opposed to market reforms targeted family planning and sex education in particular as evidence that Russia's unequal engagement with the West carries the price of moral depravity through promiscuous sex, the encouragement of homosexuality, and the rejection of family life (Kon 1995). Sex education programs were depicted as morally outrageous, foreign intrusions designed to warp Russian youth psychologically and brainwash them against bearing children (Babasyan 1999; Molodtsova 1999a; Molodtsova 1999b; Medvedeva and Shishova 2000).

Opponents have worked on several fronts simultaneously: some have used the mainstream press to convey their political messages, and not infrequently have had their opinions represented as facts. This was particularly evident in articles accusing global agencies funding family planning programs, such as USAID and WHO, of working to achieve the "genocide" of the Russian nation (Planirovanie 1999). There has also been ample street-level activity to thwart educational outreach efforts. In 1997, the Ministry of Public Health and the Russian Family Planning Association attempted a joint project to offer "counseling and assistance" in family planning through a mobile unit, aiming to teach Muscovites who were reluctant to go to a doctor about safe sex and contraceptives. On its very first stop, a group of women activists from the Russian Orthodox Women's Union boarded the streetcar and aggressively asserted that abortion should be banned, birth control was impermissible, and accused the Ministry of Public Health of corrupting minors. Protestors pelted the streetcar with an egg and sprayed graffiti on it (Kolomeiskaya 1997). Galvanized by these early events, nationalist, Orthodox opposition groups increased their use of physical violence. In one example, a Russia-wide, right wing organization called Word and Deed, set up "mobile units" of "warriors" to physically attack forms of "depravity" on the street level, including sex education classes in schools. It advertised its activism and encouraged public support in the newspaper, Russky vestnik, with the following call to arms: "Russian Orthodox believers! If you have witnessed an assault on sacred Orthodox values, if promoters of depravity with their "sex education"… suddenly appear at your school, call our pager number right away. A Word and Deed rapid-reaction group will go to the address you give us and stop the corrupters and perverts!"

Reporting on this agenda and one such attack in Moscow, a journalist from the mainstream newspaper, *Izvestia*, noted that finding the right wing publication had been difficult, and was told it was one of a number of so-called patriotic publications sold only by licensed vendors. Interestingly, the group not only has no fear of the police, but also apparently sees them as allies. When the rapid-reaction group of "warriors" burst into the sex education class, they demanded that the lesson stop and that the police be called. They then proceeded to beat the teacher conducting the class (Nekrasov 1999).

Such efforts had direct effects on the work of the Russian Family Planning Association. In the spring of 1997, a public committee called "For the Moral Regeneration of the Fatherland" sponsored by the Russian Orthodox Church, working in collaboration with the nationalist activists, submitted to the Duma batches of signed petitions asking the government to rescind funding for family planning. The Duma made the topic the subject of a roundtable discussion on "Family Planning in the Context of Russia's National Security" and consequently voted to end funding of its presidential family planning program that had been established in the early 1990s. The funding and moral support of this program has not been re-instituted (Babasyan 1999). One pilot program in sexuality education sponsored by UNESCO was targeted with vociferous protest by nationalist opponents, who depicted the project as a foreign conspiracy to pervert Russian children and promote the nation's depopulation (Baidan 1999). Their success in derailing the UNESCO project inspired more attacks and has led to the widespread de-legitimation of sex education. Projects I observed in 1994–95 in St. Petersburg were no longer offered by 2000, their supporters unable to withstand pressure from critics and public protest. The problems the RFPA and other organizations had set out to resolve – the high abortion rate, falling fertility, and infertility – had been transformed by nationalists into problems *created by* family planning services themselves. And in a move common to anti-abortion and pro-natal groups worldwide, they defined contraceptives not as a means to sustain women's health and fertility, but as a means of limiting births that would, they assumed, otherwise occur (Ginsburg 1989; Luker 1984).

In other ways, too, conservatives have gained ground. Politicians, Orthodox Church leaders, and nationalist activists have appropriated the language of global abortion opponents, defining abortion as the "murder" of an "unborn child." For example, in 2002 Duma representative Aleksandr Chuev, from the party Edinstvo, prepared a bill for the lower house of Parliament entitled "On the Introduction of Changes in Legislative Acts of the Russian Federation to Defend the Lives of Unborn Children." It sought to eliminate all abortions on the basis of "social reasons"

(Demoscope Weekly, 2 of 4). The Russian press also regularly uses such language, in what represents an entirely new framing of the procedure from Soviet era times, when the official policy of atheism precluded imagining the fetus as having a soul. As nationalism melded to religious revivalism conspires to portray fetuses as Russian persons, there is virtually no counter-discourse challenging these conceptions. Gradually, they have succeeded both in linking reproductive freedoms to national vulnerability, and in rendering abortion illegitimate.

An important aspect of this process, and one that I would argue enabled it to gain legitimacy, was that reproductive politics initially began without directly attacking abortion. Conservatives instead strove to de-legitimize the new programs in family planning and sexuality education, which could be portrayed as post-Soviet imports, clearly identified with the West, and morally ambiguous (Rivkin-Fish 2005). When they did introduce bills to restrict women's access to abortion, they first tended to do so surreptitiously, by burying the abortion issue within broader legislation concerning "bioethics," or the "protection of mothers and children" (Bateneva 1998; Ballaeva 1998), since criminalization had minimal public support. These bills failed to pass into laws, but the circumstances of their existence even as proposals proved telling: they generated no public outcry and garnered little serious attention at all. With such tepid public interest in political campaigns against abortion, the Ministry of Public Health apparently felt unconcerned that any negative fallout would ensue from its 2003 decision to substantially reduce the social criteria enabling women to access abortion in the second trimester. On the contrary, it may even have expected this move to be politically expedient, demonstrating support for conservative and nationalist parties on the eve of elections to the Russian Parliament (Duma).

Conclusion: The Paradoxical Lack of Opposition

The Russian Family Planning Association, which enjoys ties to the global reproductive rights movement, does not publicly oppose the symbolic de-legitimation of abortion; nor does it actively promote the issue of reproductive "rights." This reticence, shared with the majority of family planning practitioners throughout the country (Ballaeva 1998), stems from several factors: the resounding societal consensus that low fertility is a grave problem for the nation; the widespread success of pro-natalist coalitions to cast suspicion on the benefits of family planning programs for Russia's vitality given their close ties to the West; and the support family planning practitioners themselves express for strengthening the moral standing of families, rather than promoting "women's rights." The absence of a feminist perspective was strikingly evident in the response of Inga Gribesheva, director of the RFPA, to the recent second trimester restrictions. The *New York Times* reported that Gribesheva said that the restrictions would not greatly affect women's access to abortion and were mainly of concern due to the possibility that they would further invigorate conservative coalitions. It is curious that she minimized the strain these restrictions will place on some Russian women. One might expect organizations devoted to women's reproductive

health and rights to highlight the ways severe poverty compounds women's struggles to care for themselves and their families, and to counter the Ministry's claims
that restricting late abortion will achieve the necessary goal of "increasing women's
responsibility for their health." Yet women's groups and family planning organizations have been, paradoxically, rather unengaged in the task of defending Russian
women's reproductive rights. There are several reasons why this is so.

To some extent, this lack of an active opposition can be explained by the fact that
criminalization has not been seriously debated in the Russian public, and is thus
widely perceived as politically unlikely given the widely remembered tragedies of
the Stalin era (Borisov, Sinelnikov, and Arkhangelsky 1997). The recent proposals by
conservative politicians to ban abortion for social reasons have been disregarded as
the unrealistic attempts of extremists – although Gribesheva, at least, no longer sees
these as idle threats. Another reason for the lack of a feminist challenge to reproductive politics stems from the pragmatic difficulties organizations face. Russian wom-
en's groups work with extremely strained energies and resources. This situation has
led them to devote their efforts to women's practical and economic survival needs,
rather than on apparently more abstract issues such as reproductive autonomy
(Sperling 1999; Hemment 2000). Immanent economic crises of daily life have taken
precedence over what seems to be less immediately threatening and longer-range
struggles, such as the defense of reproductive rights and access to abortion and contraception. But even in this light, the lack of outcry over second trimester restrictions is paradoxical, for it is the poorest, least educated, most marginalized groups
of women whom these restrictions will mainly affect – sectors of society that many
women's groups around the world have felt strongly committed to representing.

I would also like to suggest that Russian women's avoidance of reproductive politics may represent an effect of the thorough hegemony achieved by pro-natalism. In a
context where citizenship is increasingly coming to be defined on the basis of ethno-
national identity, and many view the biogenetic substance of the ethno-nation at risk,
defending reproductive rights undoubtedly carries risks of appearing to oppose the
very survival of "the Russian nation." Claims that women have the "right to choose"
to reject childbearing could leave women's groups vulnerable to charges of national
betrayal, of working in concert with foreign interests against the nation. Even family
planning services in Russia represent themselves as strengthening women's reproductive health and family life, never as defending the right to abortion. As nationalists and others engage in reproductive politics to save the Russian "gene pool" from
extinction, they place the burden of national survival largely on women's childbearing and maternal obligations. Finding the means to counter these links while affirming support for national vitality remains an unresolved challenge.

Notes

1 For details on social welfare benefits intended to promote and fertility and family life, see Desfosses
   1981; Zakharov and Ivanova 1996; Jones and Grupp 1987, 275; Zakharov 1999.
2 Rasporiazhenie Pravitel'stva Rossiiskoi Federatsii 17-01-1992; Takunov 1996.

3   On efforts to restrict abortion in Eastern Europe and Germany, see Wolchik 2000; Funk 1996; Gal 2000, 16; Maleck-Lewy and Marx Feree 2000; Dölling, Hahn, and Scholz 2000.
4   Naselenie 2002, 36. For comparative figures, in 1995 Italy had a TFR of 1.17, Japan 1.42, and Denmark 1.80. Zakharov 1999, 44.

References

Alan Guttmacher Institute. 2000. *AGI Readings on Induced Abortion: A World Review 2000.*

Aleksandrovna Mishle, Nadezhda. 1998. *Iuridicheskii spravochnik: zhenshchiny i deti: semeinoe pravo, trudovoe pravo, sotsial'nye l'goty.* Moscow: Filin'.

Alekseyeva, Oksana. 2002. Yuri Shevchenko assumes responsibility for Pregnancy. *Kommersant,* October 16: 7. Reprinted in CDPSP 54 no. 42 2002, 14–15.

Antonov, Anatolii I. 1980. *Sotsiologiia rozhdaemosti: Teoreticheskie i metodologicheskie problemy.* Moscow.

Antonov, Anatolii I. 1982. *Sem'ia i deti.* Moscow: Izdatel'stvo Moskovskogo Universiteta.

Antonov, Anatolii I. 1986. *Demograficheskoe povedenie i vozmozhnosti sotsialnogo vozdeistviia na nego v usloviakh sotsializma: po materialam mezhdunarodnoi nauchno-prakticheskoi konferentsii v Vilniuse, 1985 g.* Moscow: Akademiia nauk SSSR Intitut sotsiologicheskikh issledovanii.

Antonov, Anatolii I. 1995. Sem'ia kak institut sredi drugikh sotsial'nykh institutov. In A. I. Antonov and V. V. Negodin (eds.) *Sem'ia na poroge tret'ego tysiacheletiia:* 182–198. Moscow: Institut sotsiologii Rossiiskoi Akademii Nauk, Tsentr obshchechelovecheskikh tsennostei.

Antonov, Anatolii I., and V. M. Medkov. 1987. *Vtoroi Rebenok.* Moscow: Mysl'.

Attwood, Lynne. 1990. *The New Soviet Man and Woman: Sex Role Socialization in the USSR.* London: MacMillan in association with the Centre for Russian and East European Studies, U of Birmingham.

Baban, Adriana. 2000. Women's Sexuality and Reproductive Behavior in Post-Ceausescu Romania: A Psychological Approach. In Susan Gal and Gail Kligman (eds.) *Reproducing Gender: Politics, Publics, and Everyday Life after Socialism:* 225–255. Princeton, NJ: Princeton UP.

Babasyan, Natalya. 1999. Freedom or "Life": Secular and Russian Orthodox Organizations Unite in a Struggle Against Reproductive Freedom for Women. *Izvestia,* 26 Feb.: 5. Reprinted in CDPSP, vol. 51, no. 12: 4, 6.

Baidan, Natalia. 1999. You Have to Save up to Have a Baby. *Vremia MN,* August 24: 3, cited in CDPSP 51/36: 16–17.

Ballaeva, E. A. 1998. *Gendernaia ekspertiza zakonodatel'stva RF: reproduktivnye prava zhenshchin v Rossii.* Moscow: Proekt gendernaia ekspertiza MTSGI (Moscow Center for Gender Studies).

Bassom, Ann. 1999. The Russian Press: Coverage of Women's Health. In Vicki L. Hesli and Margaret H. Mills (eds.) *Medical Issues and Health Care Reform in Russia:* 233–263. Lewiston, NY: The Edwin Mellen Press.

Bateneva, Tat'iana. 1998. Nevezhestvo pod vidom bioetiki. *Izvestiia*, October 13: 1, 7.

Borisov, Vladimir, Alexander Sinelnikov, and Vladimir Arkhangelsky. 1997. Expert Opinions on Abortion in Russia. *Choices* 26, no. 2: 23–26.

Borneman, John. 1992. *Belonging in the Two Berlins: Kin, State, Nation,* Cambridge studies in social and cultural anthropology. New York: Cambridge UP.

Brubaker, Roger. 1992. *Citizenship and Nationhood in France and Germany.* Cambridge: Harvard UP.

Daskalova, Krassimira. 2000. Women's Problems, Women's Discourses in Bulgaria. In Susan Gal and Gail Kligman (eds.) *Reproducing Gender: Politics, Publics, and Everyday Life after Socialism*: 337–369. Princeton: Princeton UP.

De Soto, Hermine G. 1994. 'In The Name Of The Folk': Women and Nation in the New Germany. *UCLA Women's Law Journal* 5, no. 1: 83–102.

Demoscope Weekly. 2003. Elektronnaia versiia biulletenia Naselenie I obshchestvo, Tsentr demografii I ekologii cheloveka Instituta narodnokhoziaistvennogo prognozirovaniia RAN No.123–124, 25 August–7 September. www.demoscope. ru 2 of 5.

Derzhavina, Olga. 1998. Russia has 100 Years to Live: The Country is Experiencing an Unprecedented Crisis. *Segodnya*, Dec. 7, 1–2. Reprinted in CDPSP, vol. 50, no. 49, 16.

Desfosses, Helen. 1976. Demography, Ideology, and Politics in the USSR. *Soviet Studies* 28, no. 2: 244–56.

Desfosses, Helen. 1981. Pro-Natalism in Soviet Law and Propaganda. In Helen Desfosses (ed.) *Soviet Population Policy: Conflicts and Constraints*: 95–123. NY: Pergamon Press.

Dölling, Irene, Daphne Hahn, and Sylka Scholz. 2000. Birth Strike in the New Federal States: Is Sterilization an Act of Resistance? In Susan Gal and Gail Kligman *The Politics of Gender After Socialism*: 118–147. Princeton.

Eberts, Mirella W. 1998. The Roman Catholic Church and Democracy in Poland. *Europe-Asia Studies* 50, no. 5: 81–87.

Feshbach, Murray. 2001. Russia's Population Meltdown. Wilson Quarterly 25 1/ Winter: 15–21.

Field, Deborah Ann. 1996. *Communist Morality and Meanings of Private Life in Post-Stalinist*. PhD thesis, Princeton U.

Field, Mark G. 1995. The Health Crisis in the Former Soviet Union: A Report from the "Post-War" Zone. *Social Science and Medicine* 41 11/1995: 1469–1478.

Finer, Lawrence B., and Stanley K. Henshaw. 2003. Abortion Incidence and Services in the US in 2000. *Perspectives on Sexual and Reproductive Health* 35, no.1: 6–15.

Funk, Nanette. 1996. The Status of Women in New Market Economies: Abortion Counseling and the 1995 German Abortion Law. *Connecticut Journal of International Law* 12: 33–42.

Fuszara, Malgorzata. 1993. Abortion and the Formation of the Public Sphere in Poland. In Nanette Funk and Magda Mueller (eds.) *Gender Politics and Post-Communism: Reflections from Eastern Europe and the Former Soviet Union*: 241–252. New York: Routledge.

Gal, Susan, and Gail Kligman. 2000. *The Politics of Gender After Socialism*. Princeton: Princeton UP.

Gal, Susan. 1994. Gender in the Post-Socialist Transition: The Abortion Debate in Hungary. *East European Politics and Societies* 8, no. 2: 256–286.

Gal, Susan. 2000. Gender in the Post-Socialist Transition. In Gal and Kligman *The Politics of Gender After Socialism*: 16. Princeton: Princeton UP.

Ginsburg, Faye D., and Rayna Rapp. 1995. *Conceiving the New World Order: The Global Politics of Reproduction*. Berkeley: U of California P.

Ginsburg, Faye. 1989. *Contested Lives: The Abortion Debate in an American Community*. Berkeley: U California Press.

Goble, Paul. 2001. *Russia: Analysis from Washington – A Demographic Threat To Russian Security* (Radio Free Europe/Radio Liberty, Feb. 16 [cited 10/4/01]), available from http://www.rferl.org/nca/features/2001/02/16022001105257.asp.

Goldman, Wendy Z. 1993. *Women, The State, and Revolution: Soviet Family Policy and Social Life, 1917–1936*. New York: Cambridge UP.

Gross Solomon, Susan. 1992. The Demographic Argument in Soviet Debates over the Legalization of Abortion in the 1920s. *Cahiers du Monde Russe et Soviétique* 33, no. 1: 59–82.

Hemment, Julie Dawn. 2000. *Gender, NGOs and the Third Sector in Russia: An Ethnography of Post-Socialist Civil Society* (Ph.D. thesis, Cornell U).

Herzfeld, Michael. 1992. *The Social Production of Indifference: Exploring the Symbolic Roots of Western Bureaucracy*. Chicago: University of Chicago Press.

Hyer, Janet. 1996. Managing the Female Organism: Doctors and the Medicalization of Women's Paid Work in Soviet Russia During the 1920s. In Rosalind J Marsh (ed.) *Women in Russia and Ukraine*: 111–120. New York: Cambridge UP.

Jones, Ellen, and Fred W. Grupp. 1987. *Modernization, Value Change and Fertility in the Soviet Union*. Cambridge: Cambridge UP.

Kak delat' detei, Peterburg znaet. No ne mozhet. *Delovoi Peterburg*, 22 June 2000, 8–9.

Khorev, Boris. 1995. Rynok: podi pri nem rodi … *Pravda*, March 30: 1–2.

Khramchikhin, Aleksandr. 2002. *Vremya* MN October 3: 6, accessed on September 11, 2003, on www.ipma.ru/publikazii/etnosotn/252.html.

Kligman, Gail. 1998. *The Politics of Duplicity: Controlling Reproduction in Ceausescu's Romania*. Berkeley: U of California P.

Kolomeiskaya, Inna. 1997. "Intimate Desire's" Journey Turns out to be Short – Radical-Minded "Mothers Foil Family Planning". *Sevodnya*, November 26. Reprinted in CDPSP, vol. XLIV, no. 47: 19–20.

Kon, Igor S. 1995. *The Sexual Revolution in Russia*. New York: The Free Press.

Kostyukovsky, Victor. 2002. "Garden Variety" Fascism. *Noviye Izvestiia*, September 17: 1–5. Reprinted in CDPSP 54, no. 38: 10–11.

Krasnopol'skaia, Irina. 2003. Novye zhertvy aborta. *Rossiiskaia Gazeta*, 12 July. Reprinted in *Demoscope Weekly*, 3 of 4.

Kuznetsova, Larisa. 1989. Glazami Zhenshchiny. *Novoe Vremia*: 33–35.

Kvasha, Aleksandr I. Akovlevich. 1981. *Demograficheskaia politika v SSSR*. Moscow.

Lepina, Marina. 2002. Krasnoarmeisk Residents are trying to drive out Armenians. *Kommersant*. July 13, 1–4. Reprinted in CDPSP 54, no. 28: 1.

Lorimer, Frank. *The Population of the Soviet Union: History and Prospects* (Geneva: League of Nations, 1946). Cited in Popov and David *Russian Federation and USSR Successor States*, 238.

Luker, Kristin. 1984. *Abortion and the Politics of Motherhood*. Berkeley: University of California Press.

Maleck-Lewy, Ewa, and Myra Marx Feree. 2000. Talking about Women and Wombs: The Discourse of Abortion and Reproductive Rights in the GDR during and after the *Wende*. In Susan Gal and Gail Kligman *The Politics of Gender After Socialism*: 92–117. Princeton.

Massell, Gregory J. 1974. *The Surrogate Proletariat: Moslem Women and Revolutionary Strategies in Soviet Central Asia, 1919–1929*. Princeton, N.J.: Princeton UP.

Medvedeva, Irina, and Tat'iana Shishova. 2000. Demograficheskaia voina protiv Rossii. *Nash Sovremennik*, no. 1.

Molodtsova, Viktoria. 1999a. Public Sin is Getting Thunderous Applause. *Rossiskaya gazeta*, Oct. 22: 25.

Molodtsova, Viktoria. 1999b. Seks: Razvrashchenie vmeste prosveshcheniia. *Rossiiskaya gazeta*, June 26: 8. Reprinted in CDPSP vol. 51 no. 24: 14–15.

Naselenie Rossii 1998. 1999. Moscow: Institut Narodnokhoziaistvennogo prognozirovaniia RAN Tsentr demografii i ekologii cheloveka.

Naselenie Rossii 1999. 2000. Moscow: Institut Narodnokhoziaistvennogo prognozirovaniia RAN Tsentr demografii i ekologii cheloveka.

Naselenie Rossii 2001. 2002. Moscow: Institut Narodnokhoziaistvennogo prognozirovaniia RAN Tsentr demografii i ekologii cheloveka.

Nekrasov, Andrei. 1999. Warriors Against Depravity. *Izvestia*, March 25: 5. Reprinted in CDPSP, vol.51, no.13: 22.

Perevedentsev, Victor. 1968. Continuation of a Controversy. *Literaturnaia Gazeta*, 12th March: 11. Reprinted in CDPSP 20/12.

Peterson, Nadya L. 1996. Dirty Women: Cultural Connotations of Cleanliness in Soviet Russia. In Helena Goscilo and Beth Holmgren (eds.) *Russia, Women, Culture*: 177–208. Bloomington: Indiana UP.

Piskunov, V. P., and V. C. Steshenko. 1974. O demograficheskoi politike sotsialisticheskogo obshchestva. In V. C. Steshenko and V. P. Piskunov (eds.) *Demograficheskaia politika*: 15–27. Moscow: Statistika.

Planirovanie nebytiia. 1999. *Novaia Gazeta*, August 30–September 5: 1.

Popov, Andrej, and Henry David. 1999. Russian Federation and USSR Successor States. In Henry David (ed.) *From Abortion to Contraception: A Resource to Public Policies and Reproductive Behavior in Central and Eastern Europe from 1917 to the Present*: 223–277. Westport, CT: Greenwood Press.

Posadskaia, Anastasia I. 1992. Tendentsii izmeneniia zakonodatel'stva v oblasti sotsial'noi zashchity materinstva. In Zoya A. Khotkina (ed.) *Zhenshchiny i sotsial'naia politika: gendernyi aspekt*: 79–88. Moscow: Institut sotsial'no-ekonomicheskikh problem narodonaseleniia.

Remmenick, Larissa I. 1991. Epidemiology and Determinants of Induced Abortion in the USSR. *Social Science and Medicine* 33, no. 7: 841–848.

RIA Novosti. 2003. 21 August, reprinted in *Demoscope Weekly*, no.123–124, 4 of 9.

Ries, Nancy. 1997. *Russian Talk: Culture and Conversation During Perestroika*. Ithaca: Cornell UP.

Rivkin-Fish, Michele. 1999. Sexuality Education in Russia: Defining Pleasure and Danger for a Fledgling Democratic Society. *Social Science and Medicine* 49: 801–814.

Rivkin-Fish, Michele. 2003. Anthropology, Demography, and the Search for a Critical Analysis of Fertility: Insights from Russia. *American Anthropologist* 105, no. 2: 289–301.

Rivkin-Fish, Michele. 2005. Moral Science and the Management of "Sexual Revolution" in Russia. In Vincanne Adams and Stacy Pigg (eds.) *The Moral Object of Sex*. Durham: Duke University Press

Rotkevich, Yelena. 2002. For the first time, St. Petersburg Police Admit Existence of Skinhead Gangs. *Izvestia*, September 18: 3. Reprinted in CDPSP 54, no. 38: 11.

Russia Faces Nationalities Question. Are Immigrants a Good Thing, or Fuel for an Ethnic Bonfire? 2002. *Vremya novostei*, Aug. 30: 1, 4. Reprinted in CDPSP 54, no. 36, 4–6.

Russian Rights Groups to Monitor Racism. 2003. *Associated Press*, September 18. Reprinted on Johnson's Russia List #7330, 19 September 2003 #1.

Santana, Rebecca. 2003. Mixed Marriages make Moscow a melting pot. Some Russian fear minorities' growth. *Atlanta Journal and Constitution* August 24. Reprinted on Johnson's Russia List #7198 25 August 2003 #6.

Semenov, S. S. 1996. Ostanovit' vymiranie natsii. *Izvestiia*, 13 September.

Shumilin, Vadim. 2000. Russians are Leaving the Volga. Change in Ethnic Balance is an Extremely Painful Process. *Nezavisimaya gazeta*, 5 Sept.: 9, 11. Reprinted in CDPSP, vol. 52, no. 36, 13.

Sperling, Valerie. 1999. *Organizing Women in Contemporary Russia: Engendering Transition*. Cambridge: Cambridge UP.

Stoliarenko, Liudmila. 2000. Roddoma Rossii vypolniaiut plan! *Novaia gazeta*, November: 23–26.

Sukhaya, Svetlana. 2002. Distressing Diagnosis – Health Problems Plague More Than Half of Russia's Children. *Trud* October 18: 1. Reprinted in CDPSP 54, no. 16: 18–19.

Sukhov, Ivan. 2002. Moscow-style deportations. *Vremya Novostei*, September 17: 1. Reprinted in CDPSP 54, no. 38: 14.

Timashova, Natal'ia. 2003. Novye Izvestiia, 19 August, reprinted in *Demoscope Weekly*, No. 123–124, 3 of 44.

Tselms, Georgy. 2002. Building Fascism in a Single Region. *Noviye Izvestia* July 12: 1–2. Reprinted in CDPSP 54, no. 28: 11–12.

Verdery, Katherine. 1994. From Parent-State to Family Patriarchs: Gender and Nation in Contemporary Eastern Europe. *Eastern European Politics and Societies* 8, no. 2: 225–255.

Verdery, Katherine. 1996. *What Was Socialism, and What Comes Next?* Princeton: Princeton University Press.

Vishnevskii, Anatolii G. (ed.). 2002. *Naselenie Rossii 2001: Deviatyi ezhegodnyi demograficheskii doklad.* Moscow: Institut narodnogo khoziaistvennogo prognozirovaniia Tsentr demografii i ekologii cheloveka.

Volkov, A. G. 1986. *Sem'ia – Ob'ekt Demografii.* Moscow: Mysl'.

Warshofsky Lapidus, Gail. 1978. *Women in Soviet Society: Equality, Development, and Social Change.* Berkeley: U of California P.

Wolchik, Sharon. 2000. Reproductive Policies in the Czech and Slovak Republics. In Susan Gal and Gail Kligman *The Politics of Gender After Socialism*: 35–91. Princeton.

Zakharov, Sergei V. 1999. Fertility, Nuptiality, and Family Planning in Russia: Problems and Prospects. In George J. Demko, Grigory Ioffe, and Zhanna Zayonchkovskaya (eds.) *Population Under Duress: The Geodemography of Post-Soviet Russia*: 41–58. Boulder, CO: Westview Press.

Zakharov, Sergei V., and Elena I. Ivanova. 1996. Fertility Decline and Recent Changes in Russia: On the Threshold of the Second Demographic Transition. In Julie DaVanzo (ed.) *Russia's Demographic 'Crisis'*: 36–82. Santa Monica, CA: RAND.

Maria Mesner

Mother-Families, Family Mothers.
Policies on Having Children in Austria

At the start of the 21st century, family policies and support for families have become issues of major political controversy in Austria. The trigger was the introduction of a new child care allowance on the 1st of January 2002. The political context implies that this move also has a high symbolic value from the perspectives of those both in favour and against the allowance. Another point of contention is how the gender relations in Austria are to be arranged in future. Participants on both sides of the conflict accept that politicians at the national level have an important role to play in this matter. The debate revolves around which gender model the politicians favour, or should give preference to. In this paper, I will investigate whether the child care allowance really does represent a new change of course in Austrian reproduction policy in a historical context, or whether it is simply an extension of an already generous – by international standards – and costly family support policy. I am especially interested in the normative perceptions of family concepts and models which shape the legal norms which, in turn, determine (and have already determined) family forms and the gender norms closely associated with them, either explicitly or implicitly.

In order to trace these perceptions, I will investigate the reproductive arrangements of political drafts and concepts which serve as both basis and objective. Here, the term "reproductive arrangements" is intended to imply the social surroundings in which reproduction should take place in accordance with each of the concepts. I could call the social form I am interested in here by its common term: "family", but would then have to question which "family" Austrian social policy wants to support. The word "family policy" does not seem neutral enough to me. The object of support, the desired standard norm, hides behind the technical term. From a historical perspective "family" does not indeed mean every private form of long-term cohabitation, but a specific heterosexual relationship. For most of the 20th century, it meant a group represented by a married couple and their children, usually associated implicitly with a gender-specific division of work where the private, reproductive and care aspects tend to be the women's responsibility, and public, productive, earning tasks belong more to the men.

So when I investigate the "reproductive arrangements" that characterise Austrian reproductive policies, it is not just the child care allowance that needs to be taken into consideration, but also the private division of work between men and women with regard to looking after children, and the division of public and private tasks. In order to make my interpretation easier to follow, I will start by outlining the key characteristics of the central policies and structures from a historical point of view in chronological order. In addition to direct transfer, this also concerns those who, in close connection with the transfer, have an opportunity to temporarily suspend employment in favour of reproductive tasks, i.e. the formulation of the intersection of work and reproduction, and the availability and financing of child care facilities.

"Family Policy" as an Innovation

Policies concerning people who have commitments to caring for children have been grouped together under the term "Family policies" in Austria since the middle of last century. As a new area of policy-making and a new concept – in relation to Austria – this happened in the 1950s. At that time the "family" became an object of support for national politics. There had been support provided for families between the world wars, but only for those in need, and in that form, it had been more of a "policy for the poor". Now "families" had become the recipients of public welfare, regardless of whether they were in need of financial assistance or not; the important thing was that children were to be taken care of.

Until that point, all allowances had been limited to people in need, and were intended to stem basic existence-threatening poverty. The one exception was the "marriage grant" introduced by the National Socialists. The intent was to increase the birth rate by means of financial support. However, only "proper" births were rewarded: the parents had to be "German", "Arian" and "genetically healthy". Whoever did not fit the bill ran the risk of being caught in the National Socialists' death machine, along with all their descendants.

Upon investigation of the prime movers in the field of family policy, it becomes clear that many of the policies defined later as family policy benefits actually stem from the area of social and labour protection policy. Since the end of the 19th century, these policies have been determined by several protagonists: Catholic social and Christian social doctrines advocated a policy which did not envision mothers going to work. The resulting clamour, which arose again and again, for a "family wage" was destined for failure as early as the 19th century due to the monarchy's lack of financial power (Grandner 1995, 169). Even during the period between the wars and then after the Second World War, wages and salaries for the masses in Austria were never high enough to support a family. Despite this, the Christian Socialists, and later the Austria People's Party, argued in favour of separating employment and reproduction. Working mothers were regarded as undesirable in this concept of society.

Compare that to the trade unions dominated by the Social Democratic party, which took an ambivalent stance regarding women at work, because it was not possible for them to coordinate the social democratic equality rule, the patriarchal attitude of trade unions dominated by men, and the fear of a cheap female workforce. Calls for equality and those advocating special action for women – either regarding gender, as in night shift prohibition, or regarding legal protection for expectant mothers and maternity leave – stood in opposition to each other. After the founding of the Frauen-Reichskomités by the Social Democratic party, gender-specific laws were heavily debated among Social Democrats, whereas in previous years the functionaries had simply demanded that such measures be implemented. At the Brünn Parteitag in 1899, the Social Democrats no longer insisted on a maximum working day of eight hours "no clauses and no exceptions" (Parteitag, 4), but also a free Saturday afternoon for working women in which they could catch up with their reproductive tasks (Parteitag, 13) – a request that can also be interpreted as acceptance of this division of roles. After the turn of the century, demographic po-litical aspects debated by the Social Democratic women's movement started to gain significance both in quantity and quality. One reason for this was gender-specific protection laws for women in general: "Because if women are protected before they become mothers then an important step has been taken to halt the degeneration of humanity." (Freundlich 1908, 40). Another reason was the special protection and support afforded to expectant and nursing mothers. Labour protection laws "are not there to protect women, they are there to protect mothers. Women have to perform the most important function in society; they have to bring the next generation into the world. The development of the people and humanity depends on the health and energy that these newborn children bring with them. In this, not only women, not only the working community, but the whole of humanity have an interest." That is why maternity leave and maternity bonuses needed to be intro-duced (Freundlich 1913, 11).

Even the civil liberal women's movement did not agree on a strict egalitarian argument that would have meant equal participation for women in employment (Grandner 1995, 174). Consequently, the gender-neutral treatment of workers (at a very low level) became a hegemonic issue only during a very short phase of the liberalisation of the economy in the second half of the 19th century. The political debate was subsequently dominated by discussions of the justification for protect-ing the rights of women in employment.

When, in the 1950s, "family policy" became established as a new area of policy making – the post-war coalition between the Catholic-conservative ÖVP and the Social-Democratic SPÖ had been in power since 1947 – certain already familiar claims were made, and existing policies were expanded and extended.

Consequently – as a modification of the previous nutrition allowance for fami-lies in need – from 1950 onwards, a child allowance was paid regardless of the social status of the parents. After 1954, the allowances were staggered according to the number of children; the more children a person had to care for, the higher the child allowance was – not as an absolute figure, but also per child. The support provided by the state was therefore higher for the third child, for example, than for the first born. In 1956, one-off payments were introduced for each birth. At around the same time, there was an extension of the legal regulations that were meant to guarantee the principle compatibility of employment and reproduction work from a gender-specific, i.e. women-specific, point of view. At the end of the 1950s, Aus-tria was "within the circle of western industrialised countries, the country with the most generous maternal protection regulations" (Neyer 1990, 41).

The social background for these measures and their political legitimisation was a medial, omni-present downturn in the number of births, which was perceived across the political spectrum as a "serious problem" (see for example "Paragraph 144", 1953). Financial support of families to increase the birth rate was meant to be the answer to this "problem". In the beginning, Austrian family policies were clearly "pro-natal". The idea was to support the small family as the only model from the point of view of the organization of reproduction within society. Lifestyles deviating from this norm – in contrast to the period between the wars, during which individual society-changing movements were represented within Austrian social democracy – no longer needed to be taken into consideration (Thurner 1992, 7).

If this form of family policy is viewed in relation to its effect on the constitution of gender relations, it can be deduced that it was neither intended nor able to change the division of work between the genders. Mothers were thought to be responsible for looking after the children, and were, at best, supported by child-care facilities which were insufficient for women in employment, or by female friends and relatives. Such a reproductive arrangement was result of a compromise of Catholic-conservative and Social-Democratic gender concepts and demographic policies.

In both the configuration of the financial support, and the development of legislation, the order of priorities indicates the relationship between employment and child care duties (for women). After the first petitions for a new "Austrian" maternity law were presented to parliament in 1952[1] and 1953[2], the law was passed in 1957, and contained the following key rules:

Work was absolutely forbidden during the six weeks prior to the expected delivery date. Expectant and nursing mothers were forbidden to work overtime, night shifts, Sundays and national holidays. Dismissal and lay-off protection laws were extended and maternity leave was introduced. The law also decreed that those concerned should not suffer a loss of income due to the working restrictions. Furthermore, nursing periods were to be granted for employees. There was a 100 percent income allowance for the period that work was prohibited before and after the birth.[3]

Maternity leave, which was limited to six months if the right to return to the place of work was to be retained, remained unpaid until 1961. In this year maternity leave was extended by one year and an income allowance was introduced, although it amounted to significantly less than an earned income[4].

The politicians maintained that women who were not financially well-off had not taken the opportunity to be temporarily away from work, because they could not afford the loss in wages. Social-Democratic politicians in particular justified giving state support to women who gave up employment to take care of their children by invoking the "Volksgesundheit" (meaning: the people's health).

With the introduction of maternity leave and partial income compensation, a critical political decision had been made in favour of family-oriented, i.e. mother-oriented, child care. To underline this connection, the relevance of the maternity allowance was to ensure that the woman lived in a joint household with her child and cared for the child more or less on her own. The setting of priorities in favour of an at least temporary "sole wage earner/housewife arrangement" was also clear from one significant detail: unlike its National Socialist predecessor, the Austrian maternity protection law included no obligatory provision of public child care facilities. This political decree did not represent a deviation from conventional everyday reproductive arrangements however; it simply strengthened, supported and rewarded practices that were already largely widespread and established.

That the law providing protection against dismissal and a relatively safe opportunity to leave a place of work when a child was born would lead to a gender-specific disadvantage on the job market was a valid argument in the debate when the resolution was passed: "Some businesses will think twice before they employ a married woman. They present the highest risk of an important post becoming vacant." This argument was advanced by trade and industry representatives (who could not be called feminists).[5]

Observing the participants in the political decision-making process, one can see that the main parties – i.e. both the ÖVP and SPÖ – exercised their function as gate keepers to the political agenda in a kind of monopoly, and became the only transmission belt (Ebbighausen 1976, 26) between the interests of social groups and the national executive and legislative branches of the state. Political representation for women existed only within these parties because the tradition of an autonomous women's organisation was in tatters after the effects of fascism.

In fact, the extension of maternal protection was borne by a wide political consensus which covered, and largely suppressed, a very wide range of gender forms and norms. In the political culture of the post-war coalition based on political consensus, maternity leave and the maternity allowance represented an acceptable compromise for everybody: employment and child care were separated, at least temporarily, which was to be regarded by ÖVP politicians and supporters as a concession to sole wage earner/housewife families. "Employment away from the home for married women as a popular phenomenon is an undesirable situation", stated Christian-Conservative politicians (of both sexes) in the first bid for an "Austrian maternal protection law" in 1948, and this represented an unmistakable continuity of the Christian-Social attitude before the war.[6] During the debates in parliament on the law, even Grete Rehor, a Christian trade unionist and one of the initiators of the new law, suggested that there would have to be "urgent reasons" for a "married woman and mother" to have to consider "working outside the home". The order of priorities in the conception of women's life plans was made clear: "After all, these women have preserved their most valuable characteristic and readiness, to become a natural mother [...]."[7] Maternity leave was provided in the service of a national issue: "If maternity leave enables us to bring the mother so close to the child that every child grows up to be a harmonious person, then we have not inflicted a sacrifice on the economy; instead we have done our people a great service, since society needs harmonious and well-balanced people in order to survive."[8]

Rehor's speech presumed a reproductive arrangement centred on the natural mother caring for her own child, which became a pivot point of collective well-being.

Social Democrats, on the other hand, believed that pregnant women and working mothers would be protected from the damaging effects of employment, so that even working class children could now be born into "healthy" families and grow up at home. As already mentioned, Social-Democratic women (the gender-specific division of political subject areas is noticeable, affecting public representation rather than decision-making) argued in terms of "Volksgesundheit" and demographic policy. They drew attention to higher premature birth and infant mortality rates among working women.[9] Female employment was indisputably part and parcel of the Social-Democratic concept for society, although this often took a back seat to reproductive tasks. Giving exclusively non-self-employed women the opportunity to interrupt their employment was part of the Social-Democratic advancement scenario, in which the gender-specific position of individuals within the work process, even when based on the allocation of reproductive tasks, was not yet an issue.

There is one notable exception outside the 1950s and 1960s period which should be mentioned: in 1969, under a Catholic-Conservative, non-coalition government, a change in the job market laws enabled the introduction of an allowance for child care for women who wanted to return to work after maternity leave. The explicit objective of this move was very different from previous family policies and did not sit well with the gender norms represented by the Catholic-Conservative ÖVP. In fact, the allowance was not of great significance, since the benefits were very rarely paid out (Neyer 1990, 46 ff.). I will come back to this and investigate how this very singular move can be contextualised.

In summarising the first wave of family policies in Austria, the following characteristics can be identified: the dilemma between child care and employment was solved at a political level – largely by consensus and without extensive political debate – by suggesting to women that they should, at least temporarily, give up employment. The solution included an encouragement for women: the opportunity to retain their job during their absence, plus partial compensation for loss of income.

The 1970s: Ambivalent Reforms

Family policies were enhanced still further in the 1970s in a new wave of political change when the post-war coalition came to an end. The Social-Democratic party, which wanted to prove its determination to bring about reform, formed a one-party government with an absolute majority in parliament. Its family policies remained ambivalent and ambiguous in regard to gender politics, however. On the one hand, previous political orientation was confirmed and reinforced to a great extent. Direct transfer payments, such as the family and birth allowances, increased significantly. The latter, a one-off payment on the occasion of the birth of a child, was linked to the "Mutter-Kind-Pass" (mother/child pass) in 1974.[10] This was arranged so that the allowance was only paid during pregnancy and after the birth if specified check-ups had been completed. The motivation was an attempt to reduce the Austrian infant mortality rate, which was well above the European average. The birth allowance was remodelled to, among other things, encourage the utilisation of medical care and/or check-ups during pregnancy. This argument, however, was also directly linked to abortion laws: those in favour had indeed argued for a liberalisation of abortion laws during the 1970s with the claim that women ought to be allowed individual rights. On the other hand, there were still individual traditional values regarding concepts of a rationalised demographic economy which had been very popular during the First Republic in sections of the Social-Democratic party. The fact that in contemporary discussion a connection is made between abortion laws and the mother/child pass – bringing to mind this earlier line of argument – should provoke some thought, without allocating any blame.

After 1970, motivated by the momentum of the booming economy, family policies underwent a change in their material services as well: great importance was placed on the direct transfer of payments. A school travel allowance was introduced in 1971, then free school travel and school books in 1972. Tax-free allowances, which favoured higher earners, were gradually abolished and replaced by write-off allowances and transfer payments. The circle of those entitled to claim benefits also grew larger. Working mothers obtained longer leave-times from work and higher payments, which were independent of their household income. Payments from the state after the birth of a child or for child care as compensation for loss of income remained linked to the mother's previous income, but never amounted to anything near that income. In 1974, the mother protection period and payment of the weekly allowance were extended to 16 weeks. This was justified with the argument that, due to an improvement in the situations of pregnant women and mothers with newborn children, access to employment would improve for women. This argument triggered a theme of the "second" women's movement, which successfully transformed gender difference and discrimination against women into issues for political debate. But it also played an important role – as mentioned above regarding the introduction of allowances to support a return to work after maternity leave – in solving the problem of a shortage of workers during economic booms, including the activation of the "hidden" labour potential of women. In addition to a relatively ineffective implementation of the allowance, which reflected the continuing ambivalence towards women in employment, in the mid-1970s, the economy took a turn for the worse, and the shortage of labour became less acute. The economic motivation to enable women with children to go to work was no longer there. At the same time, the political motivation, which had always been divided and directionless, disappeared as well. The ambivalence which had won the reproduction arrangements favour under the Social-Democratic government was highlighted by the fact that in 1972, an employee still received their redundancy payment if they handed in their notice because of the birth of a child. Because of this, it was much easier for them to decide to leave employment. Tax benefits for sole earners pointed in the same direction.

In the final analysis, during the first half of the 1970s, up until the turn of the century, the Social-Democratic party and the related trade unions developed concepts in a slightly extended form without addressing their inherent dilemma: the imperativeness of "equality" in the job world, i.e. the revaluation of the working lifestyle attributed to men, was thwarted by an extremely "unequal" allocation of reproductive tasks, which was reinforced yet again by social state regulations.

Pro-natal arguments no longer carried any weight in open debate, despite the extension of state provisions under the motto "family policies" – in stark contrast to the 1950s (Münz 1985). A corresponding reorientation occurred at the measures level as well: the graduation of allowances according to the number of children was reduced as a result of the allowance per child being increased by the same amount from 1971 onwards. This affirmed the declared objective that the child allowance should be the same for every child. As of 1 January 1981, graduated payments according to the number of children were lifted completely. Instead, the allowance was graduated according to the age of the child, taking into account the development in expenditure for each child as they become older. What was retained, however, was the tax advantage for people with more children compared to persons with fewer or no children: well into the 1990s, the amount of tax paid on the special payments (13th and 14th monthly salary per year) were highest for those without children and lowered with an increasing number of children to eventually reach zero (Lacina 1998, 27–29).

A considerable characteristic of family policies in the 1970s was that for the first time, single and unmarried mothers became a major target group for social policies at the national level: since 1974, they have received 50 percent more allowance during maternity leave. After maternity leave and up to the child's third birthday, they had the right to a separate transfer payment (the special emergency welfare benefit) if they mainly cared for their child on their own. A maintenance advance law came into effect in 1976: unmarried mothers were advanced a maintenance allowance from the Familienlastenausgleichsfonds (fund for the compensation of family burdens) after a claim had been made against the father of the child, but the claim could not be collected. The conditions for entitlement to a maternity leave allowance for women under 20 was formulated generously. That took into account a socio-political reality: after the "golden age of marriage" (Münz 1984, 6) from the mid-1950s – almost 90 percent of an age group experienced the collapse of a marriage during their lifetime – the number of marriages dropped during the seventies. The number of illegitimate children increased (again). How these unmarried mothers lived was of (socio-political) interest because they were more exposed to the risk of poverty than other people and were regarded by relevant social policies as especially needy. However, the support provided was never sufficient to provide a basis for existence, or offer efficient assistance in often precarious individual situations of need. This had an impact on the intersection of employment and reproductive work, since the duration of a possible interruption to employment was expanded in favour of unmarried mothers looking after their own children. Their specific situation was hardly covered by policies, however, because the acceptance of responsibility by society only took place in part, and private dependencies remained. The overall reproductive arrangement favoured by society and politics did not change in the slightest. The widely accepted concept of "female employment/motherhood" had been characterised by gender-specific employment taking second place to reproductive tasks. Reproductive tasks remained largely private, with their fulfilment linked closely to the female gender. Although the "second" women's movement did question this allocation, the continued dominance of social partnership institutions in which women's movements hardly had an influence was indicated by the fact that the relevant legal basis until 1990 reflected a clear gender-specific allocation (with the exception of the formulation of entitlement to nursing leave – Pflegeurlaub), in that only women were regarded as child carers.

On the whole, the tendencies in the social and tax law treatment of families or people with children requiring care have to be assessed with mixed feelings. Financial support was extended considerably during the seventies, supported by the argument that this was the best way to prevent abortion. "Assist rather than punish", was the slogan that justified child support independent of the income of those providing maintenance. It seemed as if the Socialist party, who had managed to liberalise the abortion ban in the face of fierce resistance from the Catholic church and their lay associations, were placing special emphasis on supporting "happy families" as a way of "making up" for the abortion law. As the addressee of most political measures relating to families in the seventies, it was possible to support an intact small family with sufficient although modest financial funds because it had been planned rationally. Alternative models were only rarely and marginally given any consideration.

Sieglinde Rosenberger commented that the family policies of the 1970s were directed at a deinstitutionalisation of the family and marriage (Rosenberger 1992, 139). In fact, tax law and social transfers provided for individuals entitled to make a claim – in practice, usually women seeking help with child care – and not for families or heads of households, which can be regarded as individualisation.

Family taxation was abolished in 1973, and individual taxation was introduced. (Heterosexual) domestic partnerships were granted the same rights as legally recognized marriages in some aspects, e.g. inclusion of the partner in health insurance. Single mothers received more state support.

Rosenberger's assessment is questionable, however, in regard to the 1972 introduction of the marriage allowance, a one-time financial reward for couples who decided to marry. Legal marriage was preferred and rewarded above all other forms of cohabitation, regardless of financial status.

Quantitative family policies were never designed as a vertical redistribution between richer and poorer levels of society. The only redistribution was to be between people without children and people with children who required care. Single parents were confronted with socially undifferentiated marriage grants which offered them no basic support. Although single parents were not entirely excluded from state social politics in the seventies, their existence was severely marginalised.

The reproductive arrangement favoured (politically) by the Social-Democratic elite was one in which a continuous male career opposed an interrupted female one. The "female employee/mother" was an acceptable model, providing interruptions were made in favour of reproductive tasks. The preference for mothers caring for small children echoed the attitude of a wide political consensus which, as presented below, was reflected in the structure of childcare practice and childcare facilities. The gender-specific allocation of reproductive tasks also remained uncontested in Social- Democratic concepts. Although the autonomously organised second women's movement seriously questioned the naturalness of role distribution, the resulting demands have not (yet) been transformed into legal requirements.

(Ir-)Resoluteness

The family policies of the 1980s and 1990s bore the trademarks of grand coalitions. The policies were characterised by (ultimately unsuccessful) initiatives to change the gender-specific division of labour within families and only partly effective initiatives of various ministers for women's affairs to both create additional childcare facilities and improve upon forms of flat-rate family support (which was awarded regardless of income and number of children in the family.) As of 1 January 1993, the concept that the number of children is not relevant for state support lost some ground, initially in tax law, and then in the practice of direct financial transfers. Both "social status"-related expenses for a child and the number of children in the family were taken into consideration in different ways: in tax benefits and in the form of multiple child allowances, as a direct transfer payment which was linked to a specific income.

In addition to the demand for more and better childcare facilities attuned to the requirements of working parents, the respective ministers of women's affairs turned the private division of labour in the reproductive area into a political issue – and encountered strong resistance from both parties of the coalition government. After attempts to introduce the obligation of dividing housework into matrimonial law faltered due to resistance from various quarters, these ministers decided to target public "awareness". The media campaign launched in 1996 under the title "Halbe-Halbe" (50/50) was interrupted, however, the change of the minister of women's affairs. Despite the enormous public ridicule of the advertisements, the publicity campaign was a success in the final analysis because, unlike many others, it managed to grab the public's attention. The gender-specific structural imbalance in the distribution of unpaid care work was no longer an official policy in Austria after the end of that campaign.

In 1996, motivated by an urge to reduce expenses, an initiative which required that the full maternity leave of two years (part of the "family deal" since 1990) had to be split between the parents in a ratio of 3:1 if the parental leave was to be taken full advantage of was introduced. Apart from the fact that this rule was a disadvantage to single parents since the obligation to share also applied to them, this extremely isolated incentive was not sufficient to change deep-rooted attitudes – according to statistical data which showed that the small proportion of fathers taking paternity leave was getting even smaller.

Childcare: Facilities – Everyday Practice – Financing

These factors are discussed in the following section because, in addition to socio-political influences, the standardisation, institutional environment and everyday practices surrounding childcare have a major influence on the reproductive arrangements favoured and marginalised by society. The society's attitudes towards childcare inside the family and outside of it changed over the past three decades less qualitatively than quantitatively: the proportion of children cared for outside the family has increased continually since the late 1950s/early 1960s (Faßmann, Aufhauser, and Münz, 11, ill.1). This is attributable both to changes in employment (particularly where women are concerned), and to a change in the societal attitude regarding care provided outside the family. The proportion of children between the ages of five and six who spend at least half the day in a kindergarten or other child-care facility is as high as 90 percent (Schattovits 1999/2000, 540). According to the authors of the relevant study, this relates to the high pedagogical value of childcare facilities outside the family (Kränzl-Nagl 1999/2000, 87).

The most recent family report from the Austrian State Government listed the following childcare facilities outside the family: nurseries (for children aged between zero and three years), kindergartens (for children between 3 years old and preschool age), after-school care or all-day schools for children between the first and eighth school year, and childminders, child groups, parent initiatives, including nurseries, kindergartens, after-school care centres and all-day schools – forms of care dating back to the 19th century. They are mostly organised by public groups at the national, provincial or local council level, and especially by the Catholic and Lutheran churches. Child groups and parent initiatives mostly stem from the student movement in the years after 1968 and were often motivated by an anti-institutional impetus and/or the high value of self-organisation (Schattovits 1999/2000, 553).

Assessing the utilisation of childcare facilities according to the age of the children is significant from the point of view of everyday practice in society:

Table: Utilisation of external childcare facilities

Age	usage of facilities (in %)
0–3	6
3–4	44
4–5	70
5–6	84
6–7	31
7–10	15
10–15	16

Source: Schattovits (1999/2000, 528, Table 12.13).

This demonstrates that most children are looked after at home up to the end of their third year, even at the end of the 1990s. This matches the pattern of parental leave utilised in practice. The probability of interrupting employment due to the birth of a child was and still is structured along clearly gender-specific lines: based on the micro-census in 1996 and data from the Fertility and Family Survey in the same year, it can be seen that in the mid 1990s, over 80 percent of women (Prinz 1999/2000, 115) drew a maternity leave allowance after the birth of their child (i.e. for at least six months, they did not return to work), while in only four percent of cases where couples had children under the age of 15, the mother was employed to a greater extent than the father (Prinz and Thalhammer 1999/2000, 119, Tab. 3.33).

The same source of data reports that 83 percent of men continue employment at the same level after the birth of a child. The Fertility and Family Survey established that only two percent of men interrupt their employment due to children (Prinz and Patrick 1999/2000). There was no mention in statistical sources of men who interrupt their employment after the birth of a child (let alone interrupt their employment for longer than ten years). All the same, two thirds of all women did not return to employment at the end of their maternity leave (or interrupted their career for longer than ten years), and this proportion has remained extraordinarily stable over recent decades. In 1972, a survey revealed that 67 percent of all women who received maternity leave allowances did not return to employment.[11] The Frauenbericht (Women's Report) 1995 drew similar conclusions: "The fact is that [in 1990] at the end of parental leave only around one third of all mothers decided, or were able to decide, in favour of returning to employment. Almost two thirds of women finished employment temporarily or medium-term after the birth of a child." (Faßmann 1995)

In Austria, the constitution states that kindergartens and nurseries are to be regulated by the federal provinces. Requests at the state government level to increase the number of childcare facilities are problematic because the government – quite apart from the provision of financial incentives – has little influence on policies within each province. This also applies to initiatives begun during the 1990s, usually by the relevant women's policy ministers. In the final analysis, there has been little change at the regional level in the shortage of childcare facilities to meet the needs of people in employment. Considerable regional differences – between the different provinces but also between urban and rural areas – have little to do with legal legislation, which is very similar in all areas, and more to do with the physical availability of childcare facilities (see also Neyer 1995), and the contribution of public funding towards childcare (Faßmann, Aufhauser and Münz undated, 20). Generally, childcare facilities outside the family are not available free-of-charge in Austria – unlike state-run schools. The contributions vary from region to region, as do the costs.

In some provinces, the costs of institutionalised childcare were, and still are, staggered according to family income and/or number of children. Surveys regarding the wishes of the parents revealed deficits in the area of institutional childcare, especially regarding the number of kindergarten facilities, and their short daily and seasonal opening hours. Various surveys done at the state level produced results too divergent to be addressed in detail, but the overall picture made it clear that from the parents' point of view, there are too few childcare establishments. The actual number fluctuated between 100,000 and 200,000; the differences are due primarily to the extent of childcare regarded as necessary and in the way the question was put (see Neyer 1999, 79). In an international comparison, it is clear that in Austria there is now legal claim to services in a childcare facility, which is significant for the relevant socio-political decision-making process at a basic level: absence from employment (possibly only temporarily) is generously supported, while childcare outside the family is not. Due to the structuring of childcare facilities, preference is given to a model which demands that people responsible for looking after children choose between employment and childcare. This is a disadvantage for anybody who wants to take parental leave – with the resultant negative effects on income and exclusion from participation in the employment market – and this disadvantage is clearly gender-specific.

Current Family Policies

At the start of the 21st century, a change in reproduction policy took place in Austria, and became very controversial amongst political motivators and media concerned with politics: "Childcare allowance from 2002. Family policy milestone or trap for women?" read one headline in the conservative newspaper "Die Presse" (28 December 2001, 8) thereby defining – albeit only in outline – the extremities of the debate.

So what exactly was/is the "childcare allowance"? The right to claim 436 Euro per month for a maximum of three years for each child living in Austria. Only parents who live with a child in one household are entitled to claim; if they are citizens from non-EU states, they have a right to claim only if they live in an employed situation or if they have lived in Austria for at least five years. The full time period of 36 months can only be claimed if it is divided in a ratio of 5:1 among both parents, i.e. if both claim the allowance for at least six months. The childcare allowance is not paid out to people who earn more than the annual gross limit of Euro 14,600. People who earn more must either stay at home – or work part-time, if the employer permits. Parental part-time has been on offer since 1 July 2004; although this is limited to employees who have worked at least three consecutive years for the company. The company must also have more than 20 female employees.

The probability that childcare work is divided between the parents is not high, since the gender-specific difference in income in Austria is still approximately 30 percent. On top of that, deep-rooted and widespread attitudes and behaviour patterns point in the same direction. Although the legal formulation is gender-neutral, it has the effect of reinforcing the traditional gender-specific division of work so that "parental leave" in the majority of cases is "maternity leave". Of the parents who take two years parental leave, it is nearly always women who are prepared to take the risk of losing their jobs: protection against dismissal for people on parental leave only applies for 24 months.

Parental leave legislation is aimed at parental units consisting of a man and a woman: single parents (and their children) are disadvantaged to the extent that they can only receive the childcare allowance for a period of up to 30 months. The other parent must claim the remaining six months. This applies to single-parents as well.

Both the studies carried out since the introduction of the second year of parental leave and the micro-consensus surveys and data collated by the social insurance institutes show that returning to employment is more difficult after an extended period of parental leave (see Hahnl undated). Similar results were shown by the first analysis published after the introduction of the childcare allowance: women with children left employment for a longer period (Lutz 2003). Because the proportion of men who claimed the childcare allowance remained low, the gender-specific differences became more marked in relation to the employment market and levels of income.

Coming back to the original question: is the childcare allowance really a paradigm shift in Austrian family policies, or is it a continuation of policy moulded over previous decades? If you assess this question from the point of view of the favoured reproductive arrangement, the theory can be formulated that the shift is minimal. The childcare allowance still allows an uninterrupted allocation of childcare tasks to women.

This policy also clearly promotes temporary absence from employment for anybody who undertakes childcare tasks. This form of division of work within society is still favoured in family policy as the socially hegemonic model. This setting of priorities through the childcare allowance is not singular, and is underlined and reinforced by other state policies and strategies, as can be seen by the stance on childcare facilities. None of the politically relevant motivators – neither interest groups nor political parties[12] – has proposed an alternative reproductive arrangement during the Second Republic. There was only a short time span in the late 1960s/early 1970s when the political order of priorities was orientated differently: in times of economic upsurge, there was a shortage of employees, which was solved principally by every government in office by employing foreign labour, i.e. by worker immigration. The attempts by all governments to mobilize women – the "employment market reserve" – always remained marginal by comparison, and were completely obsolete by the time the upswing subsided and the economic crises of the 1970s took full effect. From that perspective, the introduction of the "childcare allowance" was an expansion and reinforcement of previous policies. Viewed from that angle, it can be seen that largely standard practices in childcare, i.e. looking after small children up to their third year largely within the family, are supported by state policy providing better financial support.

One significant change from previous family policies was the separation of employment and financial support in cases where employment was interrupted to care for small children, and the accompanying expansion of the circle of people with a right to claim benefits, which included farmers, business people, housewives and students. The childcare allowance is a new form of financial support from the state for everybody who did not previously have a right to claim a parental leave allowance, i.e. the self-employed, farmers, the unemployed, students and housewives. On the one hand, the Austrian social insurance rights have been significantly reduced, while on the other, these groups of people receive financial support from the state to have children and care for them – providing their income does not exceed the defined limit. In this respect, the measure is distinctly pro-natalist: having children is desirable as far as the state is concerned and is promoted with relatively generous financial support. This is a shift in political rhetoric compared to the 1970s, but could certainly be regarded as having its roots in family policies dating back to the 1950s. Like then, the preparation and introduction of measures at the start of the 21st century was accompanied by clearly pro-natalist statements from leading politicians. "ÖVP alarmed by decline in birth-rate: policies for kids" (Die Presse, 20

January 1999, 7) read the headline for a report in the daily newspaper "Die Presse" on a meeting of this political party. While the necessity for a higher birth-rate was usually argued by highlighting the threat to financing state pensions, there were also chauvinistic and gender-political arguments voiced in the debate. For example, in their campaign manifesto for the general election in 1999, the right-wing, nationalist FPÖ proposed the introduction of a "childcare cheque" – from which the two coalition parties in power after this election, the ÖVP and FPÖ, wanted to develop the "childcare allowance" – for "Austrian" mothers only (Rosenberger and Schallert 2000), a suggestion which was not ultimately implemented. Andreas Mölzer, leading politician in the very same FPÖ party, regarded childlessness as egoistic and saw the "Misery of our childless society [...] in the emotional obliteration of our fellow human beings, who have never known the only truly selfless love, i.e. the love towards ones own child." (Mölzer 1997). The family bishop of the Catholic church Klaus Küng warned: "A people without a youth has no future." (Die Presse, 15 February 1996, 7). Küng wanted to raise the image of the family in previous years by introducing suffrage for children (used by their parents) benefits for their parents such as tax breaks, etc. In 1994, he summarized the family model he promoted in the following words: "It is better for children, families, and women if mothers dedicate themselves to their families full time. [Because] fewer children would be susceptible to behaviour problems." (Die Presse, 29 December 1994, 7). The heavily normative orientation of the discourse environment in which the childcare allowance was eventually drawn up shows the shift in direction of the argument: in 1993, a debate was held to discuss the possible reduction in parental leave allowance, which had been increased for sole earners. Politicians closely associated with the conservative ÖVP discussed the reductions in terms of a supposed widespread misuse of the allowance.[13] Several years later, the same group struck the "poverty" criteria off the schedule altogether: it was no longer about stigmatising sole earners, the majority of whom were single mothers, but about giving birth to children and caring for them as a behaviour deemed desirable to society.

Therefore, there is no clear-cut answer to the initial question: in consideration of the preferred reproductive arrangement, the childcare allowance represents a clear continuation of Austrian family policies with a high level of political consensus. Nevertheless, the discursive environment lends the childcare allowance implications, standardisations and orientations representing a significant shift in family and gender policies at the national level since the 1970s.

Notes

1 Petition by party members Wilhelmine Moik, Gabriele Proft, Ferdinanda Flossmann, Maria Kren, Rosa Jochmann, Marianne Pollak, Paula Wallisch, Rosa Rück and associates regarding the implementation of a national law to regulate the protection of employed mothers (maternity protection law) on 12 November 1952.

2 Petition by representatives Wilhelmine Moik, Maria Emhart, Ferdinanda Flossmann, Maria Kren, Rosa Jochmann, Marianne Pollak, Paula Wallisch, Rosa Rück and associates regarding the imple-

mentation of a national law to regulate the protection of employed mothers (maternity protection law) on 20 May 1953.

3 National law, dated 13 March 1957, for maternity protection, BGBl. No. 76.

4 For single women and women who provided the family income, the maternity allowance was equal to the unemployment benefits they were entitled to; married women received half that amount. The amount depended on income, however: above a certain household income it was reduced or cancelled (see Neyer 1990, 45).

5 Quote from Nationalrat Hans R., who was introduced as father of four and employer of five female staff. See "Mutterschutz aus der eigenen Tasche", in: Bild-Telegraf, 26. November 1955.

6 Petition Nr. 155/A from the representatives Frieda Mikola, Dr. Gorbach, Dr. Nadine Paunovic, Fink, Rainer and associates regarding the Austrian Maternity Protection Law, appendix of parliamentary correspondence from 30 June 1948.

7 Sten. Prot. NR, VIII. GP, 27th Assembly on 13 March 1957, 1182.

8 Sten. Prot. NR, VIII. GP, 27th Assembly on 13 March 1957, Rehor, 1183.

9 Moik, Sten. Prot. NR, VIII. GP, 27th Assembly on 13 March 1957, 1177.

10 This model was similar to the one introduced by the Vienna Council between the wars for baby clothes laundry service: payment was made to every mother, including those not in need financially, providing they regularly sought assistance provided by the community.

11 Report on the situation of women in Austria. Frauenbericht 1975, Vienna 1975. Volume 5: Women in the professions, 79. It is not clear from the data quoted here, taken from the survey carried out by the board of the Chamber of Labour, how long women who left their jobs after maternity leave remained away from employment. The figures cannot be closely compared except in a few cases, although the general picture is interesting.

12 The Green Party, represented in Austrian Parliament since 1986, are a possible exception here. However, family policies are not a core political agenda for the Greens. In addition, they have only enjoyed marginal representation in parliament since their founding and are therefore hardly involved in negotiations between the social partners (trade unions and employers). During such negotiations, family policy measures concerning the intersection between employment and childcare were usually actively determined in connection with the other elements of family policy.

13 See for example "Mehr Geld durch weniger Ehen", Der Standard, 9 April 1993, 4; "Erhöhtes Karenzgeld", Die Presse, 7/8 December 1993, 6.

References

Ebbighausen, Rolf. 1976. Legitimationsproblematik, jüngere staatstheoretische Diskussion und der Stand historisch-empirischer Forschung. *Bürgerlicher Staat und politische Legitimation.* Frankfurt am Main: Edition Suhrkamp.

Faßmann, Heinz, Elisabeth Aufhauser, and Rainer Münz. Undated. *Kindergärten in Österreich. Angebot – Nachfrage – Defizite.* Vienna: Federal Ministry for the Environment, Youth and Family.

Faßmann, Heinz. 1995. Belastende Lebensabschnitte. In *Bericht über die Situation der Frauen in Österreich. Frauenbericht 1995:* 70. Vienna.

Freundlich, Emmy. 1908. *Frauenwahlrecht und Arbeiterinnenschutz* (Suffrage labour protection laws for women). Proceedings of the third social democratic women's conference in Austria. Vienna.

Freundlich, Emmy. 1913. *Arbeiterinnenschutz* (Labour protection laws for women). Vienna (Lichtstrahlen 24).

Grandner, Margarete. 1995. Special Labor Protection for Women in Austria, 1860–1918. In Ulla Wikander, Alice Kessler-Harris, and Jane Lewis (eds.) *Protecting*

Women. Labor Legislation in Europe, the United States, and Australia, 1880–1920: 150–187. Urbana: University of Illinois Press.

Hahnl, Susanne. Undated. Auswirkungen der Inanspruchnahme von Karenzurlaub auf die Chancen von Frauen am Arbeitsmarkt. In *Der Ausstieg ist leichter als der Einstieg*. Conference proceedings (1994). Vienna: Chamber of Labour.

Kränzl-Nagl, Renate. 1999/2000. Außerfamiliale Angebote der Kinderbetreuung. In Maria Orthofer (ed.) *4. Österreichischer Familienbericht. Familie – zwischen Anspruch und Alltag*, Vol. 1. Vienna: Federal Ministry for the Environment, Youth and Family, Department IV/4.

Lacina, Ferdinand. 1998. Fraueninteressen und Verteilungsfragen. In Eva Kreisky and Margit Niederhuber (eds.) *Johanna Dohnal. Eine andere Festschrift*. Vienna: Milena-Verlag.

Lutz, Hedwig. 2003. Auswirkungen der Kindergeldregelung auf die Beschäftigung von Frauen mit Kleinkindern. Erste Ergebnisse. *WIFO Monthly report 3/2003*: 213–227.

Mölzer, Andreas. 1997. Wer Kinder hat, ist reich – und ein armer Teufel. *Die Presse*, 3 September 1997: 6.

Münz, Rainer. 1984. Kinder als Last, Kinder aus Lust. Thesen zu Familienbildung und Kinderzahl. *Demographische Informationen 1984*. Vienna: Institut für Demographie, Österreichische Akademie der Wissenschaften.

Münz, Rainer. 1985. *Soziologische Aspekte der Familienentwicklung und die Instrumente ihrer Beeinflussung*. Grund- und integrativwissenschaftliche Habilitationsschrift Univ. Vienna.

Neyer, Gerda (ed.). 1990. Risiko und Sicherheit: Mutterschutzleistungen in Österreich (Risk and Safety: Provisions for protecting mothers in Austria). The influence of the maternity allowance and special welfare benefits on the employment market situation for women (= research reports on social and employment market policy). Vienna: Bundesministerium für Arbeit und Soziales.

Neyer, Gerda. 1995. Childcare institutions in Austria. In *Report on the situation of women in Austria. Frauenbericht 1995*. Vienna.

Paragraph 144 und eine Grazer Ausstellung. *Wahrheit*, 1 July 1953.

Parteitag der Socialdemokratie Oesterreichs in Brünn (General Assembly of the Austrian Social Democratic Party in Brünn) from 24 September 1899. Vienna (undated).

Prinz, Christopher, and Ada Patrick. 1999/2000. Vereinbarkeit im Längsschnitt: Eine Typologie auf Basis des FSS 1996. In Maria Orthofer (ed.) *4. Österreichischer Familienbericht. Familie – zwischen Anspruch und Alltag*, Vol. 2: 124. Vienna: Federal Ministry for the Environment, Youth and Family, Department IV/4.

Prinz, Christopher, and Eva Thalhammer. 1999/2000. Vereinbarkeit im Querschnitt: Neue Ergebnisse auf Basis des Mikrozensus 1996. In Maria Orthofer (ed.) *4. Österreichischer Familienbericht. Familie – zwischen Anspruch und Alltag*, Vol. 2: 119–124. Vienna: Federal Ministry for the Environment, Youth and Family, Department IV/4.

Prinz, Christopher. 1999/2000. Berufsunterbrechung und Wiedereinstieg: Ergebnisse jüngster Erhebungen. In Maria Orthofer (ed.) *4. Österreichischer Fami-*

lienbericht. Familie – zwischen Anspruch und Alltag, Vol. 2: 115–118. Vienna: Federal Ministry for the Environment, Youth and Family, Department IV/4.

Report on the situation of women in Austria. Frauenbericht 1975, Volume 5: Women in the professions. Vienna 1975.

Rosenberger, Sieglinde, and Daniela Schallert. 2000. Politik mit Familie – Familienpolitik. *SWS-Rundschau* 3/2000: 255–258.

Rosenberger, Sieglinde. 1992. *Frauenpolitik in Rot-Schwarz-Rot. Geschlechterverhältnisse als Gegenstand der österreichischen Politik.* Vienna: Braumüller.

Schattovits, Helmuth. 1999/2000. Unterstützung der Teilzeitbetreuung von Kindern – insbesondere durch Bund, Länder und Gemeinden. In Maria Orthofer (ed.) *4. Österreichischer Familienbericht. Familie – zwischen Anspruch und Alltag.* Vol. 1. Vienna: Federal Ministry for the Environment, Youth and Family, Department IV/4.

Thurner, Erika. 1992. Frauen-Nachkriegsleben in Österreich – im Zentrum und in der Provinz. In Irene Bandhauer-Schöffmann and Ela Hornung (eds.) *Wiederaufbau weiblich.* Documentation from the conference "Frauen in der österreichischen und deutschen Nachkriegszeit". Vienna–Salzburg: Geyer-Edition.

Aurelia Weikert

In Vitro Fertilization, Egg Selling, Surrogacy. New Reproductive Technologies – the Austrian Development

In the following article I will talk about the development of New Reproductive Technologies (NRT) in Austria and comment on the political and the public discussions about these technologies. I want to discuss the development of the law as it relates to NRT, and above all I would like to highlight the impact it has on women. This includes chronological information about NRT in Austria: what happened during the last 20 years? I will also outline discussions and debates by the public and representatives of the Austrian political parties. And I would like to focus on dynamics and events within the feminist movement, at least part of it. I am aware that the feminist movement is not a homogeneous group, but I will talk about the opinion of the mainstream. I will illustrate the conflicts and ambivalences between and within different political parties and other social groups. In particular I would like to show how NRT have become an explosive force with regard to traditional family structures and how the present law concerning NRT, or rather, the political parties themselves, avoid this explosive force.

What Has Happened in Austria?

In 1982, the first Austrian in vitro fertilization (IVF) baby was born. This was only four years after the first IVF-baby worldwide was born in 1978. In 1988, the first attempt to establish so-called "surrogate motherhood" in Austria was made. An advertisement in a newspaper of a Viennese district (Bezirksjournal) read: "Ist der Kindersegen ausgeblieben – kein Grund zur Traurigkeit." (No children, no reason to be sad). These words were addressed to involuntarily childless women as well as potential surrogate mothers. To become a surrogate mother means you may receive € 7.200. Your pregnancy is induced through artificial insemination or in vitro fertilization. If more than one attempt is necessary, you will probably get more money; after three months of pregnancy, you will receive the first instalment of € 720. This is because of the Austrian abortion law, the "Fristenlösung" (in effect since 1975), under which women can have an abortion on demand within the first three months of pregnancy. The surrogate mother is obliged to undergo amniocentesis; in the case of a handicapped child, the surrogate mother should have an abortion and will get € 720. In order to give birth, the surrogate mother has to undergo a Caesarian section. The prospective parents will watch the birth and will have contact with the surrogate mother during the whole term of pregnancy. As part of the adoption proceedings, the child will be handed over to the couple who ordered the child at the time of the birth. The remaining € 6.480 will be paid to the surrogate mother only after the settlement of all adoption proceedings. In the case of twins or triplets, the surrogate mother will not receive more money (Weikert 1998).

In the same year, in 1988, the first "egg-selling" in an Austrian IVF-clinic took place: two gynaecologists, the heads of an Austrian private institute for reproductive technologies and IVF, began to use so called egg donation for IVF treatments (This was the time when the public first learned about it). The price for this kind of treatment is about € 5,100. In comparison, the costs for a sperm donation are € 2,500. The clients of this clinic are mainly couples from Arab countries, Germany, and The Netherlands. The so called egg donor, the woman who gives her eggs, receives about € 720 for each egg puncture. To harvest the matured eggs, the following procedure is necessary: one month before the operation, the woman has to start taking the contraceptive pill, on the second day of menstruation she has to take a hormone and medication for stimulation, and she gets injections of ovum-maturing hormones four or five times every day. One week before the expected ovulation date, ultrasound tests are given daily to watch the ovulation, and beginning four days before the operation, the woman has to bring urine to the clinic daily, which must have been collected every three hours. During the operation, a vaginal scanner is used to obtain the eggs. It is up to the woman to ask for an anaesthetic – like a sleeping pill or an injection – or not. In the event that no matured eggs are found, or the doctors miss the exact ovulation date, the woman receives no money except a reimbursement of expenses such as transportation (Riegler and Weikert 1988).

In 1988, there was no definite legal position in Austria concerning the selling of eggs, and after passage of the law on artificial reproduction in 1992, it was rumoured that one of the doctors, who is still running the above mentioned private institute, had or still has a branch office in Hungary.

In the Meantime – What to Do?

Politicians of all political parties became aware of the new field of human reproduction. First, proposed laws appeared. At the beginning of the discussion about laws on reproductive technologies and genetic engineering, representatives of the industry and IVF doctors, as well as some politicians, were in doubt about the usefulness of legal regulations. One of the arguments was that regulations that were too strict might be detrimental to the development of Austrian science and industry. The industry could move into foreign countries and invest their money somewhere else rather than in Austria. Some artificial reproduction specialists tried to use the threat of moving abroad in the event that laws became too strict. Later on, though, these same persons advocated legal regulations, because they wanted legitimization for what they were already doing.

Debates on different political levels began. A brief overview of proposals and ideas from different political parties or social groups follows:

In 1986, the "Österreichische Rektorenkonferenz" (Austrian Association of University Chancellors) put forward a proposal on the regulation of artificial reproduction. This group was composed of ten members: nine men and one woman! Their recommendations were quite similar to the current law on artificial reproduction. In some ways, however, it was more liberal, particularly in regard to the possibility of using donated eggs or donated embryos, if other treatments were futile, and if the husband agreed. In the meantime, egg donation was prohibited by law (Bundesminister für Wissenschaft und Forschung 1986).

Another proposal by the Ministry of Justice tried to take into account the development of a new definition of "mother": the mother is the woman who gives birth to the baby. This excluded the possibility of surrogacy (Österreichische Richterzeitung 1987, 220). However, existing definitions of "mother" and "father" no longer applied. Previous definitions of "biological" mother or father versus "social" mother or father were now – with the arrival of NRT – supplemented by the term "genetic" mother; among legal groups, the term "placentarian" mother is used (Bernat 2000).

The "Frauenstaatssekretariat" (State Secretary for Women's Affairs), headed by a representative of the Austrian Social-Democratic Party, was initially a strict opponent of all methods of artificial reproduction, and employed the argument that women would be exploited by these new technologies and that these new technologies would open the door to manipulation of human beings (Weikert 1998).

The "antagonist" reaction of the conservative Austrian "People's Party" quickly followed: if doctors are not to be allowed to manipulate an embryo, then abortion cannot be legal. The "People's Party" saw a new chance to overthrow the existing law concerning abortion, which allows women to have an abortion within the first three months of pregnancy.

Panic-stricken, the State Secretary for Women's Affairs and the Social-Democratic Party, who wanted to save the right to abortion and the right of self-determination, quickly changed course: if women are allowed to have a fertilized egg removed, then they must also be allowed to have a fertilized egg implanted. But the State Secretary for Women's Affairs opposed any kind of commercial exploitation of women like surrogacy or egg-selling; and insisted that in vitro fertilization is a means of last resort for achieving pregnancy, and therefore all kinds of manipulations of the embryo must be prohibited.

In 1989, the Green Party proposed a law (1989) that would have prohibited IVF. The arguments against these technologies were the low success rate of IVF, the physical and mental burden and stress for women, and lastly, the possibility of embryo manipulation (Weikert, Riegler, and Trallori 1989, 180).

Finally, the now current laws were enacted: in 1992, the "Fortpflanzungsmedizingesetz" (Law on Artificial Reproduction), and in 1994, the "Gentechnikgesetz" (Law on Genetic Engineering).

The Status quo in Austria

The current law on artificial reproduction is a compromise by the so-called major coalition government in Austria, i.e. the coalition government of the Social-Democratic Party and the "Austrian People's Party." Their points of agreement were:

1. IVF and artificial insemination are allowed only for couples who live together (though they do not have to be married), and in Austria "couples" refers to heterosexual couples only: this means no IVF for single or Lesbian women;
2. No egg-donation;
3. Sperm-donation only in conjunction with artificial insemination treatment, and not in conjunction with IVF-treatment;
4. No anonymity of the sperm donor (this facet of the law was quite controversial, because doctors were afraid they would no longer find enough sperm donors.)

To address different ways of handling sperm donation and egg donation according to Austrian law, in February 2003 the "Bioethikkommission" (Bio-ethical Commission) – installed by the Federal Chancellor – considered whether or not egg-donation should also be allowed (Der Standard, 14. 2. 2003). Its recommendation was seen as an important step to liberalisation and non-discrimination towards women, because under the current law women who are not able to produce mature eggs cannot undergo an IVF-treatment in Austria, and may do so only in a foreign country. This modification of the law would probably also mean more IVF-treatments at Austrian IVF-clinics. The commission's recommendation included the following planks: No surrogacy should be permitted. The mother who gives birth to the child should be the legal mother. Actually this passage was not really necessary as far as Austrian law is concerned, as surrogacy is forbidden under the law, but it is important with regard to women who undergo an IVF-treatment with donated eggs in a foreign country. The commission also voted for obligatory counselling; the IVF doctor may arrange for psychological treatment or psychotherapy. This means that an involuntarily childless woman is presumed to be ill, if not physically or somatically, then at least mentally.

The Feminist Movement

What was the position of the feminist movement (or at least certain parts of it) during these developments?

A majority of the feminist movement in Austria generally says no to NRT.

But the movement feels stuck between a rock and a hard place, in a way that is reminiscent of the positions of the State Secretary for Women's Affairs and the Austrian Social Democratic Party which I mentioned before: Do NRT mean an increase or a reduction of women's freedom and self-determination? Are women exploited by NRT or do they gain more rights? Should women be able to lease their womb and sell their eggs as a new way of earning (some) money (Weikert 2002)? As far as women's self-determination is concerned, the same slogans that have been used during the fight for the right to abortion in the 1970s were later used (although by other groups) to promote NRT:

- "Mein Bauch gehört mir!" (My womb is my own!)
- The "right to self-determination"
- "Every woman must have the right to abortion," which means the right to have no child.
- This right includes the right to have a child – including the right to use all possible forms of NRT, and the right to have a fertilized egg removed would also mean the right to have a fertilized egg implanted.

All these demands suit NRT perfectly. If my womb is my own, the surrogate mother cannot be despised for leasing her womb. Selling or donating eggs cannot be considered immoral, if women have the right to self-determination concerning their own body.

To find a way out of this dilemma, the feminist-movement responds hastily by claiming that women are exploited by these NRT and they are also exploited by gynaecologists and IVF doctors, who represent the new techno-patriarchy and are accused of being "egg-thieves". Yet suddenly, these bad guys are using the same feminist slogans! At public discussions, friendly IVF doctors, who have always supported women's demands, vote for women's rights. The IVF doctors have always supported the right to abortion as a woman's right and now they support the woman's right to choose an IVF treatment, to sell or donate eggs, or to lease her womb to become a surrogate mother.

The feminist-movement seems to be in confusion. What has happened? The new answer: the clients of IVF doctors are poor, manipulated victims of patriarchal gynaecologists. (In addition, within the feminist-movement, the desire to get pregnant or to become a mother has often been viewed as something suspicious and as a result of patriarchal manipulation.) But finally, the "victims" accompany their IVF doctors to public discussions and don't feel like victims.

What to do? What could be an alternative? Counselling and information – about the procedure of IVF treatment, about the risks, about the success rate or rather the failure-rate – instead of undergoing IVF treatment. But soon the IVF doctors will offer their own counselling, and in the meantime, there is no IVF clinic without a psychologist. However, the intention of this type of counselling probably differs from counselling in feminist information centres. In an IVF practice, the aim of psychological counselling is a successful IVF treatment, so that women are supported during the whole IVF treatment; or women are dissuaded from undergoing treatment, because the IVF treatment won't be successful and would diminish the whole success rate of the practice.

The End or New Moral Standards

I would like to return to the explosive force of NRT that I mentioned above. A side effect of using NRT would be that women could lease their womb and become a surrogate mother; and women could sell their eggs and become an egg "donor". And they could get money for that. But they are not allowed to. It is prohibited by law. In contrast, men are and have been allowed for years to sell their sperm. Throughout the entire discussion about NRT and their legal regulation, there was no doubt about the possibility of making some pocket-money by selling one's sperm.

I would like to touch on one more subject: since 2000, eight years after the law on artificial reproduction was instituted, the IVF-Fonds-Law has been in force. This law refers to the financing of artificial reproductive technologies and means that under certain circumstances, 70 percent of the costs of an IVF treatment will be paid by the social insurance system. In contrast to this, the following fact is worth mentioning: since 1975, when abortion became legal in Austria, one of the fundamental demands of the feminist-movement has been that abortion should be paid for by the social insurance system. In fact, the costs of an abortion are much lower than those of an IVF-treatment. Yet this demand remains unfulfilled – the social insurance system has never paid for an abortion.

There is a blatant imbalance here: No IVF for single women and Lesbians; no egg donation or egg-selling, no surrogacy. Nothing must be allowed to disturb traditional family structures under any circumstances. Although I am really not a fan of NRT, I think it is very interesting to look at the legal regulations of NRT in Austria concerning women and the traditional family structures. Egg-selling and surrogate motherhood – the two fields where women could profit from these NRT by earning some money – are both prohibited by law, and all political parties agree with this regulation! The most frequently used argument against this new possible source of income for women is that of immorality. All others may profit from NRT, be it IVF doctors, medical clinics, sperm-donors or even the state with an interest in increasing the population. All the risks connected with these NRT – the low success rate of IVF, the physical and mental burden and stress for women, and finally, the possibilities of embryo manipulation – take second place in comparison to the possible "immoral" behaviour of women.

References

Bernat, Erwin. 2000. Fortpflanzungsfreiheit, Privatleben und die EMRK. *juridikum, Zeitschrift im Rechtsstaat*, Nr. 2: 114–118.

Bundesminister für Wissenschaft und Forschung. 1986. *Bericht an den Nationalrat: Zu grundsätzlichen Aspekten der Gentechnologie und der humanen Reproduktionsbiologie*. Wien, August 1986.

Österreichische Richterzeitung 10/1987.

Riegler, Johanna, and Aurelia Weikert. 1988. Product egg: Egg selling in an Austrian IVF clinic. *Rage*, VOL. 1, No. 3: 221–223. New York et al.

Weikert, Aurelia. 1998. *Genormtes Leben: Bevölkerungspolitik und Eugenik*. Wien: Promedia.

Weikert, Aurelia. 2002. Wer bestimmt selbst? Neue Fortpflanzungstechnologien zwischen Gesellschaft und Individuum. *AUF*, Nr. 115: 11–14.

Weikert, Aurelia, Johanna Riegler, and Lisbeth N. Trallori (eds.). 1989. *Schöne Neue Männerwelt. Beiträge zu Gen- und Fortpflanzungstechnologien*. Wien: Verlag für Gesellschaftskritik.

Johanna Gehmacher
Re/Production of a Nation

A comparative study of reproductive policies raises a number of questions, not least the question of the implicit and explicit concepts of nationhood upon which these policies are based. How is the framework defined within which their meaning and effectiveness unfolds? To what extent do the states discussed in the essays in this book see themselves as nations and what are the consequences of this with regard to their policies for the regulation of reproduction? How does each state's specific definition of the boundaries of community affect gender relations?

The essays in this volume examine how (and with what aims and grounds) state policies attempt to structure and regulate population development. They explore the avowed interests in reproduction of state apparatuses, the technological and social measures linked to these interests and the ideological concepts used to legitimize reproductive policies. In particular they examine what consequences these policies have for women: what they (can) mean for a woman's individual right to choose, her health and her economic and political situation. They examine the conditions influencing conception, giving birth and raising children from the different perspectives of four European countries – Portugal, Finland, Austria, Romania – plus Russia and the USA, and identify two central protagonists between whom rights, obligations and costs are negotiated: these are women as (potential) mothers and the state as an apparatus articulating and enforcing social interests.

Identity Politics

When reading the texts in this book, the relevance of the concept of nationhood is not immediately obvious – the majority of the writers do not explicitly refer to it. My studies of the literature show that this reflects a common tendency of research on and discussion of issues relating to the welfare state, for which questions regarding the construction of nationality and national identity are not of central importance. When the concept of nationhood is discussed in this publication, it occurs as an ideology of legitimisation in the context of political requirements or state strategies for an increased birth rate. For instance, the Romanian contributor Adriana Baban and her Russian counterpart Michele Rivkin-Fish both refer to the discussion on the impending "death of the nation" that accompanies pro-natalist policies and propaganda. Ideologizations of this kind are an important aspect of the link between reproductive policies and the concept of nationhood; however, their function and effects can only be understood in the wider context of the discourse on the nation as a progenitor of affiliation, identity and meaning which has become so prevalent in the modern era.

The Paradox of Comparison

Because this collection of essays is structured as a comparison of countries, the concept of nationhood is an inherent aspect of it; it examines entities as nation-states, thus establishing them in advance as a framework. There are various ways in which a state can express its perception of itself as a nation or a conglomerate of several nations – discourses on a state's national identity can be dominant or marginal, homogeneous or composed of diversities, oriented towards history, cultural forms, ancestry or specific institutions such as a constitution – but all modern states need a discussion about identity, since where continuity, unity and sovereignty of a state are not legitimised by the claim to power of a ruling dynasty, the population, territory and institutions of a state must be linked by some sort of cultural construction, which is nearly always – though not out of necessity – given the umbrella term "nation". How this is accomplished in each specific context – in other words, how the relationship between state and nation is defined – must be analysed individually and cannot be ascertained beforehand.

Let us now show briefly why it could be useful to examine the issues of nationhood, nationality and national identity even though they are not immediately obvious in the source texts collected here. Let us first emphasize the reference to the specific paradox that is inherent in the comparative approach undertaken here: the formulation of comparative questions qualifies the entities to be examined while at the same time affirming them. In this way research that is designed to compare the policies of nation-states is based on the assumption that essential decisions and structures are to be found at this level. It focuses attention on a specific political entity while hampering not only the appreciation of supranational institutions, trans-national activity and the international balance of power but also of regional and local cultures.

The Language Barrier: Terminology

Discussion of the concepts of state and nation in different national contexts gives rise to a specific problem of language. At the conference preceding this publication, the lingua franca was English. This implies specific vocabulary which is inextricably linked to cultural impressions and practices as well as to political structures specific to the English-speaking world, vocabulary which cannot always meet the requirements of the wide variety of contexts just mentioned. A good example of this is the English terms "nation" and "national." In the texts on the United States, these terms refer to the level at which discussion on matters pertaining to legislation and ideology take place; they indicate the inclusion of every federal state of the USA or of a specific set of institutions common to the individual states. In discussions of European contexts, the term "nation" usually relates to specific discourses on the cultural legitimization of territorial states. In her conference paper, Michele Rivkin-Fish cited the Russian term "narod," which translates not only as "nation," but also as "people." So according to the context, the term "nation" can mean an institutional structure, a cultural construction or a specific group of people. Thus the comparative approach already has to cope with at least three definitions of nation, and matters are made even more complicated by the fact that different interpretations of the term are frequently used simultaneously within one context.

Construction Processes

The incorporation of the term "nation" in a comparative study of state policies is therefore fraught with difficulty. Any attempt to solve these difficulties by agreeing on a strict definition is, in my view, doomed to failure. Such attempts fail to recognize that it is precisely because the term *nation* is over-determined, and therefore ambivalent, that it functions as a driving force for processes of integration and differentiation. Rather than universalising a historically and culturally specific concept by finding an unequivocal definition, it therefore makes far more sense to analyse differing definitions as effects of ongoing construction processes and to examine how social processes and discussions create specific notions of the term "nation." To this end, Katherine Verdery suggests focusing the analysis on the dependency of the term "nation" on a particular context and perceiving it as a symbol that is used to further a wide variety of different interests and whose individual definitions should be studied to ascertain the respective effects and functions of this symbol (Verdery 1996, 227ff.). Seen from this angle, the question of the connection between reproduction and nationhood becomes a question of the types of interaction between the cultural and physical re/production processes in different communities – the question of the relationship between metaphorical and social practices and of the historical roots, transformations and effects of these practices.

In his definition, which has been particularly influential in the past decades, Benedict Anderson emphasizes the constructional nature of nations when he sees a nation as an "imagined community" which, as a product of a historically specific cultural construction process, achieves its reality in the discrete perception of affiliation. However, this does not mean that these constructions are socially or politically irrelevant; for Anderson it is also important to show the tremendous influence and relevance of imagined environments and relationships (Anderson 1996). However, the concept of "community" as an equivalent of nation is problematic from more than one perspective; the German term for community, "Gemeinschaft," has ideological connotations that imply the exact opposite of the perceived heterogeneity of society. On the other hand, the English term "community" also diminishes the complexity of what is imagined in a problematic manner, so that differences between the sexes such as those resulting from and emphasized by specific reproductive policies can no longer be perceived. Feminist theorists such as Nira Yuval-Davis and Anne McClintock have therefore drawn attention to the need to examine national projects and processes to ascertain what effect they have on gender relations; in so doing, they attach great importance to questions regarding the cultural and physical re/production of the nation (Yuval-Davis 1997; McClintock 1997, 89-112).

Birth, Affiliation

Ernest Gellner defines a nation as an ideological construction uniting a set of institutions (usually, but not necessarily, a state), a population and a territory. While the legitimisation of the unity of a territory (by means of administrative continuity or ethnic homogeneity, for example) is important with respect to possible military conflicts, the ideological connection between the first two terms – state and population – is especially important for the issue of reproductive policies dealt with here. The concept of nationhood forges a link between state and population that is defined by means of the specific constellation of the facts of an individual's birth. However, this does not occur in the form of distinct ancestry and its associated specific rights as in a feudal or corporate society, but aims to produce equality within a defined group (Gellner 1995). In a nation, affiliation to the community is defined by the circumstance of its members' being born into that community. This applies not only to social, political and cultural communities that define themselves by descent – the Jewish community, in which the mother's identity determines the child's affiliation, is often cited as an example – but also for every state that guarantees citizenship for all those born on its territory. It also applies, in a modified form, to communities formed by immigration, which have to regulate their internal population growth as soon as they have been established and which, in the case of colonial societies, often do so with exceptional stringency. In every case, the rights of an individual do not result from anything he or she has accomplished but solely from the fact that he or she was born into a specific context. At the same time, these rights define the boundaries of the nation, since they are shared with all the other members and exclude all those who were not born on this territory or whose parents were not born into this community.

Nationality, Gender and Reproduction

If a nation is defined primarily by the birth of its members, its boundaries, and thus its distinctness from external communities, are at issue wherever reproductive policies are negotiated. On the other hand it is at this point that the limitations of the national postulate of equality within the community's boundaries are shown, since where there is reproduction, a gender imbalance will occur and be legitimised. Thus, contrary to its fundamental objective to achieve the equality of its members, the nation produces inequality – also between those belonging to it: "Nations are contexted systems of cultural representation that limit and legitimise people's access to the resources of the nation-state, but despite many nationalists' ideological investment in the idea of popular unity, nations have historically amounted to the sanctioned institutionalisation of gender difference." (McClintock 1997, 89) Because their perception of themselves is linked to the conditions of human reproduction, nations and national projects are also always defined by gender relations. For this reason their interest in population regulation and control is genuine.

Processes of the institutionalisation of gender difference in the context of both nation-states and national projects without the state are connected in two ways with these communities' interest in influencing the reproductive behaviour of the population. On the one hand, there is regulation of population size, the reasons for which are found in a number of different contexts (military conflicts, labour market etc.). On the other hand – and in this sense it is not just a question of the reproduction of the population but also of the production and reproduction of the nation – discourses and symbolisations on the subject of human reproduction with its component elements of conception, birth and child-rearing serve the establishment of cultural identity. Where there are discussions, analyses and regulatory measures regarding who may have how many children under what conditions, and what sort of gender relationships, family types and forms of child-rearing and child-care are accepted as legitimate, there are also negotiations about what a nation is or should be, which idealisations present themselves for the purposes of identification and which kinds of behaviour and groups of people are excluded. The cultural production and reproduction of national identity manifests itself with its images and narratives at the topoi of boundaries and affiliation: war and migration are therefore the favoured settings for their discursive construction, as are conception and birth.

Controlled Sexuality and National Symbols

Because it is particular kinds of behaviour and cultural forms that are the basis of a nation's identity, the implementation of these forms is also accompanied by consent. The standardisation and sanctioning of specific gender relations goes hand in hand with this. This applies to war, which addresses men primarily as soldiers and women as guarantors of continuity and national essence; to migration, which confronts men and women with different conditions for integration; and finally, and especially, to reproduction, with which the regulation of sexual relations is linked. And although any regulation of reproduction involves male sexuality, sexuality is, in most societies, the most common means of control of women. In the context of national discourses, this control is fed from two sources: from the wish to regulate the population and the wish to preserve national identity. However, this does not mean that there is a concept of gender relations that is characteristic of nationalist discourses. Rather, it is precisely on the postulate of specific gender relations that apply only to one's own nation and are proof of national identity that the cultural re/production of nations is based; in other words, it is based on the assertion that the forms of gender relations as practised are typical of one particular nation, and of that nation only. It is for this reason that behavioural norms and idealisations of women so often act as symbolic identifiers and aim to emphasize differences, as when the typical 'modesty of German women' is praised and contrasted with the putative greater licentiousness of French women, or when the veil worn by Muslim women is defended against western norms of body covering. This means that the possibilities of integrating widely differing concepts of femininity are vast

– we need only think of the Scandinavian model, which permits a high degree of equality between the sexes – but what these concepts have in common is that unlike other definitions of affiliation (to political parties, for instance) they refer in essence to reproduction, in the broadest sense, as a regulator of the boundaries of a nation.

Against the background just outlined, it makes sense when focusing on reproductive policies to examine concepts of nationhood even where these do not occur explicitly as an ideological construct in the discourses. The question of national identity constructions as a setting for specific policies can, among other things, assist the classification of specific strategies, restrictions and requirements that enable the analysis of the success or failure of particular policies or explain the role played by women in specific forms of control. In the following paragraphs, some observations on this subject are presented, taking as their basis the texts in this publication.

Homogenisation and In/Equality

Discourses about reproduction can be interpreted as a symbolic domain in which nations are conceived and affirmed. In her paper, Michele Rivkin-Fish focuses on the shifting boundaries between the discussion about the health of individual (female) bodies and the evocation of a national body which is seen as a "biogenetic unity," the threat to which is central to nationalist discourses in post-socialist Russia. Women's bodies, as Adriana Baban postulates using the Romanian example, are being "nationalised". Such discursive constructions are not always explicit, however. Livia Popescu, for instance, refers to the structural exclusion of Romany from state benefits in Romania. Citing the example of the public discussion on teenage pregnancy in the USA, Linda Gordon reveals comparable racist implications in apparently universalist discourses. So the implications of the discussions about and policy relating to reproduction for the politics of identity are not always immediately apparent – and it is precisely for this reason that they deserve special attention.

Observation of the implicit exclusive and racist meaning of discussions about reproduction draws our attention to homogenising terminology such as "every child" or "all mothers", which do not allow us to see who is included and who excluded. We may take the Finnish paper as an example to ask a question which remains unanswered in many of the contributions: which policies of inclusion and exclusion are linked to family planning policies? Teija Hautanen describes the development in Finland of the right of "every child" to daily supervision. She describes the extensive subsidies paid by the Finnish state to guarantee child-care regardless of the profession or nationality of the mother. Hautanen explains that it is the local authorities who decide who qualifies for these benefits, an essential criterion being permanent and not just temporary residence in Finland. Hautanen discusses this development in the context of the (late and rapid) industrialisation of Finland and the changes to the fabric of society it entailed, especially with regard to female employment.

The question that remains unanswered is what the relationship is between the establishment of a welfare state in general, and state investment in child-care in particular, to migration issues: who can qualify for state and local authority benefits, and under what conditions? During the conference discussion, Virgínia Ferreira linked the question of who pays the "costs of motherhood" to globalisation processes. And indeed, the connections between migratory movement, global markets and the costs of reproduction need to be looked at very closely. Nation-states with their own specific welfare systems must therefore decide where they stand in the face of trans-national labour markets and the strategies of multinational concerns; the much-discussed outsourcing of production-lines to countries with cheap labour in order to cut personnel costs is essentially an off-loading of reproduction costs onto societies in which the state makes little or no contribution to the social security of its citizens in general and to child-rearing in particular.

Pro-Natalism and Anti-Natalism

Discourses and policies relating to reproduction define affiliation and exclusion. This affects not only state aid granted to particular parts of the population, but also the policy regarding birth itself. In many of the papers presented at the conference the evident connection between pro-natalist policies and the curtailment of women's reproductive rights was a central theme. However, exclusive reproductive policies also often refer not only to social benefits but also to the number of births. For instance, Gisela Bock (1986), by highlighting its policy of forced sterilization, showed that National Socialism – long defined as a pro-natalist regime – was actually characterized more by its aggressive anti-natalism, which was directed at specific sections of the population. So pro-natalist and anti-natalist strategies can be parts of one and the same political concept that defines who is part of the nation and who is not. From this point of view, it is extremely important to investigate implicit and explicit ethnic processes in connection with reproductive policies.

Nira Yuval-Davis identifies three different discourses with regard to the relationship between reproductive policies and nationhood. Firstly there is the policy of pro-natalism, which is based on the assumption that a large population brings economic, political and social power (Yuval-Davis 1997, 29). In pro-natalist discourses, the nation's future is linked to continual population growth. They play an important role, for instance, in communities of settlers, in the context of military nationalism and in connection with struggles for territory defined by ethnic/national concerns. Pro-natalism legitimised by nationalism often goes hand in hand with religious-ethical arguments such as the right to life of the unborn child.

The policies described by Yuval-Davis as a "Malthusian discourse" have completely different aims, regarding population control as an (inter)national necessity (Yuval-Davis 1997, 32ff.). The Chinese one-child policy is the best-known example of this. The nationalist and racist implications of this discourse result first and foremost from who is targeted by this debate about the necessity of population control. It is only ever a question of limiting population growth in developing countries, in countries of the South and in Third World countries. Terms such as "population explosion" and "population bomb," as coined by the US-American biologist Paul Ehrlich in the 1960s, are, Nira Yuval-Davis postulates, an expression of both a racist fear of non-western 'others' and Western feelings of guilt in the face of the extreme poverty that still holds sway in post-colonial societies. The policy of population control has nevertheless become a key strategy for the solution of economic and social problems in many developing societies, and is therefore described in these countries as a national project (Yuval-Davis 1997, 33).

The third discourse cited by Yuval-Davis is the "eugenic discourse", which operates with terms such as "quality" and "selection," and distinguishes within a society between desirable and undesirable groups (Yuval-Davis 1997, 31ff.). What is problematic here is the (widespread) continued use of the euphemistic term "eugenics" for talk about "good genes" in which the devaluation of all those excluded from this definition on account of their hereditary disposition remains implicit. In addition, the so-called eugenic discourses are always associated with ethnic and social racism – distinctions and selections are likewise always made between various ethnic and/or religious groups, between the educated and the uneducated, between the wealthy and the socially disadvantaged. The policies related to these discourses range from the implicit and explicit exclusion of particular groups from government benefits, to bans on abortion for women in the desirable group and forced abortion and sterilization for women (as well as forced sterilization for men) regarded as undesirable – as was the case in National Socialism.

It makes sense to analyse policies of internal selection in communities as a separate discourse. At the same time it is important, when considering Yuval-Davis's identification of three discourses relating to population policy, to bear in mind that pro-natalist and anti-natalist policies do not exist in isolation from each other at the international level either but are, through their interrelationship, an expression of the economic and political balance of power as well as of the racist (de)valuation of people.

Upbringing and Identity

Reading the contributions in this publication, it is evident that questions regarding connections to the concept of nationhood play more of a role in the debate about biological reproduction than in the discussion of state policies with respect to child-rearing and child-care. Nevertheless, the entire subject of the socialisation of the child can be interpreted as a key element of the re/production of a nation. Ernest Gellner has contended that the process of forming a nation is closely related to the centralisation and standardisation of upbringing and its institutions (Gellner 1995). However, his observations centre on the creation of national standards of school education; he too ignores the extent to which the raising and education of children in the family setting has also been changed by strategies of nationalisation. One way of gauging the importance attached to the socialization of children in national projects is to look at the propagation of a national mission of mothers in the context of cultural nationalisms. One example of this is the concept of the "matka polka," the Polish mother whose task it was to teach her children the Polish language and, in connection with this, instil them with national pride at the time of the division of Poland (Kusiak 2003). This concept is central to the process of the forming of the Polish nation. Against this background, it would be particularly interesting to look for implicit and explicit references to issues of cultural processes of identity formation in which child-rearing and child-care are discussed.

Differences, Times, Places

In conclusion, I would like to refer to a complex of questions which seems to me to be of key relevance to the development of political strategies, and which deals with the tremendous economic differences that the comparative approach of this set of essays makes particularly striking. For example, they become apparent in the comparison of the economic situation in Finland, Romania and in Russia, as portrayed by Elena Kulagina. How is a monthly child benefit of US\$ 2 in Russia – which represents 4.5% of the margin of subsistence which is fixed at US\$ 50 – to be evaluated against the extensive benefits available to Finnish families? The Romanian film-maker Lia Perjovschi brought up this difference in the discussion about *Gracious Curves*, the film made by the Finn Kiti Luostarinen, when she said in as many words: "In our struggles we have no time to watch the ageing of our bodies". In her reply, Kiti Luostarinen tried to restore the shared frame of reference by saying: "We once had the same fights as you have now."[1] Both participants tried to draw comparisons between their own specific situation and that of the other. The quest for shared points of reference is a necessary, indeed essential part of any attempt to achieve some sort of solidarity despite such differences. However, interpreting the perceived dramatic differences as (nothing more than) a consequence of development taking place at different times seems to me extremely problematic. This would imply that every society has to undergo more or less the same development, and would therefore universalise a specific (western) model.

In this connection, the question of constructions of the continuity and ending of national identification in the context of upheaval and transformation also arises. When during the conference Ceausescu's anti-abortion policy was being discussed, it seemed at one particular point as if there were no rational continuity between the Communist regime and the time following it, as if everything had quite simply changed. This made me wonder how, when a system comes to an end, people are able to reconcile their former identity with their present one. And in this context it seems very interesting that in post-Communist discourses, the reference to a country's nationhood so often unites otherwise widely differing political parties – the impression is given that an essentialist concept of national identity on the basis of a natural community becomes a guarantor of a notion of continuity which would otherwise not be possible. If this is the case, the consequences for every concept of equality (also of the sexes) with respect to reproductive issues cannot be over-emphasized.

Processes of Legitimisation, Individual and Collective Rights

When including the concept of nationhood in analyses of reproductive policies, two closely linked processes of legitimisation deserve special attention. On the one hand, there is the central ideology of nationalism which asserts that an ethnically/culturally homogeneous population on a specific territory can be the basis of a nation-state with stable borders. This means that the establishment (of the fiction) of homogeneity by means of population control is an important aim of national projects, especially when no state yet exists or when the sovereignty of an existing state is under threat. In such circumstances, specific reproductive policies – forced pro-natalism, for instance – (also) aid the legitimisation of a nationally based state. Consequently the control of women's sexuality appears as a prerequisite of the implementation of specific political requirements. At the same time, state reproductive policies can also be legitimised by nationalist ideologies. However, population control is a key argument for the control of women's sexuality. So the system of references also works the other way round: the control of women's sexuality can be legitimised by means of a specific national project. Wherever the reproductive rights of women are examined, the influence of both processes of legitimisation must also be studied. When doing so, however, it must be assumed that reproduction is always conveyed in cultural terms and can therefore also convey and stabilise identity. Because women participate in reproductive policies and practices as members of disparate and interacting collectives, their respective frameworks for action and their interests must not be seen as independent of social status, cultural traditions and collective ideological and political projects. A conceptualisation of reproductive rights as merely individual rights could therefore overlook fundamental modes of operation and contexts of reproductive policies.

Note

1   I have taken these two quotes from the notes I made at the time, so they are not word for word. I apologize to Lia Perjovschi and Kiti Luostarinen if I have misquoted them. If I have, the two sentences may be seen as a fictitious example of an often-used strategy of dealing with the differences described here.

References

Anderson, Benedict. 1996. *Die Erfindung der Nation. Zur Karriere eines folgenreichen Konzepts*. Frankfurt am Main: Campus.

Bock, Gisela. 1986. *Zwangssterilisation im Nationalsozialismus. Studien zur Rassenpolitik und Frauenpolitik*. Opladen: Westdeutscher Verlag.

Gellner, Ernest. 1995. *Nationalismus und Moderne*. Berlin: Rotbuch Verlag.

Kusiak, Alicia. 2003. Polin, Patriotin, Frau. Über die Konstruktion von Weiblichkeit in Rekonstruktionen der Vergangenheit. In Johanna Gehmacher, Elizabeth Harvey, and Sophia Kemlein (eds.) *Zwischen Kriegen. Nationen, Nationalismen und Geschlechterverhältnisse in Mittel- und Osteuropa 1918–1939*: 165-185. Tübingen: Fibre-Verlag.

McClintock, Anne. 1997. "No Longer in a Future Heaven": Gender, Race, and Nationalism. In Anne McClintock et al. (eds.) *Dangerous Liaisons. Gender, Nation, and Postcolonial Perspectives*: 89–112. Minneapolis–London: University of Minnesota Press.

Verdery, Katherine. 1996. Whither 'Nation' and 'Nationalism'? In Gopal Bakakrishnan (ed.) *Mapping the Nation*: 226–234. London–New York: Verso.

Yuval-Davis, Nira. 1997. *Gender and Nation*. London et al.: Sage Publications.

Maria Andrea Wolf

The Medicalization of Reproduction

The term "medicalization of reproduction" refers to medical interventions in the culture and nature of reproduction. These interventions, based on the medical profession's monopoly on defining health and illness, categorize physical processes that concern reproduction in pathological terms, and deal with them with a state-regulated monopoly on treatments with established medical methods. Currently, there are essentially four principal participants in this medicalization of reproduction: medical science in research and practice, pharmaceutical industries, the state, and women. Competition in the field of medical research and between physicians in order to gain competence, influence and power has lead to the medical surveillance and management of female life from gynaecology for girls to gynaecology for old women. On the clientele side, i.e. from the perspective of women, the perception of being solely responsible for the process of reproduction, the interest in planning a life career in a self-determined way, and the insecurity, anxiety and missing rituals during bodily changes dominate the motivation to medicalize one's own fertility and to hand over the shaping of reproduction to physicians. The third participant in the field of the medicalization of reproduction is the pharmaceutical industry, which manages women as a market segment with a big economic potential and vies for physicians and medical professionals as sales agents for their products, and who also finance medical research. The fourth participant is the state, which acts mainly to the benefit of men when it directs reproduction under aspects of population policies and the pressure of international competition for know-how in the field of biotechnology, when it legalizes or prohibits contraceptives, abortion or artificial reproductive techniques, and when it supports research in the field of reproductive medicine and technologies with scientific-political decisions. My comments focus only on the role of medicine, although the interests of these identified participants are mutually linked.

My comments are devoted to those lectures during this conference that address the role of medicine as regards the social shaping of reproduction. These include: first, Adriana Baban's description of the impact of abortion laws on women's health in Romania, in which she highlighted both the process by which abortions are experienced psychologically and the significance of contraception as inevitable social constructions; second, Linda Gordon's paper on "reproductive policies on abortion in the United States," which analysed both the theory and practice of the conservative reaction of "Right to Life" groups against reproductive rights, focusing especially on abortion laws in the United States; and third, Aurelia Weikert's presentation on the impact of surrogacy and "egg-selling" as regards a woman's self-determination or freedom. Additionally, the "social costs of motherhood" are influenced by medicalized practices of heterosexuality through contraception, abortion, artificial fertilization and insemination, which affect women's choices for their way of living.

Adriana Baban´s analysis of a socialist, pro-natalist population policy in the years of communist rule in Romania (1965–1989) showed the extreme manner in which women's possibilities to control their lives in a largely self-determined way was reduced to the duty of bearing children for the state. This duty was coerced by imposing economic penalties (taxes) on childless couples and those with fewer than four children, as well as by medical means of controlling women's bodies and generative potential (quarterly monitoring and compulsory gynaecological examination). In addition, modern contraception methods – taking "the pill", the insertion of IUDs and surgical sterilization – were banned. During this time of extreme restrictions and state intervention in heterosexual gender relations, women paid for the socialist-patriarchal population policy not only with their health, but also with their lives, due to hazardous methods of illegal abortion. To avoid the economic impoverishment of their families, women accepted the termination of unwanted pregnancies as a form of sacrifice for their already struggling relatives. Many women died from complications related to illegal abortion methods, and the maternal mortality rate was much higher than the average for the rest of Europe. Children became orphans due to methods of illegal abortion, as a result of maternal mortality and because unwanted children who survived were abandoned to state care in public orphanages. This "reproduction-coercion-system" bluntly shows where an extremely patriarchal control of reproduction can lead. Although the fall of the communist regime brought legislative change, and modern contraception methods and clinical abortion were introduced and allowed, the mentality towards birth control methods, which was established during these decades, continued. Women paid for their resistance to pro-natalist patriarchal state policy with their lives and health, and they continue to do so today. Romania remains what has been called an "abortion culture," according to Adriana Baban. The reasons are diverse, but the use of pills and IUDs are refused by women mainly because of their side effects. Condom use, which is a non-medical contraceptive, is rebuffed because this contraceptive practice is deemed to be incompatible with a couple's sex life in long-term relationships. However, the alarmingly increasing incidence of syphilis and AIDS recorded in recent years would make the use of condoms a choice that would protect both women and men from deadly diseases. From a feminist standpoint, I would say that women have paid the price for a patriarchal, pro-natalist state population policy, which at the same time has ensured male sexual rights. It is obvious from the data that it was a matter of course for men to continue the sexual practices through which women became pregnant, a pregnancy which women usually had to terminate due to social circumstances and the pressure to ensure the survival of the children they already had. Most women died due to harmful methods of illegal abortion. This male mentality correlates with the traditional male claim to the use of women for their sexual satisfaction under any conditions. This is not only the case in Romania, but a patriarchal attitude in general, which becomes obvious when men show no solidarity or concern for the survival of their women by changing their sexual habits. In some way, they also sacrifice their women for their male sexual rights. In order to establish an alternative sexual culture of mutual respect between women and men, as one prerequisite of self-determined choice, there is much more involved than just demanding modern contraceptive techniques and clinical abortion techniques, although the latter are indeed necessary to reduce abortion-related maternal mortality rates. However, all these techniques are not gender neutral. They make women responsible for reproduction control and they damage women's health, as feminist research and other critical clinical research have shown.

Linda Gordon's analysis of the conflict over reproductive rights in the United States focuses on the discussion of abortion laws. Her analysis clearly shows that a patriarchal, pro-natalist population policy also informs the attitude of the state in capitalist countries, where abortion laws are an arena for conflict between liberal and conservative ideas about family. She shows that within the conservative reaction to the demands for "reproductive rights for women" developed by socialist feminists, there is a traditional patriarchal anxiety regarding sexual liberation and freedom of women because it is perceived as a multi-dimensional attack on the "traditional" family and gender system. For example, the legalization of abortion is assumed to destroy the father's family wage by the mother's wage-earning work and to destroy motherhood, in which children are treated as subjects, not objects of mass-education. Only a direct path from sexual intercourse to motherhood is presumed to guarantee men's established rights to what Robert Connell has called the "patriarchal dividend". By referring to these advantages as the "patriarchal dividend", he shows how men profit from patriarchalism: by an increase in esteem, prestige and power of command, and in material profit. So the institutionalisation of motherhood, as it is done in capitalist societies, guarantees social benefits for men. But the conservative "Right to Life" movement in the United States, which Gordon characterizes as an unstable coalition with internal political differences, also focuses increasingly on the rights of the unborn. And as motherhood will gratify the demands of husbands to be the sole breadwinner, to be watched over and cared for by private women's work, motherhood also should serve the right to life of the unborn. The "right to life of the unborn" argument has become increasingly more prominent in popular consciousness. From a feminist standpoint, I would say that the anti-abortionists claimed that the state should protect the rights of all participants of heterosexual reproduction except the mother. Her bondage regarding reproductive freedom should guarantee the rights of men and their offspring. This conservative reaction affected feminist claims for reproductive rights, as Linda Gordon points out. Feminists fought for "real" reproductive choice in the 1970s, which meant that the freedom to limit their reproduction could not be a real freedom without the complementary freedom to reproduce and to be able to raise one's children in decent conditions. Then they started to play down demands from a feminist standpoint in the 1980s to facilitate a liberal coalition of feminist, family planning and population-control organizations, and to promote abortion and contraceptive rights. They emphasized individual liberty and privacy, and eventually dropped other arguments (e.g. against the eradication of infant mortality), and "implicitly they denied the validity of any social regulation of reproduction" (Gordon 2002). So the development of abortion laws in a capitalist country, whose self-image is one of liberty and freedom, showed that the access to legal abortion is constantly objected to and jeopardized by protesters who repudiate feminist aspirations for the rights of self-determination to which all women should be entitled. This claim for women rights evidently evoked much more resistance than other social views of abortion. And the feminist coalition for the medicalization of birth control, who tried to circumvent this resistance and to protect their freedom of choice, made it difficult, as I would say, to analyse the effects of modern medical contraception techniques on women's health and gender relations. Yet these effects strengthened and deepened female responsibility for reproduction and male freedom from reproduction, as I will show in my comments. These effects are typical phenomena of the "dialectic of freedom", which derive from an "instrumental reason" (Horkheimer) of modern natural sciences and have to be taken into consideration by feminist research and politics in their political theory of reproduction.

The new reproductive technologies of IVF brought this question of women's health back to feminist analyses and politics, as Aurelia Weikert has shown in her paper on the development of New Reproductive Technologies (NRT) in Austria since the 1980s. At the beginning, IVF was rejected by Social-Democratic feminists, the feminists of the Green Party and the autonomous women's movement in Austria, because it was recognized as an exploitation of women and as an open window for the manipulation of human beings. Conservative parties took advantage of the latter argument when calling into question the abortion law of 1974, which legalized the termination of a pregnancy. To avert this conservative coup, the feminists of the Social-Democratic party, and then the party itself, agreed to support artificial reproduction in 1992. At this time abortion is still legal in Austria, but women have to bear the costs of the termination, with the exception of a pregnancy after a rape or a pregnancy with a malformed foetus, which has to be verified by amniocenteses (eugenic/genetic indication). Due to the demands of conservative parties on the other side, up to 70 percent of the costs of IVF treatment is paid[1], under certain circumstances,[2] by the social-insurance-system, despite its high failure rate and iatrogenic after-effects on women. And despite the insight of the Social-Democratic feminists that all methods of artificial reproduction exploit and injure women, they accepted the negative effects of the legalization of IVF to favour self-determination of women, which they assumed would be achieved through medicalization of reproduction by the old and new reproductive techniques. However, this assumption overlooks the fact that Old Reproductive Technologies (ORT) of hormonal sterilisation, abortion and sterilisation and their widely extended use today have not lead to an alternative and respectful sexual culture between the sexes. Over thirty years after the initiation of modern contraceptive and abortion techniques, women still have to bear the financial, social and physical costs of birth control and young men obviously expect that women will be responsible for reproduction and the sexual freedom of men. Social insurance will finance the treatments only when women's decisions are in accord with the interests of population policy.

These examples of feminist struggles for women's reproductive rights in different countries pose the question of why the feminist struggles for women's self-determination by medicalized reproduction techniques (NRTs as well as ORTs) led to new dependencies and why men were liberated from reproductive responsibilities by these techniques to a greater degree than women.

One answer that I will discuss in the following is that a major social issue of gender and generational relations is reduced to a medical treatment, and that this response is a typical case of naturalizing a social question by means of its medicalization. Thereby patriarchal structures and sexism extend beyond the mere incorporation of the legal control of reproduction that has been indicated in these lectures. Indeed, I suggest that both patriarchal structures and sexism are still essential factors in the medicalization of reproduction today. They are constitutive in the mainstream of the scientific development and production of contraceptive and procreative reproduction techniques. Reproductive technologies and techniques are not gender neutral. And the utilization of these techniques impacts gender relations and society in a way that reinforces the patriarchal structures and sexism of reproduction and guarantees the freedom of man from these processes. If feminists still pursue a gender culture, where fathers share their responsibility for daily childcare and raising children with mothers, this responsibility has to begin by questioning the culture of heterosexual intercourse. Since these culturally privileged male sexual habits and reproduction technologies and techniques are not gender-neutral, it is impossible for women to handle them in a so-called self-determined way. In other words, although I share the concern about making the shaping of reproduction by contraceptives and abortion legal and affordable, I would now like to contribute a radical feminist critique of those scientifically developed technologies still in use today. In reference to the aforementioned articles I will show that mothers not only bear the social costs of motherhood, but also the health costs, because reproductive techniques are mainly developed for and applied to women's bodies. These are techniques that mostly produce iatrogenic after-effects among women due to different forms of hormonal sterilization (pill, hormonal implant; hormonal vaccine, hormonal IUD) to prevent pregnancies or hormonal hyperstimulation and surgical intervention during IVF treatments to produce pregnancies. In the first section, I will discuss the historical causes and effects of patriarchal structures in the medicalization of reproduction, which guarantee both the integration of men into the process of reproduction and their freedom from reproduction; in the second section, I will show how the historical ascent and the present power of medicine as a public institution is completely linked with population control interests of the modern state and the welfare state; in the third section, I offer a critique of the scientific development and production of contraceptives and procreative reproduction techniques, based on the idea of "freedom of research", keeping in mind the origins and history of these technologies. At the same time, I do not view medicine as a monolithic block, because there have always been differences between researchers and physicians within the field of medical research and practice. However, there is a hegemonic discourse which promotes scientific competition and determines medical research and practice. I will conclude by suggesting some demands derived from this critique.

Human Reproduction and Social Relations in Terms of Human Nature

To ensure the existence of human life and survival – in view of human vulnerability and mortality – every society has at least three functions to fulfil: 1) the care and security of the adult generation, through production and preservation of foodstuffs and the living conditions necessary for it; 2) the care and security of the species through the creation of a subsequent generation; in other words, the creation of new life by heterosexuality, fathering, procreation, pregnancy, birth, and child-rearing; and 3) the passing on of cultural heritage, customs, traditions, language, "tools" and so forth (Schön 1989, 14f). These undertakings can be defined as society's material, generative, and cultural production and reproduction. They all consist of productive as well as reproductive factors, and they are mutually dependent on one another.

In modern societies, however, this mutual dependency has become abstract; that is, it is hardly intelligible in the experience of men and women. This is the case despite the fact that differences between the sexes – determined by nature – still exist today in terms of fertility and women's capability – again, determined by nature – to give birth. These given differences are the "starting points" of socially shaped human reproduction which cannot be circumvented. This is due to the fact that neither sperm cells nor egg cells can be produced through biotechnology, and even reproductive cloning remains dependent on the existence of an egg cell.

With this, the existing and emerging orders of generation and gender, from society's need for generative production and reproduction, can be read as social responses to the existential challenge of life and death – responses with which the undertakings of human communities and societies have been organized to compensate death and to care for subsequent generations. If we discuss the term "reproduction", we call into question and theorize on all conditions and behaviours responding to the social and empirical fact of human life, mortality and transience. In addition, we seek to understand how and why a society maintains the next generation, how it shapes reproduction in respect to its realization as well as its prevention – i.e. who has the decisive power to determine this decision about reproduction; how a society organizes the care of the next generation, and how it organizes, in the broadest sense, the bodily, psychological, spiritual and intellectual needs of its membership.

The shaping of human reproduction and its established orders of gender and generation are thereby responses in which social relations to nature – and human beings themselves as part of nature – manifest themselves. This is because human life is naturally a changing, individual conditionality that cannot be circumvented. The responses to this existential challenge have evolved historically in connection with the development of productive forces, because the relationship to human nature is mediated by society. The process of reproduction – as Mary O'Brian elaborated in her 1981 historical-materialistic analysis on "the politics of reproduction", which I will refer to in the following passages – is not only the material basis of historical forms of social relations, but also a dialectical, changing process. In this way, reproduction and human consciousness of reproduction are inseparably connected to one another (O'Brian 1997, 77).

However, women and men, by nature, are and have been bound to the process of reproduction in different ways. And these differences have been – and are – important to mediate in a social context. The factors which concern women are in every way more visible and obvious than those of men. Their potency and ability consist of bearing children and knowing whether and to whom they have given birth. Their reproductive consciousness, in this light, is one of continuity. Men, by nature, are excluded from this; they do not know whether or whom they have fathered. Their reproductive consciousness is one of discontinuity.

Yet the reverse of this exclusion is for men also an experience of freedom, which, however, remains an imposed freedom. A problem first arose from this given difference between women and men, historically speaking, when that which was to be handed down had a particular, exclusive character – such as domination and property. This caused genealogies to be required that were just as particular and exclusive and, in turn, a general regulation that established who could pass on what to whom – and who was excluded.

The patriarchal structures that pervade the shaping of human reproduction in history suggest that men have devoted themselves – historically, collectively, and with concentration – to the problem of their being excluded from reproduction. The masculine genealogies and ideas of male potency, power, and superiority that have been historically developed and transmitted represent "the male triumph over the natural alienation of men from the process of reproduction. [...] 'Potency' is the name men have historically given their extensive success (over and above the individual differences among them) in working through their contradictory experiences into their reproductive consciousness" (O'Brian 1997, 86). Indeed we find this triumph in the fact that men are integrated nearly everywhere into the process of reproduction, but at the same time, they are free from caring for their children, and that women are responsible for the care of the children. The lectures of this conference have clearly shown that up until today, no interventions have succeeded in achieving the integration of men into the process of reproduction, in a way in which they become fathers who care for their children.

To counteract the experience of discontinuity in the process of reproduction, as civilization developed, men established the appropriation of the child, so that their relationships and commitments were based on contract rather than birth. In patriarchal societies, relationships and commitments through contract, as Barbara Holland-Cunz has elaborated, deny "that human life is embedded not only in socio-political culture and society, but also in natural processes" (1998, 68). This was a means of controlling the uncertainty of fatherhood, which could not be carried out biologically but, even up to our most recent century, only socially and ideologically. In order to realize this social appropriation, other men had to cooperate, "because should one man have the right to a specific child, then means must be provided to disqualify all other possible fathers." This bond among men was effectively established by forming and reciprocally controlling a "brotherhood of free appropriators" – that is, of those whose freedom was imposed upon: "Fatherhood therefore is not a natural relationship to a child but rather the right to one" (O'Brian 1997, 92).

To ensure this right, a social support system was developed based on cooperation among men who were forced to be free from the process of reproduction. Among these social support systems, the institutionalization of the heterosexual relationship in monogamous wedlock, where mothers have to bear the whole commitment to care for children and other relatives, was one of the strongest as the lectures also showed yesterday. In East and West, today's welfare policies once again count on marriage as the foundation of a successful society. And the historical development of this support system transformed the individual uncertainties of fatherhood into the triumphant universality of patriarchal structures. Thus, the term potency extends beyond its merely sexual significance. And up to today, this support system is merely driving on its own, for the benefit of men.

Against this background, patriarchy always contains "men's idea of being the ruler of nature." In fact, it means "power, with historical, man-made realities that transcend natural realities" (O'Brian 1997, 93). Men have historically and socially transformed their being, once separated from the process of reproduction into being integrated, which at the same time preserves their natural freedom: "The man as producer, who must work through his alienation by fathering is, fundamentally, the man as 'creator'" (O'Brian 1997, 94).

And this paradigm of producing, which is extremely closely related to the development of forces of production and the gender-based division of labour, becomes the paradigm of fathering. And both – fathering and producing – remain linked with nature in three ways today, forming an "organic barrier" to a male's productive ambition: in the ties to the soil, in the tie of techné (practical skills) to the body (physis), and in the female capacity to give birth. And these organic barriers are not yet overcome, even if they have been reduced in various ways: for example, the techné through automation, and the tie to the soil through industrialization (Treusch-Dieter 1990, 20ff).

Despite reproductive technologies that generate pregnancy, society's existence remains bound to female fertility and to a woman's body. And the woman as mother still remains, according to Luce Irigaray, "on the side of Nature as (re)producer, and the relation of man to 'the natural,' by virtue of this fact, will never be overcome. His 'social being,' his economy, and his sexuality will always depend on Nature's work; they continue to remain on the level of the first appropriation, that of the constitution of nature as ownership, and on the level of the first labour: namely, agrarian" (Irigaray 1977, 192).

The institutionalisation of heterosexual relationships serves the regulation of gender and generational relationships. And, through the social shaping of human reproduction, it must deal with working through the problem of the exclusion of men from reproduction. This regulation always guaranteed both the integration of men and their freedom from care. Therefore, institutionalized forms of gender and generational relations in our cultural history, at least since antiquity, as legally and economically safeguarded forms of different varieties of patriarchy, which are very strong, prove that even today, in the long run, no really alternative forms of life can be implemented.

This institutionalized network of male interests throughout much of the twentieth century has been guaranteed in marital and family laws, and in employment relations that exclude women through reproduction policies, employment policies, and education policies from paid work, with which they are able to sustain their existence economically. Through the socio-political construction of a hierarchical difference between men and women and the hierarchy between men's work and women's work, this institutionalized network of male interests has always served the supremacy of the male genus group and the appropriation of female productivity, female generative productivity and women's capacity for work. Patriarchal structures always function through the exploitation of a specific class of producers, namely women, whose products – children and goods and services – are maintained by force in a state of having no value (as a commodity). Robert Connell refers to this phenomenon as a "patriarchal dividend" which every human being who is born as a male will get (Connell, 2000, 91). This patriarchal structure has not disappeared with the repudiation of private patriarchy in the course of the construction of the modern state. Rather, it has been transferred into a public patriarchy, which is the subject that I will now address.

Modern Population Policies, Control of Female Fertility, Health of the Social Body, and Medical Advancement

An essential aim of the institutionalization of heterosexual relationships was the appropriation of female productivity and the concomitant male control of female fertility. Throughout history, women have always worked on their generative capacities; that is, they had to shape their reproduction through ecological, economic and social relations. Acts which shape reproduction, in other words, belong to the social repertoire of human history. Yet the power of decision-making regarding the use of this means legitimized patriarchal authorities – from paterfamilias of the Greco-Roman patriarch to the lords of the agrarian-based feudal societies to the state in modern times – to take advantage of women in establishing subsequent generations. This establishment of subsequent generations in family-based economies, which was founded on a private patriarchy and which individually and directly controlled reproduction, has been continued up to the modern period. The first time a familial establishment of the next generation was accomplished for a non-family economy (which emerged with industrial capitalism), it required far-reaching and drastic measures, such as the sanctioning of sexual instruction, the sale of contraceptives, infanticide and child abandonment, abortion and all forms of sexual pleasure that would not make a woman pregnant.

During the eighteenth and nineteenth centuries, industrialisation and exploitation in the capitalist economy, migration from the countryside and urbanisation, the loosening of generation- and gender bonds, and politically linked pressure to bear children (with regard to population control) led to social impoverishment and increasing morbidity, mortality, and neglect of children in the lower classes. The state's reaction to these changes engendered a "project on population technology," a new interest that demonstrated on the basis of data on population levels and conditions that the child was the most profitable investment of modern states.

This triggered the beginning of protective measures for children. The protagonists in this development were essentially doctors and educators: "The state assumes the institutional responsibility for the qualitatively sufficient development of the child, becoming in two senses the child's 'father': the state is already answerable for the child's procreation, and it now cares for the education as well. Along with the legally installed measures to force childbirth, the general obligation for children to go to school created a second pillar, which in modern times would make a 'miracle' possible – to be a community made up mostly of members without possessions, yet still able to reproduce" (Heinsohn 1979, 138).

This interest of the modern state as regards population policies – to provide people for new, non-family economies of the respective community, i. e. the labour market – led to an increased interest in health issues, beginning in the nineteenth century. In contrast to the destructive effects of social impoverishment on humans, the health conditions of the "socio-political body" were to be improved. Thus the necessary political solution to the social question was "disposed of" in its medicalization. The various public institutions, including the medical establishment first of all, were to care for the body, to help it heal and, when appropriate, also compel a healthier standard level or maintenance of it. Foucault described this change as the "guarantee of the maintenance and care of the 'labour,'" and more generally as the "political-economic effects of human accumulation" (Foucault 1996, 316).

The increase of "medical policies" led to privileging childhood and the medicalization of reproduction, in order to manage children in the best possible way, and to make the investment in this stage of life as profitable as possible. Reproduction in the family was organized as the primary and immediate authority of the individual's medicalisation: "It functioned as a hinge between general aims, which concerned the health of the socio-political body, and the desire or need of the individual for care [which] was guaranteed by a professional body of qualified doctors, who, to a certain extent, were recommended by the state" (Foucault 1996, 320). The "medicalised-medicalising family" was thus put on track in the eighteenth century. This insight is necessary to understand the function of medicine – since the nineteenth century – as an instance of the social control of life and death today: "The doctor becomes the great advisor and expert, and if not already in the 'art' of government, then in the art of observing, mending, and curing the socio-political 'bodies' and maintaining them in a permanent condition of health" (Foucault 1996, 322). From a political point of view, medicine is not only "called upon" but also feels it has a mission, "a calling," to lead the problems presented by the conditions to a solution through the advancement of its science.

And so the population policies of the modern state rely upon the advancement of medical science; the ascent of medicine is dependent on federal regulation and the financing of science and treatment. And state and medicine are fraternally bound to one another: the modern state, which is based on the power of the people, has elevated democracy to the status of a fundamental principle, but it is, from a historical perspective, an alliance of sons who wanted to share power freely, equally, and fraternally. Indeed, men were "the people", and they attempted to regulate the social shaping of reproduction according to their interests and benefits.

In this way, the private patriarchy of the feudal agrarian society transformed into the public patriarchy of the modern state and its institutions. This change transferred the division of labour between men and women to the division of labour between the state and women (see, for instance, Brown 1981; Walby 1990; Fraser 1994). This change in form from the agrarian-based feudal patriarchy is conditioned by economic change, and it is enabled by the installation of patriarchal structures in the development of public institutions. The institutions that most strongly control and shape human reproduction in the twentieth century are medicine and schools. Medicine supervises and shapes people's entry into life; schools supervise and shape people's access into the labour market, wherein the salary forms the basis of human existence. The liberation of the woman from male domination in private patriarchy, which marks the marital and family law reforms of the twentieth century, led, among other things, to the subordination of women under public patriarchy, and thereby to subordination through one of its most powerful institutions – medicine – whose ascent also simultaneously served the liberation of women.

The Male Struggle for Reproduction in the Field of Reproduction Technology

This structural history of masculine forms of (re)production and organization – which control a woman's body as a material basis for (re)production – guarantees men's integration into and freedom from reproduction and establishes childhood as an investment project, and is incorporated into the medical technologies and techniques of reproduction. Significantly, techniques for birth control as well as techniques for artificial reproduction are not gender neutral; rather, in their development and their use, they are gender and socially determined, as the lectures have shown by the examples of abortion, contraception and IVF treatment (surrogate motherhood and egg-selling). So the social, financial and health costs that women have to pay for purported self-determination and freedom of choice, which old and new reproductive technologies offer for a high price, also have to be taken into consideration in the criticism of these techniques.

Today, the medicalized shaping of fertility production can be found in reproductive technological experiments on women in the form of in vitro fertilization (IVF), egg donors (artificial insemination by donor), and surrogate motherhood. Each one consists of a hormonal treatment and a surgical intervention. The hormonal treatments can lead to iatrogenic (medical, inadvertently produced) injuries or even death. There is the so-called ovarian hyper-stimulation syndrome (OHSS), for instance, which even the journal "Human Genetics", in 1999, called "an epidemic caused by doctors on healthy female patients" (Roest 1999, 2183: cited in Kollek 2000, 58). Indeed, there are also well-known carcinogenic effects from most of the hormonal preparations. See, for example, the results of investigations by Renate Klein and Robyn Rowland on the adverse effect of hormonal treatments (Klein and Rowland 1988), which the U.S. Food and Drug Administration (USFDA) confirmed in a directive that ordered "the manufacturers of Clomid and Pergonal (two often used fertility pills) to label a warning on their products about the increased risk of ovarian cancer" (Klein 1994, 82). Besides hormonal injuries, surgical interventions can at times – though less often – lead to iatrogenic injuries: for instance, intestinal wounds, bleeding, and peritonitis (serious inflammation of the membrane lining the abdominal cavity). IVF leads to large numbers of multiple pregnancies (i.e. the possibility of twins, triplets, quadruplets, etc.), which, due to the high rate of failure, causes ever more fertile egg cells to be introduced into the womb. These multiple pregnancies present a higher health risk to mother and child and subsequently harmful psychological effects on the mother-child relationship and the relationship between the partners. With the ICSI technique (Intra-Cytoplasmatic Sperm Injection), the problem of reduced fertility of men (reduced "spermiogram") is addressed in the body of the woman (Riewenherm 2000, 5).

This entire expenditure on research and treatment – as well as the demand for and subsidies given to these technologies by health insurance companies – can only be understood against the background of the persistent, shocking failure rates of IVF as the wild obsession of masculine, self-asserting strategies in the sciences! Because IVF has failed as a reliable method of helping childless women or couples who desire a child to have one. However, the press service of the social security system in Austria announced in March 2001 that IVF is a prospering technology because in the year 2000, IVF-centres in Austria achieved the international peak in terms of success rates. That means that 2950 women underwent 4000 IVF-treatments, and 850 pregnancies resulted from these attempts[3]. However, they do not explain whether they also count bio-chemically-induced pregnancies (increase in the HCG value), clinical pregnancies (wherein the embryo nests at least five weeks in the womb) and miscarriages that aborted. There is no indication of how many couples really had a child whom they could take home. They just say that the success rate of follicle punctures which they achieved was 24 percent. In comparison to the success rate of IVF-centres in Germany[4], which publish the real "baby take home rate", it may be estimated that of the 2950 women who underwent an IVF-Treatment, approximately 2400 went home without a baby. Since 1978 – that is, for the last 25 years – IVF failure rates have improved only negligibly. Depending on how one interprets the statistics[5], 85 percent to 91 percent of women's attempts to become pregnant by IVF fail (Riewenherm 2001, 62). The admission of failure clashes, however, with the international competition regarding the export of bio-technologies, the million-dollar market of childless couples, and – as Robyn Rowland writes – "the masculine dream of quality control [in] genetic engineering" (1992, 81). The costs of this clash are borne predominantly by women. In this context, women bear not only the social costs of motherhood, but also the health costs of medical treatment.

The medical shaping of pregnancy surveillance today involves prenatal diagnostics, which permit eugenic-genetic selection and the elimination of a foetus diagnosed as disabled or defective up until the moment of birth. So-called "second nature" must, should, and can reject increasing the number of humans who upset the rationalized course of action because of their imperfections. This eugenic-genetic selection will be reduced with the aid of pre-implantation diagnostics on the cellular level. Yet this technology is once again linked with IVF treatment, with all its adverse iatrogenic effects on women. For both of these selection techniques, women have obtained a right to self-determination. This right is not granted in most countries in cases of normal pregnancies without grounds for termination, such as those Linda Gordon mentioned. As Bettina Bock von Wülfingen elaborates: "Right up until the moment of medical evaluation, it is the state that possesses the acting power of attorney for the embryo. Only in relation to a 'disabled' foetus can the woman regain the status of an autonomously deciding subject; her stomach belongs to her again, and the state apparently has nothing more to do with her further decision" (Bock von Wülfingen 2001, 150).

In regard to the medical shaping of birth control, contraception is successful in preventing pregnancies, but all of the following are a risk to woman's health: "hormonal sterilization" through the pill (which has been in use since the beginning of the 1960s), the five-year effective hormonal implant, the hormonal vaccine against pregnancy for women in the so-called Third World (in use since the 1980s), and the hormonally treated intrauterine diaphragm (in use since the 1990s). Iatrogenic injuries occur in all these hormonal sterilization methods, as evidenced in numerous studies (see Rowland 1992; Bock von Wülfingen 2001; Hicks 1994; Seamann 1995; Guymer 1998). Yet most of the commercially available pharmaceutical forms of these treatments were taken off the market only after massive protests (see Akhter 1995). In addition, it only became possible to evaluate the long-term effects of hormonal sterilization after many years. One well-known neurologist of the Kentucky School of Medicine called the pill the greatest calculated human experiment on women ever: "The pill allows experiments on the general population that would never be allowed as a planned experiment" (Clark, in Seaman 1995, 14). Even today, medicinal expertise on hormonal sterilization is extremely imprecise.

Yet it is not only the effects on women's health that are disturbing, but also the pill's social "side effects" on gender culture. The pill permits sexual relations without fear of pregnancy, and ought to liberate female sexual desires; but, at the same time, it requires that women put up with a daily hormonal intrusion in their life cycle. It appears as a ready-made, life-long contract against their own bodies, "which [also] conditions and adjusts the rhythm and the moments of passion and asserts psychological pressure toward a preference of vaginal intercourse."[6] Despite the fact that many in the New Women's Movement initially favoured this technology, the pill certainly did not contribute to the development of a sexual culture between men and women which was shaped by the wishes of the latter.

As regards abortion, when compared to "chemical" or "pharmaceutical abortion," the method developed and applied since the 1970s (the so-called "vacuum aspiration"), which can technically be used until the end of the twelfth week of pregnancy, presents a lower health risk for women, even if the abortion-pill promises more self-determination (Klein and Raymond 1992). Yet the contradictions involved in the battle for the legalization of abortion and for safer and more affordable abortion opportunities, which were evident in the New Women's Movement from the beginning, are not yet resolved. In 1975, for example, a statement by a women's group in Florence asked what a "free decision" means in a world and civilization that embodies exclusively male interests and masculine life-intentions? The analysis by "Rivolta Femminile", in 1971 read: "Men have created the cultural preconditions; on their account, a woman returns to abortion as if it were a solution that corresponded to her own reproducing nature. [...] Men know that their orgasms are not those of women, and they know that as a consequence of these orgasms, women can become pregnant against their will and therefore can be forced to abort. Men's love is a ritual of manliness. It happens that women are impregnated exactly when their specific sexual enjoyment rescinds, when the act is fulfilled, and this confines them to a sexually colonized condition. Once pregnant, women discover the other side of masculine power which, out of the conception, creates a problem for the one with the uterus – and not for the one who installed the penis-cult" ("Rivolta Femminile" 1971, 105). The demand for free abortion and for abortion financed by the social security system supports women in solving a problem for which they are not solely responsible and which strengthens "the myth of the genital act, which concludes with the male orgasm in the vagina" ("Rivolta Femminile" 1971, 105). The legalization of abortion also guarantees that man's pleasure is not disturbed by paternal obligations and overpopulation.

Against this background, it is therefore absurd to perceive motherhood as a "free decision" and to present it as a victory for feminism on the basis of the legalization of abortion, "while in reality the patriarchal structures become stronger and patriarchal rule over the world is brought up to date" ("Rivolta Femminile" 1971, 105). These contradictions, evident already at the beginning of the 1970s, accompany feminist analyses and emerge again in discussions involving the new reproductive techniques. And as these techniques are not gender-neutral, a central issue time and again is the question of self-determination and autonomy, which asserts itself in the lives of women as one of self-control and self-instrumentalisation (Waldschmidt 2002, 105ff.).

In conclusion, I would like to emphasize that there is an inherent sexism present in almost all techniques of medical reproduction (with the exception of the condom, which is not sold by doctors and is not useful in promoting the self-interests of medicine), and this sexism combines in several ways with racism and discrimination against poor women. This is because the reproduction techniques of medicine reduce reproduction to a commitment of women and guarantee the freedom of men; they medicalize the social shaping of human reproduction on women's bodies; they pathologize female fertility and maintain the ideology of male infallibility; they use women's bodies and life histories as "living laboratories" for research; they conduct reproduction of female bodies as materials and resources; they test innovations in all fields of reproduction medicine as experiments on women, because the side effects can only be analysed after long-term experience. In addition, procreative technologies are tested especially on women living in prosperous countries, while birth prevention is especially tested on poorer women and women of colour. Medical reproduction techniques also cause the majority of harmful effects on women's health and welfare and contradict the medical principle of avoiding personal injury; they educate women to make themselves into subjects and objects of the domination of their fertility as an illness; and they cause women to bear not only the social costs of motherhood but also the health costs produced by medical treatment.

Reproductive medicine is thus extremely political, since the medicalization of reproduction is, in one way, also a guarantee of male freedom from reproduction. An insult to the femininity of women and an injury to their health is inherent in the production and application of contraceptive and procreative medical reproductive technologies. Up to the present, the majority of men would not have consented to even one of the adverse side effects from hormonally directed sterilization or fertilization developed for them, because this would signify a deep insult to their masculinity. It is time for women to seriously discuss the limitations of the "freedom of science" in contrast to this pathologizing medicalization of the reproductive potential of women, which inheres to patriarchal and sexist structures, because the idea of "freedom of research" in the history of modernity emphasizes, above all, the position of the abolished God in the service of masculine domination. This critique of science should not be understood as a rejection of it, because in a society, in which all forms of the constitution and appropriation of reality are potentially embedded into and mediated by science, there are no alternatives to science but only alternatives in science. This "freedom of science" must be restricted in the area of reproductive medicine to accommodate women's rights. This is a boundary that is lacking in medical science which exposes women to medical experiments and uses them as a means for the freedom, health and welfare of others. Likewise, the financial promotion of research in the area of reproductive medicine should require an interdisciplinary review of the effects of reproductive techniques on the health of women and men, gender relations and the sexual culture between women and men. Mechanisms of discourse have to be institutionalised, with which social values and expectations and the new reproductive technologies must be mutually interconnected, as is the case in the assessment of the consequences of new techniques. The effects of these measures must be based on the analyses of the conflicts for the gender culture of a society and the consequences for women and men, which can be anticipated as a result of the intervention of reproductive technologies. All precautions must be taken in the social field of science, where these techniques are produced and which is dominated by scientific rationality and technical optimism rather than the society in which their products are used (see Weingart 2000). Essential to this criticism is a connection with the core of a socio-critical feminist theory, the concept of "sex" and "gender", because the production of new life is compellingly tied to "sex" and "nature." This core of feminist theory constrains the force of the trans-cultural association between women's bodies and the birth of new living beings: "If 'sex' is that, which we are given by 'nature,' and 'gender' that which derives from culture (i.e. the cultural representation of sex), then we need to underscore that what is left to both 'sex' and 'nature' is now little enough" (Evelyn Fox-Keller 1989, 316). And the feminist responses to that difference that has not itself been given to us by culture must struggle to save women's lives in the field of reproductive medicine, and elaborate recommendations for how women can be empowered, so that they are not solely responsible for contraception, so that their fertility is a potency and not an illness, and a potency which cannot be controlled completely, so that their sexual interests and wishes find entry into a new heterosexual culture where female generative power is respected, for how men can become responsible for their sexual habits, how men can become real fathers for their children, sharing the responsibility of caring for the children with the mothers and becoming integrated into the process of reproduction from its sexual beginning and therefore not free.

Notes

1   IVF-Fondgesetz 1999
2   70 percent of an IVF treatment is paid for by the social insurance system only for heterosexual married couples or heterosexual couples who live together, if men are diagnosed as sterile or severely infertile by a specialist of urology, if women are diagnosed to have locked or lastingly functionless fallopian tubes by a gynecologist, if women are not older than 40 and men not older than 50 when they start the treatments; and no more than four attempts will be financed.
3   http://www.sozvers.at/hvb/presseau/p2001186.htm
4   http://www.meb.uni-bonn.de/frauen/DIR_downloads/dirjahrbuch2001.pdf
5   IVF teams measure success using different parameters, which makes a clear interpretation impossible. Some count both bio-chemically induced pregnancy (increase in the HCG value) and spontaneous abortions as a success; others count "clinical" pregnancies (where the embryo nests at least five weeks in the womb); still others include stillborn births (miscarriage after 20 weeks).
6   The woman's group "Santa Croce", Florence, 1975, in Wunderle 1977, 109.

References

Akhter, Farida. 1995. Resisting Norplant: Women's Struggle Against Coercion and Violence. Narigrantha Prabartana, Bangladesh.

Baermann, Astrid. 1997. Schwangerschaft im Fadenkreuz am Beispiel von Pränataldiagnostik und "Erlanger Fall". Pfaffenweiler: Centaurus.

Bergmann, Anna. 2001. Die verhütete Sexualität. Frauen zwischen Gebärzwang und Gebärverbot im 20. Jahrhundert. In Groth Sylvia et al. (eds.) Sexualitäten. Interdisziplinäre Beiträge zu Frauen und Sexualität: 27–61. Innsbruck: Studien Verlag.

Bergmann, Anna, and Bettina Recktor. 1995. Ein Gespräch über die sexuelle Revolution und die Pille-essende Frau mit Nebenwirkung. In Ursula Marianne Ernst et al. (eds.) Rationalität, Gefühl und Liebe im Geschlechterverhältnis: 53–72. Pfaffenweiler: Centaurus.

Bock von Wülfingen, Bettina. 2001. Verhüten – überflüssig. Biomedizin und Bevölkerungskontrolle am Beispiel Norplant. Mössingen/Talheim.

Brown, Carol. 1981. Mothers, Fathers and Children: From Private to Public Patriarchy. In Lydia Sargent (ed.) Women and Revolution: The Unhappy Marriage of Marxism and Feminism. London: Pluto Press.

Connell, Robert. 1999. Der gemachte Mann. Konstruktion und Krise von Männlichkeiten. Opladen: Leske+Budrich.

Daniels, Cynthia R. 1997. Between Fathers and Fetuses: The Social Construction of Male Reproduction and the Politics of Fetal Harm. Signs: Journal of Women in Culture and Society, vol. 22, no. 3: 579–616.

Enigl, Marianne, and Sabine Perhold (eds.). 1993. Der weibliche Körper als Schlachtfeld. Neue Beiträge zur Abtreibungsdiskussion. Wien: Promedia.

Ettore, Elizabeth. 2000. Reproductive Genetics, Gender and the Body: 'Please Doctor, may I have a normal Baby?' Sociology Vol. 34, No. 3: 403–420. Cambridge University Press.

Fischer-Homberger, Esther. 1988. Krankheit Frau. Zur Geschichte der Einbildungen (2nd edition). Hamburg: Luchterhand.

Foucault, Michel. 1996. Die Politik der Gesundheit im 18. Jahrhundert. Kulturen der Krankheit. Österreichische Zeitschrift für Geschichtswissenschaften. 1996/3: 311–326.

Fox, Bonnie, and Diana Worts. 1999. Revisiting the Critique of Medicalized Childbirth. A Contribution to the Sociology of Birth. Gender & Society, Vol. 13, No.3: 326–346.

Fox-Keller, Evelyn. 1989. Holding the Center of Feminist Theory. Women's Studies International Forum, Vol. 12, No. 3: 313–318.

Fraser, Nancy. 1994. Die Frauen, die Wohlfahrt und die Politik der Bedürfnisinterpretation. In Nancy Fraser Widerspenstige Praktiken. Macht, Diskurs, Geschlecht: 222–249. Frankfurt/M: Suhrkamp.

Gordon, Linda. 2002. The Moral Property of Women. A History of Birth Control Politics in America (3rd, revised edition). Urbana/Chicago.

Graumann, Sigrid. 2000. PID: Gen-Check vor der Schwangerschaft. Gen-ethischer Informationsdienst GID Nr. 139 April/Mai 2000: 13–16.

Guymer, Laurel. 1998. Anti-Pregnancy 'Vaccines': A Stab in the Dark. Birth issues, Vol. 7, No. 3: 87–91.

Heinsohn, Gunnar, et al. 1979. Menschenproduktion. Allgemeine Bevölkerungslehre der Neuzeit. Frankfurt/M.: Suhrkamp.

Hicks, Karen M. 1994. Surviving the Dalkon Shield IUD: Women v the Pharmaceutical Industry. New York: Teachers College Press, Columbia University.

Holland-Cunz, Barbara. 1998. Feministische Demokratietheorie. Thesen zu einem Projekt. Opladen.

Hubbard, Ruth. 1985. Prenatal Diagnosis and Eugenic Ideology. Women's Studies International Forum, Vol. 8, No. 6: 567–576.

Irigaray, Luce. 1977. Frauenmarkt. In Luce Irigaray Das Geschlecht das nicht eins ist. Berlin: Merve.

Kerr, Anne, and Cunningham-Burley. 2000. On Ambivalence and Risk: Reflexive Modernity and the New Human Genetics. Sociology Vol. 34, No. 2: 283–304. Cambridge University Press.

Klein, Renate. 1989. Das Geschäft mit der Hoffnung. Erfahrungen mit der Fortpflanzungsmedizin. Frauen berichten. Berlin: Orlanda. engl.: Infertility: Women Speak Out About Their Experiences of Reproductive Medicine. Melbourne: Spinifex.

Klein, Renate. 1994. Retortenhelden und feministischer Widerstand. In Susan Hawthorne and Renate Klein (eds.) Australien der Frauen. Munich: Frauenoffensive.

Klein, Renate, and Robyn Rowland. 1988. Women as Test-Sites for Fertility Drugs: Clomiphene Citrate and Hormonal Cocktails. Reproductive and Genetic Engineering: Journal of International Feminist Analysis. 1/1998: 251–273.

Klein, Renate, and Janice Raymond. 1992. Die Abtreibungspille RU 486. Wundermittel oder Gefahr? Hamburg: Konkret. engl.: Janice Raymond. 1991. Ru 486: Misconceptions, Myths and Morals. Inst on Women & Technology.

Kolip, Petra (ed.). 2000. Weiblichkeit ist keine Krankheit. Die Medikalisierung körperlicher Umbruchphasen im Leben von Frauen. Weinheim und München: Juventa.

Kollek, Regine. 2000. Präimplantationsdiagnostik. Embryonenselektion, weibliche Autonomie und Recht. Tübingen und Basel: A. Francke Verlag.

Lyotard, Jean-François. 1993. Ein Einsatz in den Kämpfen der Frauen. Aisthesis. Wahrnehmung heute oder Perspektiven einer anderen Ästhetik (5th edition). Leipzig: Reclam.

Mathews, Henry (ed.). 1992. Schering. Die Pille macht Macht. Berichte über die Geschäfte des Schering-Konzerns. Stuttgart: Schmetterling.

Mies, Maria. 1992. Wider die Industrialisierung des Lebens. Pfaffenweiler: Centaurus.

Minden, Shelly. 1985. Patriarchal Designs: The Genetic Engineering of Human Embryos. Women's Studies International Forum, Vol. 8, No. 6: 561–565.

O'Brian, Mary. 1981. The Politics of Reproduction. Boston, London and Henley: Routledge & Kegan Paul.

O'Brian, Mary. 1997. Die Dialektik der Reproduktion. In Irene Dölling and Beate Krais (eds.) Ein alltägliches Spiel. Geschlechterkonstruktion in der sozialen Praxis: 75–104. Frankfurt am Main: Suhrkamp.

Parks, Jennifer A. 1999. On the Use of IVF by Post-Menopausal women. Hypathia. 4/1999: 77.

Raymond, Janice. 1995. Die Fortpflanzungsmafia. München: Frauenoffensive. engl.: 1993. Women As Wombs: Reproductive Technologies and the Battle over Women's Freedom. San Francisco: Harper Collins.

Riewenherm, Sabine. 2000. Wunsch und Wirklichkeit. Gen-ethischer Informationsdienst. GID Nr. 139 April/Mai 2000: 3–7.

Riewenherm, Sabine. 2001. Die Wunschgeneration. Basiswissen Fortpflanzungsmedizin. Berlin: Orlanda.

"Rivolta Femminile". 1971. Weibliche Sexualität und Abtreibung (Female sexuality and abortion). In Michaela Wunderle (ed.). 1977. Politik der Subjektivität. Texte der italienischen Frauenbewegung (Politics of subjectivity: Texts by the Italian women's movement): 103–108. Frankfurt/Main: Suhrkamp.

Roest, J. 1999. Severe OHSS: An 'epidemic' caused by doctors. Human Reproduction, 14/1999.

Rowland, Robyn. 1992. Living Laboratories: Women and Reproductive Technologies. Sydney: Pan Macmillan Publishers Australia.

Rowland, Robyn. 1985. A Child at Any Price? An Overview of Issues in the Use of the New Reproductive Technologies and the Threat on Women. Women's Studies International Forum, Vol. 8, No. 6: 539–546.

Schön, Bärbel. 1989. Anforderungen an eine angemessene Theorie mütterlicher Praxis. In Bärbel Schön (ed.) Emanzipation und Mutterschaft. Erfahrungen und Untersuchungen über Lebensentwürfe und mütterliche Praxis: 13–33. Weinheim und München: Juventa.

Schön, Bärbel. 1997. Mutter. In Wulf Christoph (ed.): Vom Menschen. Handbuch historische Anthropologie: 324–334. Weinheim und Basel: Beltz.

Schneider, Ingrid. 1995. Neue Leibeigenschaften. Wie der Frauenkörper zur Plantage und die Leibesfrucht zum "nachwachsenden Rohstoff" wird. Beiträge 37/1995: Gewalt-tätig: 127–143.

Seaman, Barbara. 1995. The Doctors´ Case Against the Pill. Alameda, California: Hunter House.

Sichtermann, Barbara. 1983. Der § 218 und das Recht auf körperliche Unversehrtheit. In Barbara Sichtermann Weiblichkeit. Zur Politik des Privaten. Berlin: Wagenbach.

Steinberg, Deborah Lynn. 1997. A most selective Practice. The Eugenic Logics of IVF. Women's Studies International Forum, Vol. 20, No. 1: 33–48.

Trallori, Lisbeth N. 1987. Die Zerstörung des Weiblichen. Anmerkungen zu einer patriarchalen Universalstrategie. In Aurelia Weikert et al. (eds.) Schöne neue Männerwelt. Beiträge zu Gen- und Fortpflanzungsstrategien. Aufriss-Buch 7. Wien: Verlag für Gesellschaftskritik.

Treusch-Dieter, Gerburg. 1990. Bios, Sexus, Psyche. Strukturprobleme der Geschlechterdifferenz. In Gerburg Treusch-Dieter Von der sexuellen Rebellion zur Gen- und Reproduktionstechnologie: 9–54. Tübingen: konkursbuch.

Waldschmidt, Anne. 2002. Leid verhindern, Autonomie sichern – Die Verheißungen der Reproduktionsmedizin kritisch betrachtet. Beiträge zur feministischen Theorie und Praxis, 25. Jahrgang, Heft 60 [Stammzellen, Stammhalter, Stammaktie]. Köln: Eigenverlag.

Walby, Sylvia. 1990. From Private to Public Patriarchy. The Periodisation of British History. Women's Studies International Forum, Vol. 13, No. 1/2: 91–104.

Weingart, Peter. 2000. Die Zügellosigkeit der Erkenntnisproduktion – Zur Rolle ethischer und politischer Kontrollen der Wissenschaft in Humangenetik und Reproduktionsbiologie. In Eva Ruhnau, Susanne Kridlo, Bernd Busch and Kurt Roessler (eds.) Ethik und Heuchelei: 106–117. Köln: DuMont.

Wunderle, Michaela (ed.). 1977. Politik der Subjektivität. Texte der italienischen Frauenbewegung (Politics of subjectivity: Texts by the Italian women's movement). Frankfurt/Main: Suhrkamp.

Contributors and Editors

Adriana Baban
Professor at the Department of Psychology, Babes-Bolyai University, Cluj-Napoca (Romania), Visiting Professor at UCLA, University of California, Los Angeles (USA).
Her research focuses on: women's health, social and behavioral dimensions of health, and domestic violence.

Virgínia Ferreira
Sociologist. Assistant Professor at the School of Economics at the University of Coimbra (Portugal).
Major topics of research are: labour market disadvantage, social exclusion, gender and work/life balance and comparative perspectives on gender mainstreaming policies.

Johanna Gehmacher
Associate Professor at the Institute of Contemporary History at the University of Vienna.
Major topics of research and teaching are: nationalism and gender, contemporary history as women's and gender history, auto/biography, politics and gender, youth cultures and youth organizations in the twentieth century.

Linda Gordon
Florence Kelley Professor of History. New York University, Department of History.
Linda Gordon has specialized in examining the historical roots of contemporary social policy debates, particularly as they concern gender and family issues. Her research and teaching areas include social movements, labor and class, migrant farm laborers, the American West, and photography.

Teija Hautanen
MSoc.Sc., University of Tampere (Finland), Department of Women's Studies.
She is a post-graduate researcher on fatherhood and violence.

Yelena Kulagina
Ph.D. in Economics, Researcher at the Department of Gender Economics, Institute of Social and Economic Studies of Population, Russian Academy of Sciences (ISESP RAS).
Research Focus: population studies, gender studies, gender approach to the problems of the families with disabled children in Russia.

Maria Mesner
Teaches at the Institute of Contemporary History at the University of Vienna, and is research director of the Bruno Kreisky Archives Foundation.
Main fields of teaching and research: Gender history, history of political culture of the US and Austria, history of reproduction and family.

Ritva Nätkin
Professor (acting), University of Tampere (Finland), Department of Social Policy and Social Work and Department of Women's Studies in the Faculty of Social Sciences.
Research topics: maternity, gendered violence and substance addiction – construction of a social problem and intervention strategies.

Ann Shola Orloff
Professor, Department of Sociology and Gender Studies Program and (by courtesy) Department of Political Science, Northwestern University; Faculty Affiliate, Center for International and Comparative Studies; Faculty Fellow, Institute for Policy Research.
Her research has focused on states, politics and gender, particularly in the social policies of the developed world.

Livia Popescu
B.A. Ph.D., Professor in Sociology and Social Policy, Social Work Department, Babes-Bolyai University, Faculty of Sociology and Social Work, Cluj (Romania).
Research interests in welfare reform in Eastern European countries, policy evaluation, gender inequalities.

Sílvia Portugal
Sociologist, Researcher at the Center of Social Studies, teaches Sociology at the Faculty of Economics University of Coimbra (Portugal).
Research interests in welfare systems, family policy, family relations and social networks.

Michele Rivkin-Fish
Ph.D. Princeton 1997, Associate Professor of Anthropology, University of North Carolina at Chapel Hill.
Areas of specialization: medical anthropology, the anthropology of socialist and post-socialist societies, Russian culture, gender, reproduction and sexuality, health development.

Aurelia Weikert
Lecturer at the University of Vienna Department of Social and Cultural Anthropology.
Research Focus: Eugenics, Population Policies, Reproductive Technologies, Genetic Engineering.

Maria Andrea Wolf
Dr. Mag., Social Scientist; Assistant Professor at the Department of Education, University of Innsbruck.
Special Research Interests in: social theory, gender and generation relations, medicalization and eugenisation of reproduction, social change of motherhood, childhood, fatherhood and family, body and biography, feminist critic of science.
2000–2003 research grant from the Austrian Academy of Science; 2001–2002 research fellow and visiting academic at the School of Social Inquiry, Deakin University, Melbourne/AUS (Prof. Renate Klein, Women's Studies/Australian Women's Research Center).

Gudrun Wolfgruber
Mag. phil., historian, main interests of research: social policy, history and theory of welfare and social work, especially child and youth-welfare.
Current research project: "Child-Welfare Provision in Vienna. Continuities and Ruptures in Theory and Practice. The City of Vienna Kinderübernahmsstelle 1925–1997." Lecturer at the fh-campus Vienna (section: social work).